PREPARATION FOR BIRTH

PREPARATION FOR

Birth

The Complete Guide to the Lamaze Method

Beverly Savage and Diana Simkin

Photographs by Mary Motley Kalergis

*Illustrations by
Dana Burns and
Laura Hartman*

Ballantine Books   New York

To Herb, who did so much for me and for everyone.

B.S.

To my husband, David, with love.

D.S.

Library of Congress Catalog Card Number: 85-90884
ISBN 0-345-31230-9

Cover design by Richard Aquan and Georgia Morrissey
Book design by Beth Tondreau

Manufactured in the United States of America
First Edition: February 1987
10   9   8   7

Contents

Acknowledgments

To Dr. Ben Pascario for reviewing and editing our manuscript and for graciously answering our many questions.

To Drs. Adam Romoff, Daniel Clement, Don Sloan, Thomas Kerenyi, Jane Galasso, Jane Holl, and James Ottolini for generously giving us their time and knowledge.

To Elisabeth Bing for sharing her experiences as a founder of ASPO/Lamaze.

To Robert Moran, director of ASPO/Lamaze, and his staff for responding promptly and helpfully to all our queries.

To Paul Placek, Ruth Lubic, Anne Rose, Joan Solomon Wise, Patricia Shimm, and Barbara Sellars for being knowledgeable and available to us.

To Dr. David Kritchman for research and sound guidance.

To James Aibel for his thoughtful intelligence and cooperation.

To Anita Wise for her flexibility, organization, and uncomplaining assistance.

To Joëlle Delbourgo for her enthusiasm for this book and her skill in guiding us.

To Mary Flynn for her availability and warmth.

To Nellie Sabin for her thoroughness and organizational skills.

To Melanie Jackson for her constant support and commitment to us.

To Concetta Gintoli for her willingness and help.

To Nancy Dalton for allowing us the peace of mind to write this book.

To all our friends and clients, who shared their birth experiences, gave us suggestions, and fueled our enthusiasm, especially Christie Smith.

To our families for special support and encouragement.

And last, but not least, to the hundreds of women who wrote us and filled out our questionnaires.

We give our sincerest thanks.

Introduction

*I*n 1982, I took my first Lamaze class with Diana and was immediately impressed by both her candor and her thoroughness. Diana is an ASPO-certified Lamaze instructor who has been teaching the method since 1976. She has attended many births and heard the accounts of hundreds of others. I felt lucky indeed to have the benefit of Diana's expertise as I neared the birth of my first child.

Six weeks later my daughter, Elizabeth, was born. However, it was only after that I realized what a good teacher I had had. Although I had been skeptical at first, the Lamaze techniques worked beautifully. The exercises were designed to alleviate pain in labor and help women achieve drug-free childbirth, and this is exactly what they did for me. The birth of my daughter was a wonderful experience, and I wanted the world to know how strongly I believed in natural childbirth and how helpful Lamaze had been.

I approached Diana with the idea of writing a book on Lamaze, and she was very enthusiastic about the opportunity to bring her teaching to a wider audience. As we worked together, however, we realized that there were many other good reasons for this book.

Diana and I share the deep belief that natural childbirth is superior for both mother and baby and that the Lamaze method is the best preparation for this goal. We are convinced that Lamaze works and that this training is one of the most important preparations a couple can make for the birth of their baby. We want everyone to have access to the techniques and information that are part of Lamaze.

Almost two million women study the Lamaze method every year. Today Lamaze is a household word, but twenty-five years ago, it was a radical departure from common childbirth practices. Doctors and hospitals originally fought against change, but through the determination of a few pioneers and the fervency of its practitioners, intervention-free, family-centered care has now been incorporated into modern obstetrics.

We have written this book because we believe the method badly needs updating. Obstetrics has undergone a revolution in the past fifteen years, transformed from the stepchild of the medical profession to a respected high-tech specialty. The cesarean rate has increased fivefold, and doctors are increasingly practicing defensive medicine under the continual threat of malpractice. Lamaze teachers have traditionally incorporated changes in their class material, but the popular literature has lagged way behind. We want to correct this deficiency and to instruct women in how to use the Lamaze techniques as effectively as possible.

We also want to make a case for using the Lamaze method to have natural childbirth. We are appalled that much of the childbirth experience seems to have reverted back to where it started. Sedatives have been replaced by Demerol, and spinals have been replaced by epidurals. Women are no longer unconscious, but they are still numb from the waist down and their babies are still being delivered by forceps. Today women are encouraged by their doctors, hospitals, and even some childbirth educators to prepare for medication and "not be a martyr." This conditioning does not acknowledge that for most women the thrill of natural childbirth far outweighs the pain of labor and that a baby is given the best possible start in life if birth is untainted by drugs, anesthesia, or instruments.

We have found that almost everyone finds the Lamaze techniques helpful. Even those women who have had the hardest time giving birth concede that they couldn't have gotten as far as they did without Lamaze. This is the strength of the method; it enables women to have natural childbirth and helps those who don't to require lesser amounts of medication and decreased intervention.

In order to present accurate information, we did extensive research and read professional journals, studies, texts, and other books about birth. We also interviewed many mothers, fathers, doctors, midwives, and other childbirth educators. While Diana's expertise provides the backbone for this book, we also tried to draw upon the wisdom and experience of as many other people as possible.

We hope you will read this book soon after you become pregnant. Your delivery may seem very far away, but it's never too soon to begin your preparations. We will help you to decide where to have your baby, how to evaluate your doctor or midwife, and how to locate an excellent Lamaze teacher. The focus of this book, however, is on birth, with complete information about the last month of pregnancy through the postpartum period. This is not a book about pregnancy; information about nutrition, fetal development, and the experience of pregnancy will have to be found elsewhere.

The information here is meant to complement your Lamaze classes, not to replace them. By reading this book early you can get a head start on learning the exercises, relaxation techniques, and breathing patterns. But only an instructor can give you personal attention, correct any difficulties, and answer your questions. Seek out an excellent instructor and attend Lamaze class as well.

Another purpose of writing this book was to provide reassurance. There's no getting around it: Having a baby is frightening and just about every woman needs support and information. While useful generalizations can be made about labor and delivery, it is also true that there is simply no such thing as an average birth. One woman can have a short, pain-free labor while another may require a cesarean section after many hours of hard work. Two women may have labors of similar length and intensity, but one ends up feeling exhilarated and enthusiastic, the other disillusioned and resentful. Each experience is as unique as the woman herself. Both circumstances and perceptions vary tremendously.

To help us describe this wide range of experience, as well as to bring you both the theory and the reality of childbirth, we have included the words of hundreds of women and their partners. These you will find throughout the book, particularly in chapter 16, which is composed of comprehensive labor reports. The source of the majority of this material was a questionnaire we created and distributed at the suggestion of our editor, Joëlle Delbourgo. (It is reproduced in the back of this book, on page 429.)

In 1984, we placed an ad in *Parents* magazine, asking women to send for a questionnaire about childbirth. It read:

> Was your birth experience memorable, or was it something you want to forget? We are a childbirth educator and a mother writing a book on the relationship between natural childbirth and current obstetrical practice. We'd like to hear about your experience. Please send for our questionnaire.

We didn't specifically mention Lamaze because we wanted to hear from women who used other types of childbirth preparation and discover the percentage of women who studied each method. We also kept the description of our book as neutral as possible because we wanted to learn about all types of birth experiences, the positive as well as the negative.

We expected that perhaps two hundred women would reply; when the post office called to ask us to come to pick up our mail, we assumed the box was getting full. Instead, there was an entire mailbag waiting for us, packed with long letters and requests for the questionnaire. In all, we received more than three thousand responses to the ad, and from these, nearly one thousand women (and most of their partners) filled out five long pages of detailed questions.

Our request touched a nerve, and women seized the opportunity to talk about one of life's most important experiences. We were overwhelmed, to say the least, but we quickly became absorbed in the hundreds of different and fascinating birth stories. We heard from women living in trailer parks and on army bases, from small towns as well as from the biggest cities. Many included comments about more than one birth. Answers were crammed into the spaces provided and often spilled onto the backs of the pages and onto added sheets. Some generous women even included photographs of their births and their babies. We laughed and cried as we read. The women and men who wrote to us were funny, courageous, exuberant, and extremely canny about current birth practices. We selected hundreds of their comments and descriptions for inclusion in this book; to our great regret, we had to put aside thousands of others because there simply wasn't room.

The majority of the women who filled out our questionnaire had studied the Lamaze technique, and they described their teachers and the method in glowing terms. This overwhelmingly positive response fueled our enthusiasm for the book. A large percentage studied Lamaze in order to experience natural childbirth, and many of them succeeded. We were pleased and surprised at the range of choices available throughout the country and the number of women who had the opportunity to deliver at home, in alternative birthing centers, and in delivery chairs or beds. We were amazed and appalled to learn that doctors were still insisting on enemas and full pubic shaves—practices we thought had long been abandoned.

As expected, there was unequivocal praise for the partners' support, and over and over again we read, "I couldn't have done it without him." The descriptions of the highlight of the birth experience brought tears of joy to our eyes and made us want to get pregnant ourselves.

In order to have a great birth experience, we think you need as much preparation as possible, a good doctor or midwife, the strong emotional support of your partner, and motivation. We hope our book will help you achieve all of these. We also hope that during labor, you will reflect on the words of the women in our book and feel less alone.

We wish you an absolutely fabulous labor, an easy delivery, and a gorgeous, healthy baby who sleeps through the night from the first day home.

How to Use This Book

♦

If you are like most pregnant women, you will buy or borrow several books on pregnancy and childbirth and browse through them all. You may dip into each one at different places or read them cover to cover in one sitting.

We've designed this book so that it works best if you read it systematically from beginning to end. Each chapter builds on the information in preceding ones, in chronological order, so that the information will make the most sense if you read the chapters in sequence. We encourage your partner to read the entire book, too, but if time or inclination prevents this, he can simply read the partner's chapter.

We've organized the material so that there is a minimal amount of repetition. If you browse through the book at random, you may think a particular topic has been glossed over, when in fact, a more thorough discussion may be elsewhere. There has been some cross-referencing within the text, but if you need more information on a specific subject, you should check the index. Rather than continually redefining medical terms, we have included a glossary. It's located at the back of the book beginning on page 441.

Certain other information is summarized in chart or list form. For example, you will find a review of labor at the end of chapter 5, a description of drugs used during childbirth at the end of chapter 11, and suggestions for packing your Lamaze bag in chapter 7. As you near your due date, you may want to review the summaries or cut out some of the charts (such as "The Partner's Guide to Labor") and pack them into your Lamaze bag.

We have tried to present detailed and up-to-date information as much as possible, but medical practice varies widely from location to location, and in general, the field of obstetrics is quickly changing. This book will help clarify the issues and present current thinking, but it should never be used as a substitute for talking to your doctor or midwife about the specific nature of his or her practice.

Lastly, a note on gender. Some may accuse us of sexism, because throughout the book we refer to mothers as *she* and doctors and babies as *he.* Since the mother is always female, we use the pronoun *he* for everyone else. This is not meant as a slight to female obstetricians, but simply as a means of preventing confusion. The repeated use of *he or she* for every reference to the doctor or baby is cumbersome. A neutral pronoun would be ideal, but has yet to be invented.

PREPARATION FOR BIRTH

chapter 1

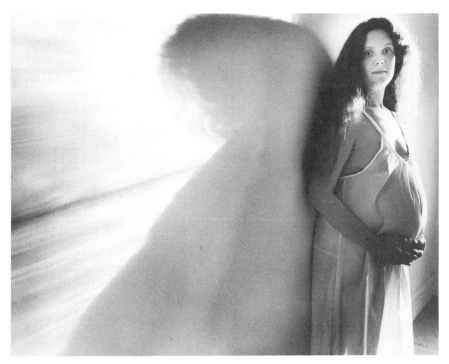

The Lamaze Method

O ne of the most profound changes that has taken place in the twen-
tieth century concerns the manner in which women give birth.
Today women are knowledgeable about the processes and procedures
of childbirth. They prepare themselves mentally and physically ahead of
time, and they expect to exercise a certain amount of control. Women

once accepted all kinds of medication and intervention; they now assume that these measures will be taken only if medically necessary. Husbands, once banished to lonely waiting rooms, now play an active role in a joyful celebration of life.

The Lamaze method helps women in every stage of childbirth, from pregnancy to the postpartum period. You probably know that Lamaze involves certain kinds of breathing patterns, but there is more to Lamaze than learning how to pant-blow through a contraction. Lamaze's goal is to enable women to experience natural childbirth. To accomplish that, Lamaze teaches you what to expect from labor, how to cope with pain, what options are available if complications occur, and how to achieve your fantasy birth, whatever that may be. Lamaze expects you to play an active role in the management of your labor and delivery, to work hard, and to be *assisted* in giving birth, not *delivered.*

The Lamaze theory is founded on several principles. The first is that education dispels fear. The Lamaze technique educates couples about the realities of labor and delivery so that they will have an idea of what to expect. Couples are taught relaxation techniques, which are used to counteract muscular tension, the natural response to pain. In addition, the Lamaze method teaches a series of breathing exercises designed to distract a laboring woman's mind from pain. These breathing techniques work on a sensory principle called the gate theory. When attention is focused on one specific thing, such as breathing or a focal point, the transmission of pain signals is blocked. The theory is that the brain is capable of receiving only one kind of stimulation, and pain messages are stopped by the gate.

There are many pitfalls in the road to a good birth experience: long labors, intrusive hospital procedures, unsympathetic doctors, and a natural fear of giving birth. But in almost every case, the Lamaze method is helpful. The strength of the method is that it enables many women to have natural childbirth and helps those who can't to use minimal amounts of medication and accept minimal intervention.

BEFORE LAMAZE

Thirty years ago, obstetric wards were filled with women whose only positive expectation about birth was to emerge with a healthy baby. Labor was often painful and lonely and usually heavily medicated. Elective inductions were performed routinely, and many women knew in

◆

"Was so glad we had taken the classes. I really felt my husband and I were as ready as we could possibly be."

◆

"I felt I had been well prepared and had control of what was happening around me and to me."

◆

"It helped, but I was still scared in labor."

◆

"I felt wonderful—ready to have another one!"

◆

"Although I didn't follow all of the prescribed breathing, it was still wonderful."

◆

"A laboring woman is in no position to have to make an uneducated choice or decision. For people who want to participate as a couple and want to minimize medication and medical intervention, Lamaze is the way to go!"

◆

"At first, I felt uneasy about natural childbirth, thinking I could never withstand the pain. But once I got to the hospital and calmed down and started the breathing techniques, I realized how wonderful this experience could be. My daughter is now almost a year old, and hardly a day goes by that I do not think of when she was born and what a truly wonderful experience it was to have given birth to her the natural way."

◆

continued

◆

"I was somewhat skeptical beforehand about whether or not it would really work. After labor and delivery, I became a firm supporter of Lamaze."

◆

"My main criticism of Lamaze is the way it gives you the idea that childbirth is mind over matter and that everything will work the way you want it to if you do your homework. This is facile to the point of being damaging. I could never have had a natural birth, but part of my sense of guilt and failure are because the Lamaze mystique says, 'Anyone can,' and I can't. The labor was long and difficult, and the cesarean was a colossal disappointment, but I was glad that I had the courage to stay awake for the surgery and that my husband had the courage to stay with me. Perhaps Lamaze training helped give us the strength for that."

◆

"I am usually a very nervous person when it comes to new experiences. Thanks to Lamaze preparation, I was calm and relaxed. Without the breathing techniques, I probably would have been one of the screaming women in the next room. I was prepared, and I knew what to expect."

◆

"Although nothing can prepare you for the pain, I think I was ahead by knowing how to work with the contractions."

◆

"God bless Lamaze!"

◆

"I felt misled, to some extent, by my Lamaze instruction, which had emphasized the ease of natural childbirth. This was complicated by my perfectionistic desire to 'do it right,' to be in control, and to match the success stories I had heard about or seen (mother does breathing flawlessly, pushes a few times, and delivers a baby

continued

with a smile on her face and no sweat, pain, or tears). I *was* able to use the Lamaze technique and stay in control of the pain for the most part, but I hadn't expected labor to be so painful and wished someone had told me it could be. I was surprised that it was so difficult.''

♦

"The Lamaze method is wonderful. It got us involved and prepared us in a very positive way for the great and scary unknown. I have heard complaints from mothers that the actual labor and birth was far harder than they had been led to believe, but I don't think that criticism is valid. We were not told it would be easy or painless. If all of us went away confident that we could lick it (even if we later discovered we couldn't completely), well, it waylaid most of our fears and stress, and at least we went through a portion of our labor fairly calm. That can only help, especially since facing childbirth for the first time is terrifying. For those of us who experience less than textbook-perfect childbirths—I had a cesarean after five hours in transition—or who couldn't continue the Lamaze techniques, an unprepared childbirth would have been that much more horrific, physically and emotionally. Both my husband and I feel that Lamaze made the birth of our son the most beautiful experience of our lives.''

advance exactly the day their babies would be born. Childbirth itself was not particularly joyful, and it was merely a means to an end.

Consider this typical scenario: A woman in labor was dropped off at the hospital by her husband. After being admitted and sent to the labor floor, the mother-to-be was put into a hospital gown, given an enema, and subjected to a complete pubic shave. She might have been given a pill to hold under her tongue. This was Pitocin, known in this form as buccal-Pitocin, and it stimulated labor contractions. As labor intensified, she was given scopolamine, a drug nicknamed "twilight sleep" for its tendency to induce a hallucinogenic haze. She was confined to a bed, forced to use a bedpan, hooked up to an intravenous, and her hands were often restrained to prevent her from harming herself. When she was fully dilated, she was wheeled to the delivery room and tied down again. Her doctor performed an episiotomy and then delivered the baby by forceps. The baby was taken immediately to the hospital nursery without being seen or touched by his mother.

The next day this woman probably thanked the doctor profusely because scopolamine is an amnestic and she didn't remember anything. In the 1950s, most women expected to be unconscious during childbirth. The average hospital stay was about five days. Breastfeeding was discouraged, and babies spent most of their time in the hospital nursery.

HOW LAMAZE BEGAN

All of that began to change, however, one summer's day in 1951 when an unknown French doctor named Fernand Lamaze attended the International Congress of Obstetricians and Surgeons in Russia. Lamaze had heard about a new method of pain control used by laboring women called psychoprophylaxis, literally meaning "mind prevention." In Leningrad he was able to witness a full labor and delivery during which this technique was employed. His reaction was one of utter amazement. "I had, at the time, thirty years of experience as an obstetrician. I had never been taught anything like this. I had never seen it, nor had I ever thought it could be possible. My emotional reaction was therefore all the stronger. I made a clean sweep of all preconceived ideas and, now an elderly schoolboy of sixty, I immediately began studying this new science."

When he returned to Paris, Lamaze became a proselytizer for the psychoprophylactic method of childbirth. Interestingly, his middle-class patients were less than enthralled with his new approach and Lamaze's practice shrank. This turned out to be a blessing in disguise for it afforded him the time to refine the technique with the patients at a local metalworkers clinic where he was chief of obstetrics.

Today Lamaze's name is a household word. The psychoprophylactic method of pain control is taught in every hamlet of North America and Europe. Lamaze has become part of the rite of passage to parenthood along with decorating the nursery and choosing names.

The Lamaze theory is founded on several principles: The first is that education dispels fear. During the 1940's British obstetrician Grantly Dick-Read wrote about the fear-tension-pain syndrome in relation to childbirth. He surmised that fear caused tension which created unnecessary pain which caused more fear, then more tension and so on in a vicious cycle. The Lamaze technique prevents this syndrome by preparing couples for the realities of labor. In addition, Lamaze students are taught relaxation techniques which are used to counteract muscular tension, the natural response to pain. The Lamaze method also includes a series of breathing exercises designed to help women cope with the pain of labor.

Lamaze was popularized in the United States largely through the efforts of two women, Marjorie Karmel and Elisabeth Bing. We met with Mrs. Bing in her New York apartment and she shared with us her memories of the early days of the Lamaze movement as well as those of her deep friendship with Marjorie Karmel.

Both women had had their first children in 1955: Karmel had a beautiful birth experience in Paris, using the Lamaze method with her husband, a labor coach, and Dr. Lamaze in attendance; Bing, attended only by her doctor in a New York hospital, received a spinal anesthetic, which left her with an eleven-day headache.

For the next few years Bing continued to teach preparation for childbirth at Mount Sinai Hospital, using the Grantly Dick-Read method (the earliest method of childbirth preparation and a precursor to Lamaze and Bradley). Her own experience convinced her, however, that the method was flawed, and she was casting about for a more effective technique. Karmel had her second child in America, using the Lamaze method (an induced labor), and in 1958 *Harper's Bazaar* published her article, "A New Method of Painless Childbirth."

Bing kept hearing of the Lamaze method but she couldn't find anything to read about it. At last in 1958 a Cleveland doctor, Isadore Bonstein, wrote the first book in English about the technique: *Painless Childbirth Through Psychoprophylaxis.* "Just after getting the book, I had a private patient come to me to prepare for her second baby," Mrs. Bing recounted to us. "I told her I had just received it and couldn't teach her the method, but I told her to take the book and read it. She did and then had her baby. A few days later, she called and said, 'It works! It works! It works!' "

The following year, in 1959, Karmel's book, *Thank You, Dr. Lamaze,* was published. It was immediately recommended to Bing, who read it and was very impressed. "I wrote to the publisher for Marjorie's address and found she lived just across the park (Central Park in New York). Her oldest son was a few months older than mine," Bing said, "and we became great friends."

The two women immediately began to organize a campaign to promote the Lamaze method in the United States. They geared their approach to doctors because they felt that without medical support the technique would go nowhere. They began educating people about the Lamaze technique, using a French film, *Naissance* (birth), which had to be smuggled into the United States so that it wouldn't be confiscated as pornography. The film was shown and reshown at Marjorie Karmel's apartment. Hundreds of people saw it, some of them receptive, others hostile. Many people were impressed with the film simply because they weren't used to seeing women give birth without forceps.

From the people who saw the film, a small group emerged—ten doctors, plus Karmel, Bing, and Elly Rakowitz (a mother who successfully used Lamaze)—to form the American Society for Psychoprophylaxis in Obstetrics (ASPO). Dr. Benjamin Segal was its first president, and membership was initially limited to doctors, nurses, and physiotherapists, those people who could most easily put Lamaze into practice. Elisabeth Bing and Marjorie Karmel were not happy about this organizational arrangement, but felt it was necessary if Lamaze was to be widely accepted. A year later, in 1961, the organization was restructured into its current form of three separate-but-equal divisions: one for doctors, one for childbirth educators, and another for parents.

USING LAMAZE FOR NATURAL CHILDBIRTH

We define *natural childbirth* as birth that takes place without the influence of drugs or anesthesia (except, of course, the local anesthetic for an episiotomy).

We believe that most women, given the proper emotional support, can use the Lamaze method to have natural childbirth. Often there is confusion about the difference between "natural" and "prepared" childbirth. *Prepared childbirth* is an ambiguous term because it can mean preparation for just about any type of birth experience, ranging from a scheduled cesarean to homebirth.

We advocate natural childbirth because it is the ideal way to have a

◆

"After the first meeting, I realized that I didn't know as much about labor and delivery as I thought I did. I learned *everything* that could happen and what we could do to make it easier."

◆

"Lamaze made my baby's birth the most memorable moment of my life."

◆

"I didn't want to end up like my mother-in-law, who was drugged so much she didn't know she had a baby until the next day."

◆

"Afterward I realized that the class was very helpful in preparing me for both back labor and a cesarean, neither of which I thought could ever happen to me."

◆

"The coping techniques gave me something to hold on to and got me through the worst parts of labor. Instead of going over the cliff (as I felt I might), Lamaze gave me the footholds to keep going and reach the top."

◆

"Several times during labor I would think, 'What would I have done without Sara's class!'"

◆

"Without Lamaze we would have been at sea. It really opened our eyes to alternatives."

◆

"As a labor and delivery nurse, I learned that Lamaze-prepared couples accomplished their stated goals more often than couples with alternative preparation."

continued

"I wanted to understand childbirth better than I had during the births of my two sons, where I was drugged and anesthetized and totally out of control and frightened. After this time, I was very pleased that I'd had a drug-free labor and delivery and was *proud* of myself."

"I felt that it was the thing to do."

"To get a better understanding of the delivery process."

"I took Lamaze so that I could share the experience of labor and delivery with my reluctant husband and so that I could play a more active role in the birth process."

"To have a birth that was meaningful, unmedicated, and safe, and to involve my husband in the entire pregnancy and birth process."

"I wanted to be a participant, not just a patient."

baby. Ever since its inception, ASPO/Lamaze has considered one of its primary goals to be decreasing the need for medication during delivery. We're not implying, however, that if you take medication during labor, you can't have a wonderful birth experience. Drugs and anesthesia have their place, and medication is sometimes the best solution to a problem in labor. The Lamaze method teaches you to make an informed choice about your options. If medication is needed, you should not allow guilt and regret to overshadow the positive emotions of childbirth.

We believe that a woman's ability to have natural childbirth is influenced by her motivation. Some women come to Lamaze class and say their goal is to handle labor until they can receive pain medication, whereas others say they want to experience birth without any drugs or anesthesia. The beauty of the Lamaze technique is that whatever your goal, you can use and benefit from the training.

We were really impressed by the women who filled out our questionnaires. Most of them said they wanted unmedicated births, and many of them accomplished this goal. Those who did have drug-free births perceived their babies to be especially alert immediately after birth and attributed this to the absence of medication or anesthesia. They also expressed great pride in giving their babies the best possible start in life. But interestingly enough, these mothers also expressed genuine understanding and compassion for women who did receive drugs and anesthesia.

One of the biggest recent changes in the Lamaze technique is its overdue recognition that childbirth can be painful. The earlier attitude stemmed in part from Dr. Lamaze's name for his method: *"accouchement sans douleur,"* which means literally, "childbirth without pain." Because labor is a natural body process, just like digestion or breathing, he couldn't believe that it had to be so intensely painful. Lamaze found that women approached birth frightened by old wives' tales and general misinformation, but that after proper training and education, many of them could use the breathing techniques to avoid pain. Childbirth without pain is possible in some cases, but not in most, and usually not for first-time mothers. Lamaze no longer claims to be a technique to achieve painless childbirth, but rather an effective method for coping with the pain.

Childbirth educators do women a disservice when they avoid the word *pain* and substitute *discomfort.* Granted, there is a fine line between educating people and frightening them, but we don't think anyone will be surprised to hear that labor is painful. Besides, pain really can't be measured; it boils down to a matter of perception. A demonstrated low or high threshold for pain has little to do with the way a woman handles labor; it's attitude and support that count.

Most women are afraid of the pain of childbirth. Pain is a part of giving birth, but it doesn't have to define the experience. Marathon runners or weight lifters push their bodies to the limit, experiencing pain and fatigue, and their efforts are something to be admired. Why can't we have the same sort of respect for women in labor? Labor pains are more productive than any other kind because at their end lies a new life, not just a new statistic.

Lamaze works beautifully because it constitutes only one-third of the time spent in labor. You spend one-third of your time breathing through pain and the remaining two-thirds relaxing. If you're motivated and you can relax, labor should go well because the breathing gives you something to do, altering your perception of the pain's intensity. Every physical discipline uses special breathing, and labor should be no exception. After doing Lamaze breathing for several hours, many women reach a kind of transcendent state that removes them from the physical experience. This is analogous to the kind of high, dreamy feeling long-distance runners often achieve. It's a beautiful sensation, and it should be your goal.

Lamaze works best under ideal conditions. You're obviously going to feel a lot more relaxed if you're in a comfortable position, if you can move about freely, if people are helpful, and if your partner is with you. Your ability to use Lamaze is bound to be compromised if you're immobilized by an intravenous and a fetal monitor and you're worried because your doctor hasn't shown up yet. If, for whatever reasons, the breathing techniques aren't enough and you need pain relief, that's okay. At least your Lamaze course will have familiarized you with different types of medication and their effects (see chapter 11). If things go well, Lamaze will enable you to have natural childbirth. If things don't go as smoothly as you hoped, Lamaze should nonetheless provide you with some measure of relief, as well as preparation for the unexpected.

THE LAMAZE TEACHER

We hope that couples can learn the Lamaze method by reading our book. But we also believe that a book is no substitute for a good teacher. Ideally you will use this book to complement what you learn in class. As one woman said in response to our questionnaire, "No matter how much I read, I wanted an instructor to give me individualized attention."

You may think you can get by without going to class and learn the

♦

"The day she 'delivered' Bert the Muppet from a dryer pipe kept us laughing during many tense moments."

♦

"She had a marvelous positive attitude and seemed genuinely concerned about each couple. But I think her positive attitude went a bit too far and that she did not present a realistic picture of the pain involved."

♦

"She wanted to help all of us, but she was a mouthpiece for hospital policy, as if there was no other way to do it."

♦

"She was extremely positive and supportive. I liked the fact that she didn't stress a 'right' or 'wrong' way, but encouraged us to feel that what would be most comfortable would be the best."

♦

"She had several children and had used Lamaze in their delivery. She was very honest about what had worked for her. All of us were first-timers, and her success was encouraging."

♦

"Our instructor was an R.N. She was knowledgeable, approachable, and enthusiastic."

♦

"We had two instructors. One was kind, loving, and supportive. I could ask her anything, and she would have an answer both clinical and personal. The other was extremely knowledgeable, but she was so antihospital it was frightening. She

continued

often made remarks that made me uncomfortable, as if my child's birth would be ruined by having a medical person available."

♦

"Her biggest strength was her faith in the Lamaze method. She didn't tell us that this would be painless childbirth, but instead told us that through Lamaze we would learn to gain control of the pain and have it work *for* us instead of *against* us."

♦

"She gave me so *much* of a positive outlook that I had no open mind for anything but a beautiful, easy natural childbirth—which I did not have at all."

♦

"Really tops. She knew her material and covered it in a friendly and informative manner—and she had had four children using the Lamaze method!"

♦

"We had four instructors, who took turns leading the class. I appreciated the variety of leadership offered, and I felt that was a strength of the class."

♦

"My instructor has been a nurse for at least twenty years. She was very informative and stressed that every woman is different; you can't all expect the same experiences."

Lamaze techniques from our book, but it's not the same. We know it's a lot of trouble to rush home from work, gulp down dinner, and then run off to class, especially in the third trimester, but you won't learn the method nearly as well without some expert instruction. A teacher can demonstrate the right rhythms for the breathing patterns and can offer corrections if you're breathing too slowly or too fast. She's also there to answer any questions either of you may have.

The women who filled out our questionnaire overwhelmingly found their Lamaze teachers to be knowledgeable, helpful, and enthusiastic. Many women could not point out a single weakness in their instructor. We discovered, however, that people have different expectations about what a teacher should do. Some complained because their teachers glossed over possible complications, while others were dissatisfied because pain was not discussed. Many were pleased to have a pregnant instructor or one who was a mother herself.

How Lamaze Teachers Are Certified

All Lamaze teachers are certified by the ASPO/Lamaze organization (which is accredited by the Council for Noncollegiate Continuing Education), and they must satisfy rigorous standards before becoming teachers. To qualify, a person must be a registered nurse or hold a baccalaureate diploma. Then, the candidate is interviewed by a three-member committee, one of whom is a certified ASPO teacher. If the committee approves the candidate, she then pays a nonrefundable fee, fills out an application, and begins the training. This consists of taking an exam in four subjects—the physiology of pregnancy, the psychoprophylactic method, community relations, and instructional methods—observing five complete births and submitting detailed birth reports about each one, and then observing two full series of Lamaze classes.

At that point, the candidate is required to attend a twenty-six-hour seminar taught by faculty from the national ASPO/Lamaze office. Then, within sixty days, she must submit an original syllabus for her own six- or eight-week Lamaze course. If the syllabus is satisfactory, the candidate practice-teaches one series of classes. The next step is a test on instructional methods. If she passes and the supervising teacher recommends her, she then becomes a certified Lamaze instructor with the letters ACCE (ASPO-Certified Childbirth Educator) following her name. The entire program usually takes from eighteen months to two years to complete. This is the primary way Lamaze teachers are trained, although in some cases a teacher may be certified by a chapter with the approval of the national organization or by completing a university program.

How to Select a Lamaze Teacher

What can you do to find one of these well-qualified teachers? Well, it's not difficult. You can call the ASPO/Lamaze national office at (703) 524-7802 and inquire about instructors in your area. The mailing address is 1840 Wilson Boulevard, Suite 204, Arlington, Virginia 22201.

Your doctor or midwife or friends can probably recommend a good teacher. It's advisable to speak to a prospective instructor either by phone or in person, and it may also be helpful to speak to graduates of her classes.

When you query prospective instructors, you should be looking for enthusiasm, candor, accessibility, and for someone who will prepare you for variations of normal labor and delivery. Questions to ask include:

♦ *Is the instructor ASPO/Lamaze certified?*
  If there is any question, call the organization for verification.
♦ *How large will the class be?*
  Class size usually ranges from five to ten couples. A larger class is unwieldy.
♦ *How many sessions are held?*
  The course usually runs about six weeks. Be suspicious of any course that claims it can teach you about childbirth in two or three sessions.
♦ *How long is each session?*
  In general, one class should last from one and a half to two hours.
♦ *What are your feelings about childbirth?*
  Look for an answer that seems consistent with your beliefs.
♦ *Is an early-bird class available?*

There are several pitfalls in this selection process of which you should be aware:

First of all, make sure that any course you sign up for, especially if it is taught through your hospital, is really a Lamaze course, taught by an ASPO/Lamaze-certified instructor. The ASPO/Lamaze organization receives many complaints from people about hospital "Lamaze" classes. Hospitals frequently run programs that consist of a hospital tour and a talk by a labor nurse. This is billed as a prepared-childbirth course, and while the term *Lamaze* may be bandied about, it is not a Lamaze course. To avoid this deception, make your own check to see if the instructor is certified.

Hospital classes tend to be large and are usually taught by a labor and delivery nurse who works at the hospital. She is therefore very familiar with the policies of the institution and is unlikely to encourage rebellion against her employer. She may prepare you to face the standard hospital procedures, not to exercise your rights. Although your hospital teacher may be trained and certified by ASPO/Lamaze, she doesn't have the freedom of expression that a private teacher does. We believe private teachers are best because there's no question that their allegiance lies with the client. In addition, private classes are usually smaller, so you are able to receive more individualized instruction.

Private Lamaze classes, most commonly held in the homes of instructors, are often slightly more expensive than those offered by hospitals. We know this is a consideration for many people, but we encourage you to spend the extra money. Women who filled out our questionnaire repeated over and over that a good instructor made a tremendous difference in reducing their fear and helping them cope with the stresses of birth.

Second, it is vital that your Lamaze instructor be both *honest* and knowledgeable about medical procedures. Lamaze teachers are discovering that couples today have a great many questions and concerns about the use of technology during labor and delivery. Instructors must inform their classes about all the newest monitoring and appliances, such as fetal-scalp sampling. This is important because it touches on the malpractice issue. It's critical that your Lamaze teacher tell the whole story about these devices and that she not be one-sided in her presentation. Lamaze takes a position of advocacy for new parents, and there are always several sides to every story.

Third, be especially cautious if the Lamaze instructor is your doctor's wife or works in his office. While there's nothing inherently wrong in an obstetrician's wife being a Lamaze instructor, it's much more difficult for her to be objective about the way her husband practices. For example, if he does a lot of forceps deliveries, she's likely to tell you this is a very good way to have a baby. Lamaze instructors are not doctors' adversaries, but they should feel free to exert a healthy independence. This freedom is sometimes hard to achieve because just about every Lamaze teacher depends on doctors for referrals. The dependency is certainly exacerbated, however, if the instructor is married to the source of her referrals or depends on him for her weekly paycheck. The doctor may feel that by sponsoring Lamaze training he is offering comprehensive care, but you are actually being deprived of a choice.

THE LAMAZE CLASS

Lamaze courses usually start at the beginning of the eighth month of pregnancy. The reason for this timing is that you'll enter labor with the breathing and relaxation techniques fresh in your mind. It's to your advantage if the Lamaze series includes an early-bird session to discuss exercise and nutrition during pregnancy, as well as how to choose a doctor or midwife (see chapter 2), which is one of the most important decisions you will make while you are pregnant. If an early-bird session is not a standard part of the course, you will have to research these issues on your own.

Some courses require that you sign up well ahead of time, often months in advance, so start researching your options early.

Classes provide a format for expressing ideas and fears about giving birth. You don't have to speak in class if you don't care to, but you'll probably be surprised how much you end up contributing to class discussion. Even if you don't want to talk about your personal experience, you'll enjoy just being in the company of other very-pregnant women and their partners. Many people who filled out our questionnaire remarked how much they liked the camaraderie classes provided.

We have noticed that men tend not to read about pregnancy or childbirth during their wives' pregnancies, so they often pick up the bulk of their knowledge in Lamaze class. Also, by attending the classes, the imminence of your baby's birth may become more real to your husband.

THE FUTURE OF LAMAZE

In 1985 ASPO/Lamaze celebrated its silver anniversary. The occasion seemed the perfect time to ask its executive director, Robert Moran, what the next twenty-five years held in store. The organization is strong at this time, with more than 6,100 teachers, and approximately 500 additional teachers being trained each year.

One trend Moran sees and doesn't like is the movement of hospitals into the childbirth-education business. "In the past, we could pretty much rest on our image as the good guys and we didn't have any problem with business. Now, hospitals want to capture the obstetric market from the earliest possible point," he said. "Hospitals are trying to be comprehensive, saying, 'Look, we have an entire package: childbirth education, baby care, labor, and delivery, and it's all here.' There

THE LAMAZE CLASS

◆

"Since it was difficult to keep from laughing while practicing in class and at home, I thought Lamaze would not be much help—we were not serious enough about it. I was amazed at how the practice sessions came back to me when I needed them."

◆

"I would have liked a more personal class. There were twenty couples in ours."

◆

"I was afraid while taking the class. The film made me even more afraid, and I was ready to chicken out at any moment. After giving birth, however, I was so glad I had taken the class and had had a natural delivery."

◆

"It was a hospital-sponsored class, so all they taught us was what they wanted us to know so that it would be easier on them."

◆

"Lamaze classes made the last two months of my pregnancy an active time. We enjoyed learning and practicing our exercises. It brought my husband much closer to what was happening to me."

◆

"I found out later that it wasn't actually a Lamaze class, though they showed us a few breathing techniques."

◆

"We enjoyed the classes tremendously. I was familiar with all the materials before taking the classes, but after our positive experience with our first child, we felt the classes were an important part of preparing ourselves for the birth experience. We needed the involvement to get mentally 'up' for the birth."

continued

"At first, the classes confirmed my worst fears about childbirth. As the classes progressed, I began to relax more because I knew I would have a lot of help and support from nurses, doctors, and husband. After birth, I was thankful I had attended classes."

◆

"Since the hospital gave the course, they told us exactly the hospital policies and procedures, which did help. However, I resented their assumption that medication would be needed."

is concern that couples are not receiving good preparation for childbirth in hospital courses. We've been using a little slogan for the past few years, 'All childbirth teachers are not created equal,' and it's quite true."

ASPO/Lamaze is pleased with the growing cooperation among health-care professionals. "We're happy to see the maternal child health team growing to include midwives, nurse practitioners, and, of course, our instructors," said Moran. "And the doctors are really beginning to share information with all these people. We think this is all to the good, helping provide healthier babies and mothers and better birth experiences for everyone."

We couldn't agree more and think Mr. Moran has succinctly stated the goals of Lamaze training: a healthy baby and mother and a memorable birth experience.

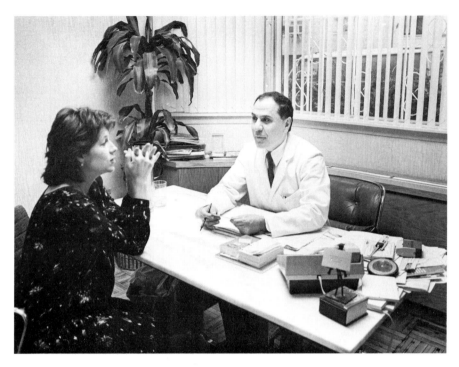

CHAPTER 2

Choosing Your Doctor or Midwife

A CRITICAL CHOICE

*E*very couple fantasizes about their baby-to-be, and those dreams are one of the most pleasurable parts of pregnancy. It's understandably difficult to pull yourself away from the imaginary realm of cooing babies in order to begin thinking about the real world of labor and delivery.

Right now, your baby's birth may seem remote, but in just a short time it will be more real than you can imagine. If you want to have some measure of control over your birth experience, you and your husband must plan ahead.

If you want natural childbirth, choosing an obstetrician or midwife will be the most important decision of your pregnancy. The quality of a couple's birth experience is primarily determined by three factors: your labor, your attitude, and the person who attends you. You don't have much control over the first variable, but you can improve your mental approach and you can have a supportive obstetrician or midwife. Many women say they want a fabulous birth experience but are quite casual about finding the person who can make it possible. The likelihood of a cesarean or forceps delivery can actually be determined when you select the person who will help you deliver your baby.

The Lamaze method is an active one. There will be many important decisions and you will need a doctor or midwife who is receptive to the idea of your involvement. To find the proper person, you should educate yourself about your options.

It seems only logical that upon beginning any new endeavor, whether it's buying a car or building a greenhouse, you would want to do some research into the available choices. Yet, most couples attend their first Lamaze class in the eighth month of pregnancy, completely unaware of many current obstetrical practices and their choices regarding these practices. Lamaze classes often become consciousness-raising sessions, in which standard hospital procedures surrounding childbirth are discussed. Consequently, many students don't know to ask about these issues until a few weeks before delivery. At that point, those who find their doctor's responses to be inflexible or vague usually wish they had brought up these topics months ago.

Midwifery and natural childbirth go hand in hand, and you will have an excellent chance of having a natural birth if you are able to use a midwife. Because midwifery is poorly understood, we have devoted a special section to it at the end of this chapter. We know, however, that 98 percent of you will be attended by a doctor. Therefore, this chapter concentrates on helping you find the best possible doctor.

From the outset, you've got to understand there's no such thing as perfection. Don't expect to find the perfect doctor or to have the perfect birth experience. There are always variables, such as fatigue or faltering contractions or an odd presentation, that can prevent you from achieving

A Critical Choice

♦

"In the office, the doctor had somewhat of a patronizing attitude. In the hospital, we realized how important the choice of a doctor is. He was in control, and the nurses basically did what he wanted done."

♦

"My doctor said that women need to start telling doctors what they want and fighting for it before the doctors will change. But first, we need to educate the public."

♦

"He was not supportive of my decision to try for a natural birth and took it for granted that I would require strong painkillers (which I didn't)."

♦

"The one thing I've learned, especially after having my second baby, is that you need support. You need a deeply committed doctor."

♦

"We had discussed my goals fairly extensively, and I thought I had made it clear that I wanted to go natural and generally just be left alone unless there was a medical emergency. But my doctor walked in and tried to take control immediately. He wanted to speed things up. I became very angry and told him so. After that he pretty much let me go at my own pace, but his attitude really stank."

♦

"I was lucky enough to have found a doctor who liked to see himself as a midwife —very noninterventionist, did perineal massage. I couldn't have asked for a better birth experience."

♦

continued

"My informed sources were limited. I asked everyone I knew about obstetricians and got a few names. But none were enthusiastically recommended. I was surprised how many women told me, 'I can't recommend my obstetrician. I was not happy.' "

♦

"I knew what I was looking for in a doctor. I wanted a woman obstetrician who had had a child of her own. I felt I could be most relaxed with someone who would know about pregnancy, labor, and delivery from the inside and the outside."

♦

"I got exactly what I wanted in medical care. My doctor was caring and patient and supportive. He didn't insist on prepping and didn't push any medication."

♦

"He turned down the lights, spoke softly, did not use stirrups until the last few stitches, and gave me my son as soon as he was delivered. I even pulled him out after the shoulders were delivered."

♦

"I felt totally let down because he went back to his office when I was fully dilated and forgot about me. He called the hospital three hours later and then ordered X rays. When he showed up, he decided to do a forceps delivery without any anesthetic. It was traumatic and painful."

♦

"The doctor let us do everything our way."

♦

continued

"My doctor was more attentive than I ever would have guessed. He was with me constantly, even held one leg while I pushed for forty-five minutes. He was very in tune to where I was, and he was just great!"

♦

"I was very happy with my doctor. He always had time to answer questions and treated me like a well-informed, intelligent individual who was in charge of her pregnancy."

your fantasy. But that doesn't mean you shouldn't try for everything you want.

A doctor's attitude can have a tremendous impact on your birth experience. It's the difference between a doctor who is supportive during labor and one who arrives once you're fully dilated. If you plan on a natural delivery, you've got to choose someone who understands the risks of medical intervention during childbirth. If you don't want a cesarean, you've got to find someone who performs them with great reluctance.

Although it's never too late to start a dialogue with your doctor, your bargaining position is much stronger in the first trimester of pregnancy than in the third. Don't save all the hard questions until the last minute. Your ninth month of pregnancy is not the time to realize that you and your obstetrician have different ideas about childbirth. Although the idea of interviewing a doctor ahead of time may make you nervous, it's the best way to find out how he practices. If you're unwilling to ask your doctor a few hard questions before you retain him, there's no real way of knowing if this is the right doctor for you. It is possible to fall into the hands of a great obstetrician by chance, but why leave it to luck?

Finding a doctor is like hiring any professional, for example, an architect, contractor, or accountant. You will be looking for someone who is competent but shares your philosophy. You want a person you can talk to comfortably and who is sensitive to your needs and desires. It's important to remember, however, that you are the one in control, the one who is making the choice.

SELECTING A DOCTOR
Getting Recommendations

In order to get the kind of doctor you want, you must actively seek recommendations and then interview those doctors who sound promising. We realize it would be more enjoyable to think up baby names or plan a nursery at this time, but in order to have a chance at the birth experience you would like, you must take control now. Soliciting recommendations is not difficult. We suggest you start with friends or neighbors who've recently had babies. Be sure to get as many details of labor and delivery as you can and ask specific questions about the doctor's involvement, so that you'll have an idea of how he practices. Also, you could inquire about the amount of time spent with the doctor during office visits, because this seems to be an area in which women frequently feel shortchanged. And you may want to ask your friend's husband, assuming he participated in the birth, about their doctor.

Take these recommendations with a grain of salt and keep in mind that different women need different things from their doctors. Sometimes a husband and wife have divergent ideas about the obstetrician, and it might be worthwhile to hear both opinions.

Another source of recommendations may be your internist or family doctor. Don't feel guilty about pressing your doctor for information; it's part of his job to recommend specialists. If you happen to know any nurses, ask them for names or for an introduction to a labor and delivery nurse, who will certainly have preferences among local obstetricians.

There are two excellent organizations that can help you find a doctor. Both train and certify childbirth educators. The first is ASPO/Lamaze (ASPO stands for the American Society for Psychoprophylaxis in Obstetrics), and you can usually find its local listing in the phone book. If not, contact the national ASPO/Lamaze office. The other group is the ICEA, or International Childbirth Education Association. See page 435 for both listings.

The Interview

The next and hardest step is interviewing the doctors from your list of hopefuls. When making an appointment, be sure to say exactly why you are calling so that the receptionist or nurse will schedule enough time for the visit. Some doctors will charge for the consultation, whereas others will give their time freely. To find out, simply ask about the doctor's policy concerning interview appointments when you call. If there is no precedent, we advise offering to pay so that it doesn't appear you're just window-shopping.

Many women report that they were glad their husbands went with them to interview prospective doctors. You are in this together, so your husband's opinion does matter. In addition, he may pick up on things you overlooked. The fact that the two of you are spending your time on a consultation also shows that you are serious. To help you find the right doctor, we've developed a list of questions you may want to ask. We don't expect you to storm into the office, clutching our questionnaire like a list of demands, but we do encourage you to ask every question you want. In general, we hope you won't be scoring doctors on their number of correct answers, but will be looking instead for an overall feeling of flexibility as well as a commitment to natural childbirth. The interview should help you discern the doctor's attitude and style of practice. We realize that some of you will be going to general practitioners and family-practice specialists instead of obstetricians, but you should screen them as closely as you would an obstetrician.

In order to make your interviewing easier, we're also providing what we consider to be appropriate answers to these questions. Again, don't take them too literally. There are any number of good responses to most of the questions, and an interview is not a test, but a chance to meet and evaluate someone you may be working with for nine months.

The following questionnaire contains technical terms and presents situations that we will discuss in much greater detail later. If you are unfamiliar with a term, refer either to the glossary in the back of the book or to the appropriate chapter.

THE DOCTOR'S QUESTIONNAIRE

Questions About the Practice

1. What is your hospital affiliation?

Obviously you'll want to know where your baby will be born. If your doctor has privileges at more than one hospital, you might ask which one he prefers and why. The answer may give you significant information. For example, the doctor might prefer hospital A instead of hospital B because A has an alternative birthing room and the nurses are well versed in Lamaze techniques. (See chapter 3, "Home, Hospital, or Birth Center.")

2. What is the fee and the payment schedule?

Fees vary from doctor to doctor and between cities and rural areas. In general, city obstetricians cost more. Some doctors charge a flat fee, no matter what type of pregnancy you have, while others will charge extra if you are high-risk or if you have a cesarean. Payment schedules and insurance arrangements differ from doctor to doctor. Do not make the mistake of believing that the most expensive obstetrician is the best. Doctors' fees are not an indication of skill.

3. Who covers for you in case of illness or vacation?

This question is applicable only to solo practitioners, because members of a group practice always cover for each other. At your first visit, an obstetrician should be able to tell you when vacations are scheduled, so that you'll know if his plans conflict with your due date.

4. Can I meet your backup?

There's no reason your doctor can't arrange to have you meet or talk to the person who replaces him in case of emergency. Even if the chance of your getting the backup doctor is slim, you don't want to run the risk of being with someone you haven't met.

5. How many times will I see you?

The standard schedule is usually a monthly visit until the eighth month, then a visit every other week until the ninth month, when you are examined weekly. Of course, there are variations—for example, if you are late or have a special medical problem—but normally you should be seen about twelve times in all, not counting postpartum checkups.

6. How long does an average appointment last?

A good answer might be: "As much time as necessary, depending on your physical condition and the questions you have." You want to know that the doctor will have the interest, and therefore the time, to discuss any of your concerns.

Questions About Labor

1. What are your feelings about natural childbirth?

It is essential that the answer to this question not contain any jokes or be accompanied by grimaces or other strange body language. If a doctor attempts to make a humorous remark about childbirth in the fields, you know you're not sitting in front of your future obstetrician. There are lots of acceptable answers to this one, but a really good doctor might say, "The less medication the better," and then ask how *you* feel about natural childbirth.

2. How do you view the role of the partner?

Look for an answer indicating some enthusiasm for the father's active participation. At the delivery, the doctor's attitude will influence your husband's experience as well as your own.

3. What percentage of your mothers receive drugs or anesthesia for labor and delivery?

If more than 50 percent of a doctor's patients receive medication, find out why. Some doctors consider natural childbirth to be a delivery in which a woman is awake and cooperative but numb from the waist down so that she can't feel the forceps pulling out her baby. If most of a doctor's patients receive some kind of medication, this could indicate a lack of commitment to true natural childbirth.

4. What medications do you normally use and under what circumstances?

When asked, many doctors respond that they use medication "when indicated." This is meaningless, so press on. Some doctors give medication as soon as a patient asks for it, others routinely give it at a certain point of dilation, still others would rather not give it at all. There's a world of difference here, and it's important to get a specific answer.

If a doctor says you won't have to feel a thing and that he uses "twilight sleep" (scopolamine), leave right away and forget about the rest of the interview. (For more on medication, see chapter 11.)

5. How much time do you usually spend with a woman in labor?

Obviously you can't expect a doctor to tell you exactly how many minutes he'll be with you at the hospital, but from the answer to this question you should be able to glean whether he'll be on the golf course, in the hospital, or actually in your room as you labor. What you don't want is a doctor who will arrive just in time to catch the baby. You're paying him to be with you for the "just in case," and that's where he should be.

6. What is your policy concerning such routines as the intravenous, enema, and pubic shave?

These procedures are totally up to the individual doctor's discretion. Most doctors have modified or omitted the enema and the shave, but many still insist on the use of the intravenous. This is a point you may be able to negotiate, but there are lots of caring *and* skillful doctors who insist on the IV "just in case." (See chapter 3 for a discussion of hospital routines.)

7. What percentage of your patients receive Pitocin?

We're against the routine use of Pitocin to speed up labor. A skillful doctor might say he relies on Pitocin as a last alternative, for example, when twelve hours have elapsed since the water has broken and there are no signs of contractions or if early labor drags on and on. A doctor who uses it with 50 percent of his patients is probably manipulating labor to fit his schedule.

8. How do you feel about fetal monitoring?

Fetal monitors are invaluable for high-risk pregnancies, but unfortunately some doctors insist that every patient be monitored continuously throughout labor. During your interview, try to determine how and when a doctor uses an internal or external fetal monitor. (For more on fetal monitors, see chapter 9).

9. Do you use fetal-scalp sampling?

Fetal-scalp sampling is now considered the most valid check on fetal distress because it accurately measures oxygen supply to the baby. Scalp sampling is not performed at all hospitals, so this is worth asking about.

10. What is your cesarean rate?

The national cesarean rate is more than 20 percent, and some doctors have rates as high as

35 percent. This is appalling. A doctor should have a cesarean rate of approximately 10 to 15 percent. If it's higher than that, ask why. Some doctors, for example, specialize in high-risk women with diabetes or hypertension, so it's important to interpret the doctor's answer correctly. Be skeptical of a doctor who equates better babies and the relief of unnecessary suffering with cesareans. (For more on cesareans, see chapter 12.)

11. Do you perform cesareans routinely for women who have had a previous cesarean section?

There used to be a saying, "Once a cesarean, always a cesarean," and unfortunately many doctors still practice by that outmoded axiom. More and more, however, are adopting a wait-and-see attitude, and a doctor familiar with the latest studies will generally let you attempt a normal delivery, depending on the reason for your previous cesarean.

12. If a cesarean is necessary, may my partner be with me for the operation?

Once men gained entrance to the delivery room, the next logical step was into the obstetrical operating room, where cesareans are performed. Unfortunately, there are still many hospitals that do not permit fathers to witness the cesarean births of their children. While it may be the hospital's policy to exclude fathers from cesarean births, exceptions can sometimes be made in advance if you are insistent. A caring doctor can tell you how to go about getting the necessary clearance.

13. If a woman's water breaks before labor begins, what do you do?

What you're trying to avoid is a doctor who will insist that your baby be born twenty-four hours after the membranes have ruptured, regardless of the progress of labor. Some doctors may try to scare you about the dangers of infection, but if you stay at home and use commonsense precautions, there shouldn't be a problem. Obviously, it's not ideal to have your water break and then have nothing happen, but—except for certain unusual situations—this shouldn't be treated as an emergency. Think twice if a doctor says he would put you in the hospital immediately and induce labor. On the other hand, if the doctor mentions the possibility of using natural methods to get labor started, you should be encouraged. (For more on induced labor, see chapter 8.)

14. What is your policy regarding a woman who is past her due date?

Here you are looking for flexibility and a basic trust in nature. Any doctor who routinely induces labor on or before the due date should be avoided. Bear in mind that a due date falls within a twenty-eight-day range, and any date within that period should be considered normal. (See chapter 7 for more on the significance of your due date.)

Questions About Delivery

1. Where do most of your deliveries take place?

Lying flat on your back on a delivery table is the worst possible position for delivery, defying the law of gravity, putting you at a mechanical disadvantage for pushing, and possibly interfering with the blood supply to the baby. Any doctor who doesn't insist on using the delivery room and will use a birthing room sounds promising. (See chapter 3, Choosing a Birth Site.) Any mention of sitting up, squatting, or side-lying is encouraging. Look for a doctor who takes your comfort and choice of position into consideration.

2. How do you feel about episiotomies?

All American doctors are trained to do episiotomies, and only an exceptional doctor will consider not performing one. A doctor who is flexible regarding the episiotomy will almost certainly be flexible about other procedures. Most midwives never perform episiotomies routinely and believe they are necessary only in unusual situations. (For more on episiotomies, see chapter 9.)

3. What are your feelings about the Leboyer birth method?

Many progressive doctors are now doing a modified Leboyer delivery, which means allowing the cord to stop pulsating before it is cut and dimming the lights. It seems to be a rare doctor who allows the Leboyer bath, but if you feel strongly about this, ask how it could be arranged.

4. How much time do couples usually spend with their baby immediately after the birth, assuming there are no problems?

There is no reason that you can't all be together for an hour or so after the birth, if everything goes well. You have certainly earned the reward of seeing and holding a healthy baby, and your doctor can make it possible.

An Alternative to the Interview

If you don't have the disposition to interview doctors, and not everyone does, there is one other way to determine if an obstetrician is really committed to natural childbirth—by talking to women (other than your friends) who have been his or her patients. This concept is analogous to providing references, and you shouldn't have any problem obtaining the names of a few recent patients. We got this idea from a friend, a doctor, who warned us that many obstetricians can sound as if they believe in Lamaze but practice very differently.

Other Considerations

SOLO OR GROUP PRACTICE?

We personally prefer a doctor who works alone, although we realize it is becoming increasingly difficult to find this type of obstetrician. We don't like the concept of a group because it is designed for the convenience of doctors, and personalized care suffers. However, there are two

RED FLAGS

◆

Sometimes it's hard to know when someone's putting one over on you, particularly if that someone is a doctor. We hope you'll interview your doctor using our questionnaire, but even with that, you could still be snowed by a warm smile and a rush of reassuring clichés. There's nothing we can do about the smile, but we have composed a list of expressions that should send up a red flag of danger. If you find a doctor you like and he makes one or two of these remarks, don't be alarmed. If, however, the doctor tosses off more than two, he is probably a real smoothie, and you should beware. Here are our favorite red flags, in no particular order of vagueness or overuse:

◆

"I only use medication when I think it's necessary."

◆

"Lamaze, schlamaze. Whatever you do is fine with me."

◆

"You're the only one who ever asked me that."

◆

"Of course you want an episiotomy. Don't you want to be nice and tight for your husband?"

◆

"It's for your safety."

◆

"Let's cross that bridge when we come to it."

◆

"Don't worry about a thing, I'll take care of everything."

continued

♦

"We can't take chances."

♦

"I don't think your husband should be with you for delivery because it might ruin your sex life. Do you want him thinking about the birth every time you have sex?"

♦

"It's a hospital rule."

♦

"There's no reason for women to suffer."

♦

"Don't worry, I only do it when I have to."

♦

"The episiotomy won't hurt the way I do it."

♦

"You have to think of your baby."

♦

"You should have faith in me. After all, I'm the doctor."

advantages: Your appointments are never canceled because of a delivery, and you don't have to worry about your delivery coinciding with your doctor's vacation.

Doctors in a group often share an approach to childbirth, but there can be a great deal of diversity within the practice. Therefore, if you choose a group, it's essential that you meet all the doctors during the course of your visits to discuss the kind of birth experience you want.

Childbirth can be approached with more confidence and control if you know exactly who will be delivering your baby and if you've gotten to know that person during the past nine months. If there are no competent solo practitioners where you live, we suggest finding a group compatible with your philosophy and as small as possible. Two or three partners is manageable; five or six can be overwhelming.

OLD OR YOUNG?

Another factor you may want to think about in selecting your doctor is his age. This is a fuzzy issue because there are pros and cons for both older and younger doctors. Some women like young doctors because they are often less patronizing and more approachable. They also tend to get more emotionally involved because they have fewer patients and because they are often experiencing the excitement of having babies themselves. On the other hand, young doctors are sometimes more apt to rely on machines and surgical intervention, because that's the way they've been taught. They also lack the wisdom brought by experience. A thirty-five-year-old doctor would probably do a cesarean instead of a mid-forceps delivery, whereas his fifty-year-old counterpart would be more skilled in the use of forceps. Older doctors are more experienced and therefore often calmer, having learned that most labors proceed uneventfully. But age can bring burnout and a lack of patience in dealing with the day-to-day concerns of normal pregnancies.

MALE OR FEMALE?

We don't think a doctor's gender is related to the way he or she practices, but we know this is one preference some people feel strongly about. With more and more women going to medical school these days—it's expected that by the year 2000, 20 percent of all doctors will be women —you may well be interviewing a woman obstetrician. You can't assume, however, that she'll be terrific just because of her sex. Although she is like you in some ways, she has also had the same technological training as her male counterpart. And, the fact that she is a woman doesn't mean she'll necessarily practice like a midwife. In general, you have to scrutinize a female doctor as closely as you would a male.

FOLLOW YOUR INSTINCTS

You may find a doctor who answers all of your questions beautifully but for some reason rubs you the wrong way. Unless there are no other

SOLO OR GROUP

♦

"Unfortunately, I got the only doctor in the office that I didn't like. He was arrogant and cold. I was very disappointed."

♦

"I don't think he even knew what my name was. The primary doctor knew me, but he wasn't the one to deliver me."

♦

"The obstetrician induced me because he was going on vacation and didn't want me to have the baby while he was gone. The baby was five weeks early."

♦

"Even though he wasn't 'on call,' he came in for my delivery as we had agreed."

♦

"There were four doctors in the group. It was like a factory."

♦

"I wanted a doctor in solo practice and that's what I chose. My gynecologist told me that if you go with a group, you invariably get the guy you like least, and I believe that. In a group, consistency of care is lost, the doctor always has his nose in your file, seeing what happened last time. With only one doctor in charge nothing gets overlooked and you develop a real close relationship."

♦

"It made more sense to go to a group. One doctor can't possibly deliver babies 365 days a year. So common sense told me, if my doctor gets a lot of vacation, terrific! I at least have somebody who's not exhausted in the delivery room."

♦

continued

"I chose a group practice because I wanted to know the physician that would be attending the birth. I was worried that if I used a single physician, he might be ill or on vacation or totally exhausted when the baby chose to arrive."

♦

"I used a group practice. They had me rotate with all four doctors so that I would know everyone. I had confidence in them all and had terrific care. I felt the practice was very unified in philosophy and approach. I'd hate to have to depend on only one doctor."

♦

"I had a backup doctor, who was totally against my using the birthing room and made very sarcastic statements the moment he entered the room. I will definitely check into the backup doctors next time so that this will not happen again."

♦

"I didn't choose my obstetrician on the basis of single or group—I just stuck with the single doctor I had. As it turned out, he was on vacation when I had the baby, but I liked his backup even better. I liked seeing one doctor throughout who knew me, even if he wasn't there for the big event."

obstetricians in your area, it would seem best to look for someone else. A critical component in selecting a doctor is whether you like him. It's essential that you feel comfortable when you are being examined, talking, and, most importantly, asking questions. Unless you've had a chronic disease, you've probably never visited a doctor almost fifteen times in ten months. This frequency gives you an excellent chance to get acquainted, but it also allows a mild dislike to grow into something much more negative. Today many people seem to believe that a doctor can be either medically competent *or* emotionally supportive but that they can't have it both ways. We don't agree, and know many doctors who are nice people as well as skillful obstetricians.

Some women look for a fatherly type in an obstetrician. Others want someone they can chat with easily. We think both of these priorities are fine, and it's great if you can clearly identify your needs. There are, however, women who expect too much from this relationship and invariably end up disappointed. To avoid this pitfall, we have drawn up a list of what we feel you can reasonably expect of an obstetrician:

- To answer your phone calls promptly;
- To share all knowledge about your pregnancy;
- To welcome your husband or partner at all office visits;
- To be attentive to your feelings (but that doesn't mean being as excited as you are about your pregnancy);
- To be there while you labor.

In general, you want your obstetrician to be friendly and respectful, but you don't want him to act like your best friend or take the place of your husband. You must remember, this is a professional relationship.

CHANGING DOCTORS

Suppose you've chosen a doctor, but for one reason or another (you're moving or the two of you are incompatible) you need to find someone new. Don't despair. You're not married to your obstetrician, you're merely seeing him for medical care. Until the moment of delivery, it's never too late to switch doctors. We know several women who changed doctors in their ninth month, and all of them were happy they had done so.

We're not encouraging you to change doctors frivolously. Unless there is a true personality conflict, you should try negotiation first, making yourself perfectly clear about why you're not happy. Doctors aren't mind readers and don't always know why you're dissatisfied. Go to your next visit with a list of questions and ask the receptionist to schedule extra time. Bring your husband along so that you can present a united front as well as gain his impressions of the doctor. Be willing to compromise somewhat, bearing in mind that no relationship is perfect. Also, try to come to terms with what you really want. Women frequently revise

CHANGING DOCTORS

♦

"We moved out of state in my eighth month and had to find a new doctor. We inquired about birthing procedures at a few hospitals, then went to the hospital we liked best and asked them to recommend a younger doctor who was comfortable with natural childbirth. We were lucky because we immediately liked the doctor they recommended."

♦

"Much bitterness is aimed directly at my doctor. I have sworn never to use him again and have very few good memories of the man. I should have known right from the beginning that our relationship would be poor. At my first prenatal checkup, I felt like I was just another uterus. Things did not improve over time, but I was afraid to change doctors mid-pregnancy. As it turned out, he handled my labor very poorly and ultimately did a cesarean. My daughter was born at 4:39 P.M., and to this day I believe that he took her then so that he could be home in time for dinner."

♦

"I decided to change doctors in my seventh month. It would have been easy just to continue and say, 'It's out of my hands,' but I was tired of feeling like a victim."

♦

"He would laugh at me sometimes and say I was trying to undo what the medical community had already achieved. He did not do enemas or shave, but he insisted on an IV and monitors. I now wish I had changed doctors, but I didn't."

♦

"When we moved, I had to scout around for a new doctor. When I spoke with one doctor, who was quite young, about natural childbirth, his response was something like, 'If you like pain, you'll like natural childbirth.' Needless to say, I found someone else."

continued

♦

"The awkwardness of changing doctors was of surprisingly little concern to me. I didn't know how I would deal with the good-bye explanation, but I knew I had to be able to trust completely whoever would be with me during labor and delivery. I had done my reading and I had an inkling of the intensity of the birthing experience. It made sense to try to decrease stress as much as possible in preparation for that effort and to try to arrange to have competent, warm, supportive people with me.

"As silly as it may sound, I think this decision to change doctors was a watershed for me. I grew up some. The 'obedient girl to authorities' took a backseat. I took responsibility to make what effort I could for me to have a positive birthing experience and for my baby to have a pleasant entrance.

"My delivery was problem-free, and my doctor was terrific. If I have another child, I would want her to be there again."

♦

"There were four doctors in the group. They had a very good medical reputation, but I didn't particularly like the two I had met. If I had had a good pregnancy, I might have been able to deal with their lack of sympathy and poor bedside manner, because in my mind, medical competence was number one. But I was getting all of one and nothing of the other, and I needed lots of number two.

"I felt one doctor had been in the business too long. He was very pleasant, but also very egotistical. He'd answer yes or no to my questions, but he never offered any information. There was some concern for my constant nausea, but only from a strictly medical point of view. Appointments were very short; I was in and out in five minutes.

"I hesitated to change doctors for yet a third time. I was eager to find somebody who was just right for me, but I had little confidence in my ability to make decisions. Luckily, someone I respected very much came along and said not only that I should change doctors (I had heard that a lot), but that she had a suggestion and handed me the name and number. It was a godsend, something handed to me on a silver platter, out of the blue. All I had to do was make the phone call.

continued

"The consultation went very, very well. I had a chance to speak about concerns I had, and by the end of the appointment I really felt good about being pregnant. I then arranged to meet my new doctor's associate, and that meeting went equally well. They were able to make pregnancy exciting and less scary. In just one or two visits I had a lot of my concerns cleared up, I was much happier and much more at ease."

their idea of a good obstetrician in the middle of pregnancy because their needs change or they didn't know what to look for in the first place. For example, you might select a surgical/technical whiz and then feel disappointed several months later because you're not being supported emotionally.

Most pregnant women aren't in the mood for a confrontation with their doctor, but we can't emphasize enough how important it is to have an obstetrician you like and trust. If, after thinking the whole thing through and discussing it with your husband, you're still unhappy, change doctors. Don't worry about causing an upset. You have a professional relationship that just isn't working out, and you must do what's right for you. Your doctor will not be devastated—but you might be if you have a bad birth experience with someone you neither like nor trust.

A letter is usually the best way to extricate yourself from the relationship. If you've paid the fee in advance, ask that the cost of your visits be prorated and that your new obstetrician be sent your medical records. Getting your money back shouldn't be difficult, because you can always enlist the help of the state or county medical society, and your doctor knows this. We recommend explaining the reasons for your dissatisfaction, even though this can be painful. Perhaps if enough people tell a doctor why they aren't happy, he may try to change. If it weren't for couples who complained and asked for what they wanted fifteen years ago, mothers would still be strapped to delivery tables while their husbands paced the floors of waiting rooms.

MIDWIVES

As mentioned before, you will have an excellent chance of having natural childbirth if you are able to work with a midwife. Midwives have an inherent trust in the natural process of birth and are committed to a policy of nonintervention. We've never heard of one who arrived just in time to catch a baby, or offered an epidural in place of emotional support, or routinely performed an episiotomy. In a normal birth a good midwife is always better than an indifferent obstetrician, provided there is no medical emergency.

There are two basic types of midwives. You can have either a certified nurse-midwife (C.N.M.) or a lay midwife. The difference between a lay midwife and a C.N.M. is formalized training. A lay midwife may have gone to school, but her expertise is based largely on practical experience, and she can assist only at homebirths. A C.N.M., on the other hand, is a registered nurse, trained as a midwife, and is certified by the American College of Nurse-Midwives. She generally has a good deal of practical experience and can deliver babies at home, in an alternative-birth center or in a hospital. This type of midwife is sometimes in practice with an obstetrician and usually handles prenatal visits and routine deliveries. There are approximately 2,500 C.N.M.'s practicing in the United States today, and they assist in about 3 percent of all births, delivering about 100,000 babies a year.

With a midwife, you receive more personalized prenatal care than you would with most obstetricians. Checkups are not rushed, and you are encouraged to ask questions and voice your concerns. Midwives place a great emphasis on teaching, especially nutritional counseling. In addition, you will probably get more emotional support throughout pregnancy and labor. Midwives are concerned about your feelings at every stage, and they are renowned for staying at your bedside, not at the nurse's station, during your labor.

Under a midwife's care you will be assured that everything done to you is essential. Midwives advocate nonintervention in obstetrics, and that means a midwife will be more likely to allow labor to proceed along its natural course. If a midwife decides your labor needs to be stimulated, you can be assured it's for your benefit, not hers.

Midwives cost approximately half as much as ob/gyns, and with a routine pregnancy and delivery you'll get much more care for your dollar. In addition, more and more insurance companies are covering their costs.

Another bonus is that your family will be treated as a whole. The

CHOOSING A MIDWIFE

♦

"Giving birth is a natural process that midwives seem to be more in tune with than the medical profession. Also, being in control at the start will begin the confidence necessary for childrearing."

♦

"I was extremely happy to have had the option of using a midwife for prenatal care and birth because I feel that pregnancy and childbirth should not be treated as medical emergencies. Unfortunately, medical training in this country deals with trauma (very well) and is not good with cooperative, educational, and preventative work with the client/patient. My fears of medical emergency are alleviated by the fact that my midwives practice at a large hospital. Being with women is great."

♦

"Pregnancy is one of the most insecure periods of my life, and I felt I needed to be with other women, to be 'mothered.' I wanted as little interference as possible and to be able to let things proceed naturally."

♦

"I come from a family of nurses and doctors, but I chose midwives for both of my deliveries. A midwife in private practice in a hospital—the best of both worlds."

♦

"My midwives have given me much more time, information, and intelligent caring than I could have gotten from the vast majority of obstetricians. Because I will be informed during birth, I'll have control over my body, and I'm sure that no difficulties will arise due to a doctor's need to use technology."

♦

"I think I made the right decision about using a group-midwifery practice for my first birth, but I'm not sure I'd make the same choice again. I had a C-section, but

continued

the circumstances were quite unusual: I dilated beautifully to eight centimeters and then stopped. I continued to have strong contractions, but after three more hours of labor I was still in transition, the cervix had begun to swell, and I had regressed to five centimeters.

"If I had selected an obstetrician instead of the midwives, I know the outcome would have been identical. The only difference would have been that I would have been spared those extra three hours of labor. I approached the birth of my first child from a fairly radical viewpoint, but now I think I'm more aware of some of the risks associated with childbirth and I'm more inclined to try to find a doctor I trust."

midwife will be instrumental in getting the three of you off to a good start. She will allow generous time after birth for introductions and will help you with breast-feeding. Midwives welcome your husband's involvement, and you'll both be encouraged to get acquainted with your baby for as long as possible.

If you think you would like a midwife, we hope you'll use the questionnaire we developed for screening obstetricians. Obviously, some of the questions are not applicable, but we think the interview can be useful in determining how a particular midwife practices.

There are dangers in having a midwife deliver your baby at home, and it should never be considered unless a doctor and hospital are backing her up. (See chapter 3 for more on home delivery.) We think the best place to have a baby is in a birth center attached to a hospital, but unfortunately there are just a handful of these scattered around the country. Alternative-birth centers, run by midwives, are becoming increasingly popular, but if complications develop, you must be transferred during labor to a hospital. We feel the midwife practicing in a hospital offers the best compromise between the high-tech delivery room and the more risky home environment.

If you select a midwife and then develop any sort of complication during pregnancy, you'll probably be transferred to a doctor's care. Moreover, midwives are prohibited by law from performing cesareans or forceps deliveries. For this reason many people prefer obstetricians, who can promise continuity of care, come what may. Also, some couples just can't feel comfortable with a midwife—they may be from a family of doctors, or they just may be particularly anxious about childbirth.

New York City has several successful midwifery programs. One that has received national attention began in 1977 at the North Central Bronx Hospital. In five years of operation, the midwives lowered the hospital's overall infant mortality rate so dramatically that it now out-ranks the average for the city's municipal and private voluntary hospitals. This is remarkable because 30 percent of the patients at North Central Bronx are considered high-risk—teenage mothers, Medicaid recipients, and women with little prenatal care. Even with this population, the midwives have a cesarean rate of only 9 percent. As you might expect, the midwives have also greatly decreased the use of forceps, medication, and anesthesia. They handle 87.7 percent of all births at the hospital, or roughly 2,600 deliveries a year.

Selecting a doctor or midwife is a decision only you can make. There are many accomplished and compassionate doctors and there are also hundreds of dedicated professional midwives practicing in the United States today. There is no one choice for everyone. We hope you will take the time to consider which alternative is best for you and to choose carefully the person who will make your birth experience the best it can be.

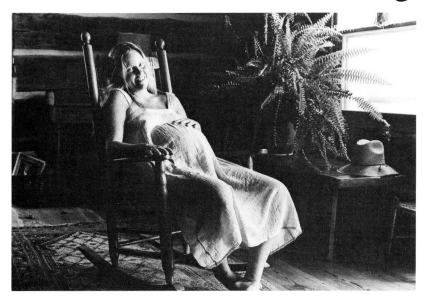

CHAPTER 3

Home, Hospital,
or Birth Center

*A*lthough both homebirth and birth centers are enjoying great popularity today, approximately 98 percent of all couples choose a hospital delivery. This is because a hospital is perceived to be the safest place to have a baby (women who filled out our questionnaires repeatedly stated this belief). Most doctors would argue strongly that a hospital is the *only* safe place to have a baby. As more and more studies appear, however, there is growing recognition that homebirths and birth centers are safe alternatives if there is proper screening, expert care, and hospital backup.

The foundation of hospital birth is not as old or as solid as you might think. Jimmy Carter was the first U.S. president to have been born in a hospital, and today it's not unusual to meet a senior citizen who was born at home. Before 1930, most women gave birth at home, but after World War II, the national birthplace shifted from home to hospital. In the span of two generations, birth moved from the family circle into the medical marketplace.

THE IMPORTANCE OF YOUR CHOICE

Whatever setting you choose, there is no guarantee of absolute safety. Each option has benefits and hazards. If you select a hospital, you are faced with the possibility of many types of medical intervention, including the use of intravenous, enema, pubic shave, fetal monitoring, labor stimulation, and routine analgesia. In addition, you and your baby may be exposed to bacteria that can cause infection. If you deliver out of the hospital, unexpected complications can become life-threatening because precious minutes must be spent in transport to a hospital. Neither alternative is completely safe. Each one carries different risks, and you must decide which ones you prefer to take.

Many observers believe that American obstetrics is being pulled in opposite directions. On one side are the high-tech obstetricians, who order interventions at an astounding pace. On the other side stand the homebirth advocates, who trust a woman's ability to give birth. Although it seems ironic, the obstetrical technicians have helped to fuel the alternative movement because they've made hospital births unattractive to so many people. In a foreword to *Home Birth: A Practitioner's Guide to Birth Outside the Hospital,* Dr. Phillip Stubblefield explains this impetus for out-of-hospital birth. "It's harder to change an existing setting than to create a new one. Couples having babies right now want a better birth experience; they have no time to change the system, except by voting to stay out of it. Hence, the growing homebirth movement and the rapid rate of establishment of out-of-hospital birth centers." One woman responding to our questionnaire had a choice between a hospital with a 50 percent cesarean rate and a homebirth. She decided to have her baby at home.

Most women, however, never consider alternative options and simply assume they will go to the hospital. These women often have a long-standing relationship with an obstetrician/gynecologist, and it is taken for granted that he will deliver the baby at the hospital. Although this choice of a birth site may not seem important, it will greatly influence the quality of your birth experience. Before deciding where you will give birth, we strongly recommend investigating all options.

There are many variables that will affect your decision: your health, your feelings about previous births, your financial status, your husband's attitude, your philosophy about childbirth, the facilities available to you, and whether this is your first baby. It's impossible for us or anyone else to tell you what to do. Only you can consider all the interrelated factors and choose the place best suited to your needs and desires.

It's human nature to want to improve upon experience. The women who filled out our questionnaires showed a strong desire to change each subsequent birth for the better. For example, many of them were disappointed because the hospital's one birthing room was in use; next time they hoped it would be available. Some of them also mentioned they would like to try an alternative-birth center instead of the hospital. Only a few were interested in trying homebirth, but the ones who had experienced a homebirth were adamant about never having anything else again.

It's very likely you'll have a great birth experience wherever you have your baby if you have carefully selected your doctor or midwife. No setting provides guarantees, so it's critical that you trust the person who attends you. Many people believe you have better control if you first choose the person who will deliver the baby and then choose the birthplace. But sometimes circumstances dictate that these steps must be reversed. For example, if you live in an area with two hospitals, one a modern, well-equipped teaching hospital with a high cesarean rate and the other a small community one, dedicated to family-centered care, you'd select the hospital first and then try to find a doctor you like who practices there.

Although a hospital is regarded as the best place to be "just in case," the hospital setting actually promotes unnecessary medical intervention. In 1976 Dr. Lewis Mehl conducted a comparison study of 1,046 women who planned a homebirth with the same number of women who planned hospital deliveries. The two groups were well matched, but Mehl found a striking difference in the degree of obstetric intervention each required. The hospital group had more analgesia, oxytocin, forceps deliveries, and episiotomies. It is important to note that the birth attendants shared the same philosophies, so that differences came as a result of being in the hospital. The increased likelihood of medical intervention in the hospital may result from a lower motivation for the women to have natural childbirth, or from more readily available analgesia, or from pressure on the birth attendants to intervene sooner and more aggressively in the hospital than at home. There were no significant differences in birth weight, newborn mortality, neurological abnormalities, or other major complications between the newborns of the two groups.

In evaluating the risks of the different birthplaces, you should take into consideration the size and quality of the hospital that would provide backup emergency care for a birth center or home delivery. In *Home Birth,* Dr. Stubblefield notes that all hospitals are not alike:

> There is great contrast between the kind of technically high-quality care that can be provided in the best hospital setting and that which can be provided in the home, but how much contrast is there, really, between a small hospital's care and the well-trained and equipped home delivery team? If the mother can be transported to a hospital within ten minutes where a team awaits capable of performing an emergency cesarean section, the outcome of an emergency at home may be better than if the mother were laboring in a small hospital where it would take half an hour to assemble the cesarean section team.

The bottom line on this question is your ability to feel relaxed and assured. Labor will proceed most smoothly if you are at ease emotionally. If a hospital would give you the proper peace of mind, that's where you belong. If you really want a homebirth, but your husband would be too anxious, then perhaps a birth center is a happy compromise. It's good to have choices, and today there are some new alternatives. The only situation we can't sanction is a homebirth with only your husband in attendance. Although you may have complete faith in natural childbirth, your husband is inexperienced at delivering babies. A problem easily handled by a midwife can turn into a disaster at the hands of a novice. If you choose to deliver unattended at home, you are setting yourself up for the riskiest of all obstetrical situations.

HOMEBIRTH

No one really knows how many planned homebirths take place every year in the United States. Estimates range from two to three percent of all births in the nation. Oregon, where homebirth is popular, claims a rate of four percent. The national figure is believed to be inaccurately low, because home deliveries are illegal in many states and therefore are not always reported.

Homebirths did not become scarce because they were unsafe, but because hospital births were more cost-efficient. To manage a homebirth properly, a doctor or midwife must spend hours at a woman's bedside patiently observing the course of her labor. In a hospital he or she can rely instead on nurses, residents, interns, and fetal monitors to chart the progress of labor. By performing all deliveries in a hospital, a doctor can also manage the labors of two or more women simultaneously and can save countless hours traveling to and from different locations. Homebirth is often a long, drawn-out affair, and most practitioners simply don't have the time.

Most doctors believe homebirth is patently unsafe. Dr. Warren Pearse, past president of the American College of Obstetricians and Gynecologists (ACOG), has labeled the homebirth trend maternal trauma, as well as child abuse. In 1978, ACOG attracted considerable press attention when it released a statement claiming that the risk to a baby's life was two to five times greater if he was born out of the hospital. This estimate was based on data gathered from eleven state health departments. What ACOG failed to explain, however, was that included in the out-of-hospital category were many late miscarriages, premature and unplanned deliveries, and unattended homebirths.

The Centers for Disease Control conducted a major study of homebirths in North Carolina from 1974 to 1976, which was published in the *Journal of the American Medical Association.* This research strongly demonstrated the necessity of eliminating confusing variables in comparisons between birth sites. The study concluded that "deliveries occurring at home ranged from lowest to highest risk of neonatal [newborn] mortality depending on planning and the attendant present." Neonatal mortality rates were 3 per 1,000 for planned homebirths attended by a lay midwife, 30 per 1,000 for planned homebirths without a lay midwife, and 120 per 1,000 for unplanned homebirths. It's clear that homebirths without proper emergency arrangements and obstetric care are unsafe and should never be attempted.

An expert on homebirth, Dutch obstetrician G. J. Kloosterman, estimates that for a well-screened, low-risk population the probability of an emergent complication that would make loss of time in transit to the hospital a serious problem to be less than one per thousand. This

HOMEBIRTH

◆

"I wanted to be able to use my own kitchen, my bathroom, and to eat whenever I wished. I felt very comfortable at home. I also wanted to get in my own bed with my new baby. It was special."

◆

"I wanted to be in my own surroundings, have a happy, unmedicated birth, and care for my baby myself and not have her taken from me. I just feel that hospitals are for sick people and unusual situations, and that birth is a natural, normal process."

◆

"I wanted a natural delivery, without interference because of someone else's routine or schedule. I think homebirth is the safest way."

◆

"While I often toyed with the idea of homebirth, I feel the risks are too great."

◆

"I felt happy and comfortable in my own setting, and had a lot of support and help from family."

◆

"I had my first three in a hospital, and the fourth in a home setting. There is no comparison. As long as qualified help is with you, and a hospital nearby just in case, you are in control. We need to get away from assembly-line delivery."

◆

"After the birth it was a wonderful feeling to snuggle up with my family in our bed. As long as the pregnancy is normal, I'm convinced that homebirth is safe and natural."

continued

"We had a homebirth, and it was the most meaningful thing I have ever done. I feel very fortunate to have birthed this way. I don't advocate homebirth for every woman, though I do believe that more women could successfully have their babies at home and have an easier, more rewarding experience than in a hospital. I myself am not against hospital birth for others. Many women could not feel safe outside this setting—but I could not feel safe within it.

"I think society has brainwashed us into believing that childbirth is a horrible, dangerous condition that can be handled only in a hospital by medical personnel. While many problem pregnancies and births are best dealt with in a hospital with its technology, there are many more births that would be best left alone. Too many procedures are for the convenience of the doctor. Women need to know that they needn't simply surrender their bodies to their doctors—that the choice is theirs."

risk must be considered by couples contemplating a homebirth and it should be weighed against the different sort of risks found in hospitals.

In general, home is where we feel most relaxed and secure. A common compliment is to say we feel "at home," or to describe an environment as homey or homelike. To give birth at home for many is simply to settle for nothing less than the real thing—your own environment. There's also a lot to be said for not having to be transported during labor, and when it's all over, for being able to fall asleep in your own bed. In addition, homebirth represents a holistic philosophy and, often, a way of life. It works best for people who have faith in the normal workings of their bodies and who don't fall prey to the "what if" mentality that characterizes much of American obstetrics.

According to the women who filled out our questionnaires, the decision to have a homebirth was often based on the desire to be in charge. The issue of control is a compelling one. At a homebirth the doctor or

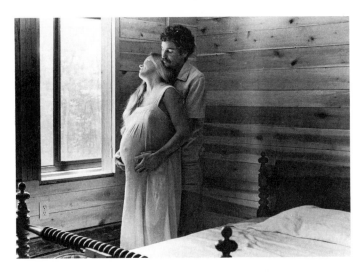

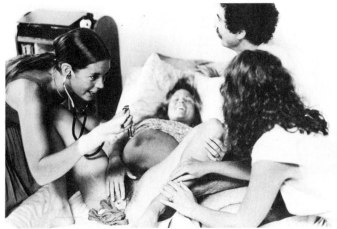

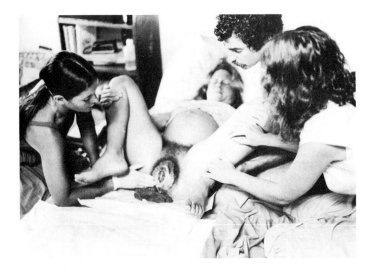

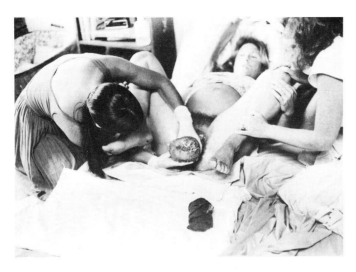

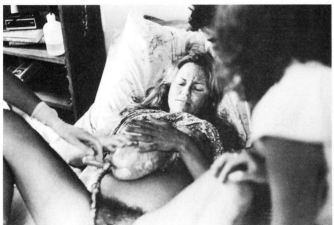

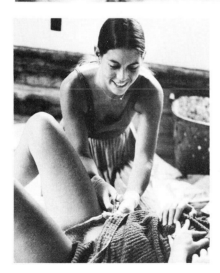

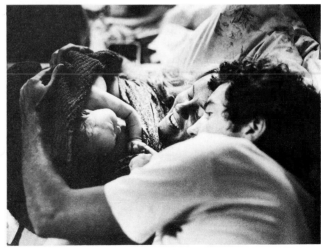

midwife is in your home at your invitation, and there's much less chance of running up against authoritarian attitudes.

Author Barbara Katz Rothman discusses her decision to have a home-birth and her struggle with the issues of social acceptance and responsibility in her provocative book *In Labor: Women and Power in the Birthplace:*

> There were some risks I knew I could take that were totally acceptable socially. I was not held responsible, for example, for how I chose a doctor. Had I taken just the local doctor because I hated traveling on the subways, that would have been considered legitimate. And if he/ she screwed up, that wouldn't have been my fault. Back in 1973 I could still ask to be drugged out of it completely and would not have been held socially accountable for whatever risks that entailed. A friend of mine went to a doctor I know to be something of an idiot and asked that she be knocked out when she got to the hospital and not brought to until they had a clean, preferably diapered baby to show her. And she got that. And that was socially acceptable. A friend's mother took diet pills all through her pregnancy twenty years ago because the doctor prescribed them. The pills have since been taken off the market for everybody, not just pregnant people. . . . But none of these women are responsible, because they followed doctor's orders. The moral was that the more control I gave up, the more responsibility I gave up for the consequences and the more socially acceptable my behavior would be.

Many people equate homebirth with a primitive sort of experience, like childbirth in the fields. We're not talking about that kind of thing here. Homebirth should be a well-planned and carefully executed event. In order to have a safe birth at home, you should have the following:

- An experienced and qualified doctor or midwife, with a backup birth attendant in case of illness or emergency
- A hospital ready to accept you in case of complications
- A reliable means of transportation to the hospital
- A normal pregnancy with no unusual symptoms as labor begins
- A special caretaker for other children during your labor and delivery
- Help with household duties during the immediate postpartum period

Your doctor or midwife will bring certain supplies but will expect you to have others. All preparations should be made well in advance of your due date.

BIRTH CENTERS

A birth center can be a doctor's office, a building adjacent to a hospital, or a facility all by itself. Officially, birth-center deliveries are categorized as out-of-hospital births and they are the fastest-growing trend in the obstetric business. Today there are more than 120 birth centers scattered around the nation, with at least 300 additional ones currently planned.

Birth centers—sometimes called alternative-birth centers, or ABCs— are popular because they are a compromise between home and hospital birth. Emergency supplies, such as IV or resuscitation equipment, are hidden out of sight, and typically all that meets the eye is the homey environment of bedrooms, a playroom, and a kitchen. Birth centers encourage natural childbirth, free of intervention, but they are equipped to handle most emergencies short of cesarean section. Birth centers often provide complete prenatal care and nutritional counseling as well as a site for labor and delivery. Families return home within twelve to twenty-four hours.

Care is provided by midwives or doctors, although some centers are staffed by both. Birth centers are designed for low-risk deliveries, and approximately 25 to 30 percent of their prospective clients are determined to be unqualified. Multiple births, anemia, hypertension, or unusual presentation of the baby would prevent you from having birth-center delivery. During labor, another 15 percent of all women are transferred to a hospital because of complications, such as previously undiagnosed cephalo-pelvic disproportion, severe meconium staining, or failure to progress.

Most childbirth experts believe birth centers to be extremely safe, but there are very few studies to document this opinion. A study by Ruth Watson Lubic, C.N.M., director of the Maternity Center Association, and Anita Bennetts, C.N.M., Ph.D., attempted to compare the outcomes of mothers and babies at birth centers with similar low-risk mothers who delivered at hospitals. This wasn't possible, however, because they were denied access to hospital data.

Instead of a randomized controlled study, Ms. Watson and Ms. Ben-

BIRTH CENTERS

◆

"We live in a rural area, and the clinic was the closest—thirty-five miles, instead of sixty-five miles to the nearest hospital. I preferred the nonhospital setting, and at $800, the delivery was also much cheaper."

◆

"I think the setting of a birth is important, and the birth center room was great. The curtains, rocking chair, dresser, lamp, walls, bassinet, and birth bed were all color-coordinated in soft peach. No green tile walls and stainless-steel machines."

◆

"The birth center was in a hospital, near emergency equipment if needed. The birthing suite was very cozy and comfortable, with an adjoining bathroom and a tape cassette player. Homelike, yet in the hospital."

◆

"My husband would not agree to a homebirth, so the hospital birth center was the next best thing. It's nice to know that if any medical help is needed for yourself or the baby, it's right there."

◆

"The hospital didn't allow the Leboyer bath, but otherwise the birth center was ideal. Our five-and-a-half-year-old daughter attended the birth, and the room was darkened and very homey. The baby never had to leave the room, which was nice."

◆

"I think it's the safest way. It's in a hospital setting, I could have whoever I wanted to attend, yet hospital care was only seconds away."

netts settled for a study of the outcomes of two thousand women who gave birth at birth centers during the period from 1972 to 1979. Of this group, 15 percent had to be transferred to hospitals during labor; 5 percent were delivered by cesarean section; 5 percent required the use of forceps or vacuum extraction. The death rate for infants, including those whose mothers were transferred, was 4.6 per thousand live births, which compared favorably with those at many prestigious hospitals.

For those who can safely use birth centers, there is much to enjoy. Women in labor are encouraged to walk around, to eat and drink lightly, and to relax in a warm shower. Siblings are permitted to be present, and whole families are often assembled after the birth for a real celebration. Some women dislike the early discharge. Hospitals can be impersonal institutions, but they do provide service and an opportunity for rest, which can't always be found at home.

We think birth centers are great and have summarized why they are the perfect solution to the home-versus-hospital dilemma—provided you are eligible and have access to one. A birth center

+ Has an established backup arrangement with a hospital. The facility is experienced in transferring women with complications. You don't have to worry about calling an ambulance or relying on your own car.
+ Frequently provides prenatal care, so that when labor begins, there is comfort in the familiarity of the surroundings and personnel.
+ Has emergency equipment if you need it.
+ Costs roughly half as much as a hospital birth, and many insurance programs are now reimbursing for birth-center deliveries.
+ Encourages personalization of care and choice of procedure. There are no set routines.
+ Encourages the participation of whomever you want at your side. You are not limited to a single support person, so if you want friends or relatives to join you, that's fine.
+ Gives you an excellent chance of having natural childbirth. You can be relaxed because you know you're in a safe environment where you're unlikely to encounter unneeded intervention.

Many people believe birth centers are the wave of the future, and even doctors are buying them. The National Association of Childbearing Centers (a trade organization) is currently considering a proposal to offer some centers for franchise ownership. In 1983, ten thousand babies were born in birth centers, but there are now enough centers to accommodate as many as twenty thousand births annually. By providing an alternative to hospitals birth centers are indirectly pressuring them to be more accommodating to the people they serve.

You should scrutinize a birth center as closely as you would a hospital. Make sure that

+ It is staffed with experienced and accredited doctors and/or midwives.
+ There is a hospital backup and proper transportation to get there, should transfer be necessary.
+ The facilities are clean and well maintained.
+ There is professional prenatal care, and referrals to appropriate specialists when indicated.
+ There is basic emergency equipment available, such as blood expanders, resuscitation equipment, and an infant warmer.

HOSPITAL BIRTH
Hospital Procedures

Though homebirths and birth centers have recently received much media attention, the fact remains that most births today occur in a hospital. Many women aren't comfortable with the idea of homebirth, and for one reason or another do not use a birth center. Often women select a certain doctor and then without question follow him to the hospital. If you are high-risk or have an emergency complication during labor, the hospital is the only place to be. The only problem is that many hospitals treat *all* women as if they were high-risk.

Hospitals tend to view a woman in labor as an accident waiting to happen, and their actions are governed by the "what if" school of thinking. Continuous fetal monitoring is justified just in case fetal distress develops. An intravenous is called for just in case surgery is required or hemorrhage occurs. Food and liquids are withheld in case an emergency cesarean is needed. A pubic shave is performed to facilitate an episiotomy. People justifiably expect hospitals to be concerned for their safety and prepared for intervention, but hospitals tend to assume that intervention is required by all.

Many couples don't realize that the shave, the enema, the fetal monitor, and the intravenous are really all optional procedures, ordered by

HOSPITAL BIRTH

"Our insurance covered only a hospital delivery. I would have preferred a more gentle atmosphere."

"I thought it was the safest, but it proved to be most impersonal and lonely."

"Have you ever been in a happier part of the hospital? Have you heard the wheels on the carriers bringing all the babies? It's the neatest sound—here come the babies. It was special, a wonderful time."

"I knew my husband and I could still maintain our support and relationship, with the backup of professionals if something were needed."

"I am a labor-room nurse and have seen how women, including myself, can be manipulated and intimidated in a hospital. The medical community has a way of doing things and turning your wishes around to suit their needs and practices."

"I was all set to butt heads with the doctor and hospital staff about how I wanted the birth to go, but I was pleasantly surprised to find they all wanted to cooperate with me."

"It was most important to me to have great attending obstetricians; the setting was secondary."

continued

"All went according to my wishes. The baby had a Leboyer bath and was not separated from me. My four-year-old and my mother were allowed in right after the baby was born."

♦

"I chose a large teaching hospital with a neonatal intensive care unit, where there were experienced personnel and adequate staffing for both myself and the child."

♦

"The nurses are terrific and very helpful. I loved the hospital stay and the way they treated the baby."

♦

"The atmosphere was terrible, and the intrusions were upsetting. I felt an awful lack of privacy. The doctor badgered me, and even after birth the nurses were ever present to correct me. The worst part was having to fight for every inch of territory. I seemed to have no authority in making decisions that ultimately affected only me."

their particular doctor. There are very few ironclad hospital policies—such as visiting hours—that are nonnegotiable. Most everything else is left to the discretion of individual doctors, and each doctor leaves standing orders concerning the care he wants for his patients. What happens, however, is that at each hospital, standards of practice evolve. Obviously, the hospital will run most smoothly if each obstetrician practices similarly and the staff doesn't have to make exceptions, which can be time-consuming. For example, it's a lot easier for a nurse to set up a fetal monitor and run it continuously than it is to attach it and detach it several times so that a woman can walk about and be monitored periodically.

It is possible to receive individualized care at a hospital, if you make arrangements in advance. You must talk to your doctor during an office visit and discuss with him what you want (see chapter 8 for a discussion of the pros and cons of the enema, pubic shave, intravenous, and fetal monitoring). If he agrees, he then becomes your advocate for changing standard procedure and must leave orders concerning your particular treatment with the staff. It's really quite simple. If a breakdown in communication occurs, and a nurse attempts to give you, say, a pubic shave, you say, "No, I'm Dr. Smith's patient and he left orders that I'm not to be shaved." If the nurse is persistent, you must say no again and ask her to recheck the orders or call the doctor.

We know we sound like firebrands, but the idea is that you do not have to allow unnecessary procedures. Obstetric departments have changed dramatically in the last twenty years because people got angry and asked for what they wanted. Women demanded that their husbands be allowed to stay with them during labor and delivery and that their babies be treated gently after birth. The recent addition of birthing rooms to obstetric wards has had a profound influence on practice, bringing about greater flexibility in delivery and more time for families to enjoy one another after birth. Many labor nurses are now trained in Lamaze breathing techniques and provide compassionate support to laboring couples. These days, hospitals have become more flexible, but you still have to know what you want and you must ask for it.

The Hospital Tour

Part of your preparation for birth should be a tour of the hospital. Tours tend to be regularly scheduled a couple of times each month. If you're studying Lamaze at the hospital, the tour will probably be part of the series. If your doctor delivers at more than one hospital, you may want to scrutinize each one before you choose. Some tours are excellent and cover every possible point; others are not, and you must ask many questions. To help you make an evaluation, we've put together a list of things to look for and ask about:

1. Are the labor rooms private or semiprivate? Are any of them equipped with birthing beds?
2. Are women encouraged to be mobile during labor? If so, where can they walk?
3. Can I have more than one support person?

4. Is there an anesthesiologist available at all times? If not, how quickly can one be summoned?

5. When does the hospital's fiscal day begin, so that I may gauge the time of my arrival and possibly save some money?

6. Are there separate entrances for the daytime and evening?

7. Where can we park? Is there a twenty-four-hour lot available?

8. Can we register in advance in order to save time when we arrive and prevent being separated?

9. Are there any birthing rooms? How many? What is your policy regarding eligibility? Do they contain birthing beds?

10. Is a birthing chair available?

11. What is the policy regarding fathers in the delivery room for cesareans?

12. If the baby has any problems, will he be transferred, or can my baby be treated here? Can my pediatrician be granted privileges, or will the baby be treated by the staff physician?

13. What are the visiting hours for the father, other guests, and siblings?

14. What is your policy on rooming-in? Can I have the baby examined and cared for in my room so that we never have to be separated?

15. If I want a private room, what are my chances of getting one? Do cesarean patients get private rooms for recovery?

16. If I have a private room, can my husband spend the night with me?

17. How many beds does a semiprivate room contain?

18. Are there classes on breast-feeding and baby care?

The Delivery Rooms

A delivery room is really an operating room, and for that reason sterile procedures are maintained. It is kept cold to inhibit the growth of bacteria, and everyone who enters, except you, must wear a surgical cap and gown. It contains a baby warmer, as well as all the instruments and emergency equipment that might ever be needed. It's usually a large room and it is brightly lit. There is a mirror attached to one of the lights over the delivery table, and you can request that it be positioned so that you can see your baby's birth.

Most women are brought to the delivery room just as the baby's head is crowning. You will spend most of your time pushing in your labor bed in the labor room. You will be transferred to the delivery room when you're only about three pushes away from actually giving birth. The

THE DELIVERY ROOM

♦

"I wanted to be in the delivery room and was relieved when we finally went and everything was handy if needed."

♦

"At the time, I would have delivered on a roller coaster just to get it over with! But I think I would have preferred to be in a more upright position."

♦

"The rush to the delivery room was a horrible experience. My hands were actually strapped down. I had to ask them to untie me so that I could hold my son."

♦

"My feet were tied, and I was constantly told not to move my hands or they would be tied, too. I hated it!"

♦

"Had no problems. Was propped up on a foam wedge, could see, and was as comfortable as possible."

♦

"Lying on your back to give birth is utter nonsense."

♦

"It was more like a freezer than a delivery room."

♦

"The only problem was getting from the labor bed to the gurney to the delivery table. I was very tired, in a lot of pain, and not in the mood to move."

♦

"I felt so helpless and vulnerable, lying with my legs up like that."

moment of transfer can be quite frenzied and your husband is apt to forget the camera and your glasses, if you wear them.

Many women describe the worst moment of labor as the one in which the baby's head was bulging, but they were instructed to stop pushing while being draped and prepared for delivery. Changing beds can also seem heartless at a time like this. Sometimes, the transfer is directly from the labor bed to the delivery table, but sometimes a gurney is used, necessitating two uncomfortable switches. Most people would never dream of moving an animal about to give birth, and it seems crazy to subject women to this inhumane disruption when it's unnecessary.

The delivery table is narrow and made of metal. The foot of the table has a retractable shelf, and when you climb on, your feet will first be placed on this shelf. After you are situated, the stirrups are put into place, your legs are placed in them, and the shelf is tucked under the table. The back of the table is sometimes adjustable—if it's not, you can request to be propped up with pillows. You'll be asked to slide your buttocks down to the end of the table (as you do during a gynecological exam). Your stomach and legs will be draped with a sterile sheet, leaving open a small square from which the baby will emerge.

For the final pushes, women frequently grip the handrails of the table to gain extra leverage. The table may also have leather straps attached to the handrails to secure your hands and prevent you from touching the sterile field. Their presence is a reminder of the days, not so long ago, when women were heavily medicated and out of control. You shouldn't permit your hands to be strapped down, and you can assure your doctor you can be trusted not to disturb the drapes.

Your husband can take pictures, using a high-speed film—flashes are not permitted because of the presence of oxygen. You may feel quite uncomfortable and vulnerable perched on this cold table, but it may console you to know that this is the way most women in the United States give birth today.

Delivering in Your Labor Bed

The choice of the room where you actually give birth is something you should discuss in advance with your doctor or midwife. Many of the women who responded to our questionnaire were delighted with the birthing room because they were able to labor, deliver, and recover in the same bed. Many other women expressed unhappiness with the delivery table, complaining about having to push uphill and being cold and uncomfortable.

As an alternative, we suggest giving birth in your labor bed in the labor room. If your doctor has an immediate negative response to this idea, don't acquiesce right away. Lots of babies have been born in labor rooms. This is an issue that can be negotiated—you're not asking him to do a cesarean in the back of a covered wagon, although he may react as if you were. Every labor room is equipped with oxygen and a fetal monitor, so you should have everything you need, and the delivery room is nearby in case a problem develops. Some doctors object because the labor room is usually very small, and a few special accommodations must be made. But if your labor is going smoothly, there's really no reason why you can't have the baby there. The actual issue is your doctor's comfort—he won't be able to sit on a stool with you conveniently displayed in stirrups before him. A classic excuse for transferring you to the delivery room is that the lighting is better there. If you discuss the idea in advance, offer to provide some extra lights. If your doctor says that there's no instrument table in the room, ask him how many he usually uses and whether there isn't enough room for them near your bed. Make it clear that if complications arise, you assume you will be moved to the delivery room. If your doctor insists on using the delivery room, you may be able to compromise by suggesting you be permitted to deliver in your labor bed in the delivery room. This solution minimizes your disruption and discomfort while allowing him the familiar atmosphere of the delivery room.

The Hospital Birthing Room

Birthing rooms are the biggest thing to hit hospital obstetrics in years. People want them badly, and hospitals are fast converting labor rooms into birthing rooms. The beauty of a birthing room is that labor, delivery, and recovery can all occur in the same place. In addition to this convenience, birthing rooms are designed to simulate a homelike atmosphere, something like a cross between a bedroom and living room. You're likely to find flowered sheets, plants, a television, a rocking chair, and pictures on the walls. This is great, because it is an acknowledgment that environment and comfort do matter.

The Hospital Birthing Room

◆

"My sister used a hospital birthing room, but she still had a pubic shave, episiotomy, IV, internal fetal monitor, a paracervical, and had her waters broken. I can't see why this had to happen. It certainly wasn't home style."

◆

"I really wanted to use the birthing room, but chose not to when I felt something was wrong. I was told I could not have *any* medication, and that scared me."

◆

"The birthing bed was fantastic—100 percent better than the delivery table."

◆

"I was very pleased that I did not have to use a delivery table or be moved from room to room. The room was lit only by sunlight, and it was very private, with just my husband, the doctor, and one nurse present."

◆

"The birthing rooms are beautiful and new. I felt at home there, yet safe with qualified hospital personnel nearby."

◆

"The hospital has one lovely birthing room, with a brass bed, plush carpet, elegant wallpaper, soft lamps. They are very proud of it, and it is advertised heavily. But it's first come, first served—they take you in when you're ready to deliver and whisk you out quickly to let the next one use it. I never got to use it at all."

◆

"The hospital birthing room was great. I enjoyed the atmosphere, space, and privacy; loved the rocker and the shower."

continued

"It was the greatest. My husband, his sister, and the doctor were all on the double bed with me at the end! The whole room was so comfortable, I'd hate to have to deliver in a cold delivery room."

"I loved it. Having everything in one room seems more private and personal and keeps you from being shuffled around."

"We had signed up for the hospital birthing room but were told that Susan wasn't advanced enough to use it. They offered to move us to the birthing room when her labor was almost over. Rather annoyed, we stayed in the labor room for delivery."

Ideally, birthing rooms stand for nonintervention and should be limited to normal labors. Birth in this setting is supposed to be a natural event, and it's not the place for epidurals or forceps deliveries. It is a misuse of birthing rooms when hospitals employ them as public-relations gimmicks, heavily advertising their availability and convenience. The net effect is that there is great demand for the one birthing room and no one is able to spend an entire labor, delivery, and recovery there. It becomes nothing more than a decorated delivery room, to which women are transferred to have their babies. The solution is to have enough birthing rooms for all women desiring natural childbirth and to use the regular labor and delivery rooms only for those requiring special care.

Different hospitals have different standards of qualification for use of the birthing room. Normally, a woman must be low-risk with an uneventful pregnancy and early labor. Usually no Pitocin or anesthesia (including epidurals or spinals) can be used, although a local anesthetic for an episiotomy is permitted.

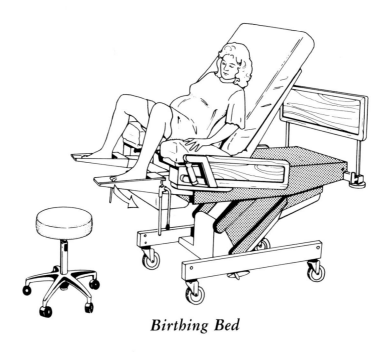

Birthing Bed

A distinctive feature of a birthing room is a special birthing bed, which can be used for both labor and delivery. Run by a motor, its top and bottom sections move, allowing for great flexibility of position. It has adjustable foot supports and the bottom of the bed breaks away so that your doctor or midwife can sit facing you. Women can deliver while sitting, squatting, or lying on their side. Not all birthing rooms have these beds, because they are very expensive, but if you are lucky enough to get one, you can instruct your husband to position it in any number of ways.

Even though it can't be seen, there is emergency equipment in the birthing room. Hidden behind cabinets or curtains are resuscitation material, oxygen, an episiotomy kit, and perhaps a baby warmer. And if necessary, there's more equipment close by because you are right on the obstetrics floor. Sterile drapes are not routinely used in birthing rooms, and your husband will not have to wear a scrub suit. This means you can look down and see your baby's head as it emerges and you can touch it if you want.

The Birthing Chair

Another option for delivery that has recently become available is the birthing chair. This is actually a revival of an ancient birthing stool. The Greeks used a chair with a crescent-shaped opening, while sixteenth-century Venetians sat on V-shaped stools. Today's model is a bit more functional, made of high-impact plastic with molded knee braces and adjustable footrests. It can be raised, lowered, or tilted because it is motorized.

Frankly, we were dubious about the birthing chair until we sat in it and were instructed in its use. We realized then that the birthing chair is only as effective as the person at its controls. Most of our negative impressions were refuted by our saleswoman, who expertly demonstrated its versatility.

We still have certain reservations, however. The size of the leg rests cannot be altered, and women with heavy thighs may find their flesh spilling out somewhat uncomfortably. The plastic seat was also a bit rigid because it's not padded. More importantly, a woman's autonomy is limited because she cannot adjust her own position in the chair; this must be done for her.

The most frequent criticism of the chair is that it promotes serious

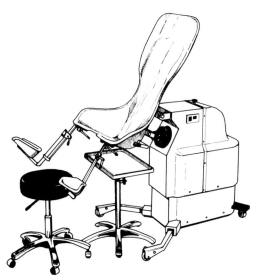

Birthing Chair

perineal tearing. This is not the fault of the chair, however, but of the pushing technique. Births aided by gravity require less forceful pushing and a more controlled delivery than those in the lithotomy position. A doctor must be able to guide a woman through a gentle delivery, and she must be responsive to his instructions.

We would prefer a birthing bed to a birthing chair, but the latter might be a practical addition to a busy obstetric department with only one or two birthing rooms. In that case, the birthing chair would provide a welcome alternative to the delivery room if the birthing rooms were occupied.

THE BIRTHING CHAIR

♦

"I thought it gave good support for my back, legs, and arms."

♦

"I loved it! I was a little intimidated at first by the idea of it and I didn't like the way it looked in the pictures I had seen, but my doctor preferred it to the birthing bed, and I went along with him."

♦

"It was a little awkward to go from the bed to the chair, but not painful."

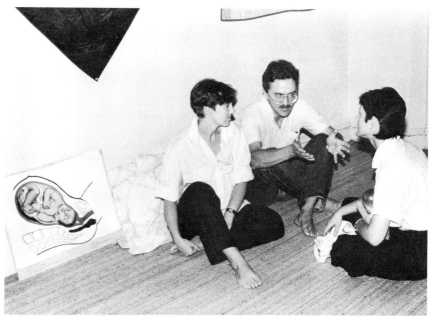

CHAPTER 4

Understanding Labor

An important part of the Lamaze method is understanding pregnancy, labor, and delivery—learning why you feel a certain way, understanding the terms your doctor or midwife uses, and familiarizing yourself with the physical process of birth. In the past, much of the fear surrounding childbirth was generated by ignorance. Women had only the most elementary knowledge about their bodies, and once they became pregnant, they had no classes to attend or books to read. Instead, they relied on information from their doctors or from friends and relatives who counseled them with personal anecdotes and old wives' tales. Women frequently heard about labors that were difficult, rather than about those that were easy or free of complications. Pregnancy myths abounded—a baby with a lot of hair causes heartburn; stretching your hands over your head creates cord entanglement—and it's no wonder women approached childbirth with dread. Knowledge about birth can help you distinguish fact from fiction in the stories you are told. It also helps to alleviate your fears and apprehensions about pregnancy and birth.

KNOWING YOUR BODY

Every field of study, whether it's Chinese cooking or car repair, has its own special vocabulary. Birth is no exception, and if you understand its terminology, the experience will seem less strange and intimidating. To start, there are several parts of the body you must be familiar with to better understand the workings of your body and share common language with your doctor or midwife (see illustration). They are:

Internal Organs

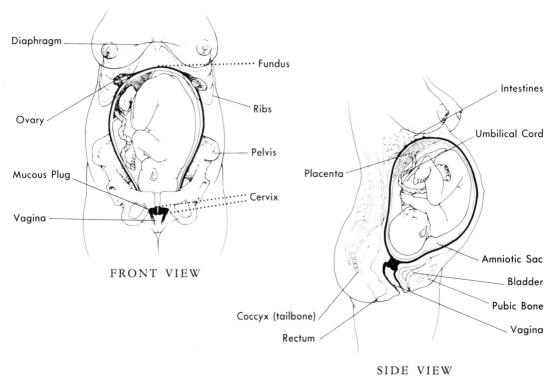

FRONT VIEW

SIDE VIEW

Diaphragm. A muscular sheath that controls respiration, the diaphragm lies underneath the lungs, like an opened upside-down umbrella. It lowers during inhalation and it relaxes back to place on each exhalation.

Pelvis. This bony structure encloses and protects the pelvic organs—rectum, vagina, bladder, and uterus. The back of the pelvis is called the *sacrum,* which is composed of five fused segments of the spine; the front of the pelvis is the *pubic bone.* The top of the pelvis is called the *pelvic inlet;* the bottom is referred to as the *pelvic outlet.* The pregnancy hormone *relaxin* causes the pelvic joints to soften, thereby allowing the pelvis to widen. The *coccyx,* also known as the tailbone, is the very last vertebra on the spine, located just below the sacrum.

Uterus. This muscular organ encloses the baby, the amniotic sac, the amniotic fluid, and the placenta. In a nonpregnant state, it is the size of a clenched fist.

Cervix. The cervix, or neck of the uterus, can be seen and/or felt at the very top of the vagina. It is oval in shape and a little more than an inch in length. It has an opening in the middle called the *os,* which is the size of a very thin soda straw.

Mucous plug. This is a mass of capillaries and mucus that fills the cervix during pregnancy. Its function is to seal the cervical opening and thereby protect the baby from infection.

Amniotic sac. Forming a lining inside the uterus, the amniotic sac encloses the baby and the amniotic fluid. It is also known as the bag of waters or membranes.

Amniotic fluid. This clear, odorless, sterile liquid surrounds the baby and is completely replaced every few hours. The baby will swallow the fluid, urinate into it, and be kept warm and protected by it.

Placenta. This organ begins to form in the fourth week after conception and grows to weigh about a pound at birth. Because mother and baby have separate circulatory systems, the placenta is necessary to transfer oxygen and nutrients from the mother to the baby and then waste products back from the baby to the mother. Since almost everything the mother ingests or inhales passes through it, the placenta has been described as a "bloody sieve."

Umbilical cord. This is the vital cable that connects the baby to the placenta. It's a two-way lifeline, containing three blood vessels. Oxygen and nutrients travel to the baby through the vein, and waste products are conducted to the placenta through the two arteries. The cord is about three-quarters of an inch in diameter, is semitransparent and jellylike in appearance, and has an average length of twenty-two inches.

THE PHYSICAL PROCESS OF BIRTH

Physiologically, the process of labor and delivery is quite simple and straightforward. The cervix opens to accommodate the widest diameter of the baby's head, the baby descends into the vagina, and then the baby is born. The placenta follows several minutes later. This process is divided into three stages. The first stage is labor, the second stage is the delivery of the baby, and the third stage is the expulsion of the placenta. Chapters 8, 9, and 10 fully describe the physical and emotional aspects of these stages. They will be easier to read, however, once you have a general knowledge of the process of labor and delivery.

THE FIRST STAGE OF LABOR

Dilation and Effacement

The first stage of labor begins with regular uterine contractions and ends when your cervix has effaced 100 percent, and dilated ten centimeters. Once your cervix has thinned and opened fully, the first stage of labor is completed. This can take as little as three hours (even for a first labor) or as long as thirty hours. The average for a first birth is twelve hours.

Normally, the cervix is long, thick, and almost closed, separating the uterus from the vagina. Late in pregnancy or during early labor, however, uterine contractions pull upward on the cervix, causing it to thin out and flatten, or efface. Effacement can only be determined by means of an internal examination, and depending on the changes felt by your doctor or midwife, you will be told you are 25, 50, 75, or 100 percent effaced. Your cervix is fully effaced once it is completely flat and thin as a tissue (see illustration).

Dilation occurs when the pull of the uterine contractions causes the cervical opening to expand. This process is somewhat like the dilation of the pupil in your eye, which opens wide in the dark to allow the maximum amount of light to enter. Like effacement, the extent of your dilation can be determined only by an internal examination. Progress is

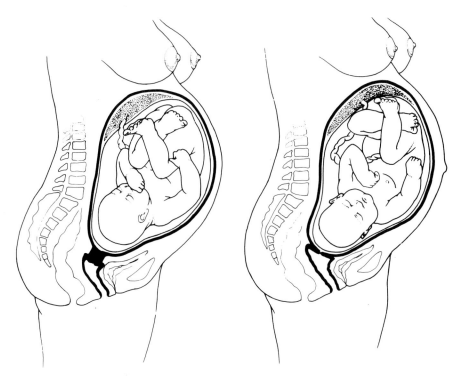

ZERO EFFACEMENT   FULL EFFACEMENT

measured in centimeters or "fingers," with two centimeters equaling one finger. Dilation is complete at ten centimeters or five fingers (see illustration). This is a very subjective measurement, however, since no one introduces any instruments into your vagina to get an exact reading. You may be examined by a resident and told you are five centimeters dilated. Then, half an hour later, you are checked by your doctor and told you are only four. There is no reason to be discouraged or worried. Cervical checks are not an exact science. Whether your baby is six pounds or nine pounds, you will have to dilate to "ten centimeters" before you will be permitted to start pushing. Even at full dilation the baby is still high in your vagina. The baby can be seen only after you've been pushing for a while and are well into the second stage of labor.

Effacement and dilation can occur separately or in unison. You can be 50 percent effaced and two centimeters dilated, or 100 percent effaced and not dilated at all. In any case, you will probably be 100 percent effaced by the time you are about five centimeters dilated. Sometimes dilation and effacement occur prior to labor, which is lucky, since it can decrease the length of labor. However, this does not always happen. Many women efface to 50 or 100 percent and dilate to one or two

Dilation of the Cervix

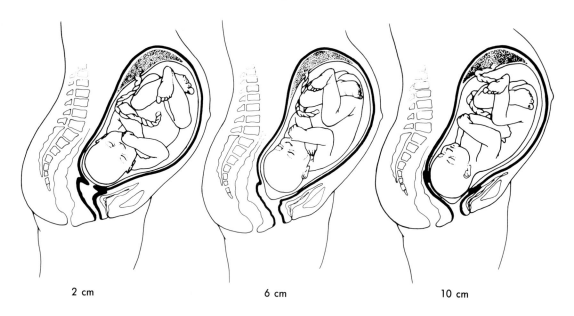

2 cm   6 cm   10 cm

DILATION RINGS

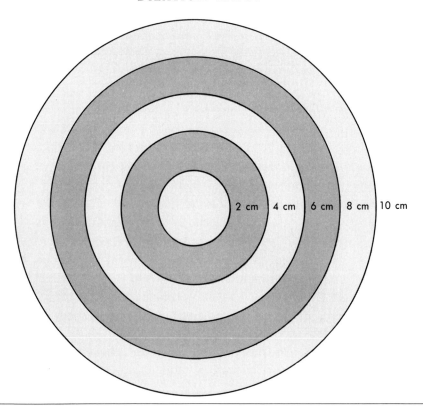

2 cm | 4 cm | 6 cm | 8 cm | 10 cm

centimeters prior to labor, but it is rare for a woman having her first child to dilate past three centimeters and not be in labor.

Early dilation and effacement can be exciting, but should not be used to gauge the accuracy of your due date. You can go into labor at any time, regardless of whether you were two centimeters dilated or showed no progress at all during your last checkup. Try not to be discouraged if you're a week late and are told, "Nothing's changed from last week." Conversely, don't drop everything if you discover you have begun to efface or dilate. Cervical change is only one indicator of readiness for labor. Unless you are induced, labor begins when the baby is ready to be born, and no one can accurately predict when that will happen, including your doctor or midwife.

Engagement and Station

To describe your readiness for labor, your doctor or midwife may use two additional terms: *engagement* and *station.* Engagement occurs when the baby's head moves deep into the pelvis. This event is commonly referred to as the baby dropping. If this is your first child, engagement usually happens several weeks before your due date. If this is a subsequent pregnancy, it usually doesn't occur until labor begins. Once the baby is engaged, the upward pressure of the uterus on the diaphragm, lungs, and stomach is somewhat relieved, and it's easier to eat a full meal or breathe deeply. On the other hand, engagement puts extra pressure on the nerves emerging from the lower back and bladder, creating soreness in the groin and thighs and a greater need to urinate.

Station refers to the baby's position in relation to the pelvis (see illustration). When the baby's presenting part engages, it rests at zero station. Anywhere above this point is a minus station, anywhere below is a plus station. The numbers range from one to five, and each digit is equivalent to a centimeter. Minus five is the very top of the pelvis; plus five is the bottom of the vagina (crowning). The position of the baby is related to, but not dependent upon, cervical dilation. The true progress of labor includes cervical dilation and effacement and the descent of the baby.

Rotation and Presentation

During the first stage of labor, the baby will engage more deeply in your pelvis. He should also turn anywhere from 90 to 180 degrees

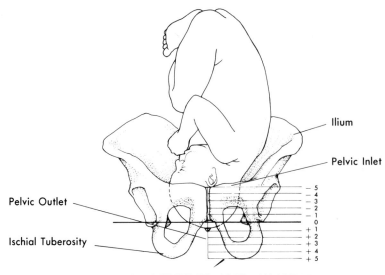

Ilium

Pelvic Inlet

Pelvic Outlet

Ischial Tuberosity

ENGAGEMENT AND STATION

within you, moving to a position that is either face-down or face-up. This movement is called internal rotation. In over 96 percent of all births the baby is positioned head down. In approximately 75 percent of these cases, the baby rotates to a normal anterior position, which means that he faces the mother's spine. In the remaining 25 percent the baby rotates so that he is facing the mother's stomach and the back of his head rests against her spine. These babies are said to be in a posterior presentation. (See illustrations.) Many babies begin labor in a posterior position or become posterior as labor progresses. Most of them reposition themselves, however, before delivery.

The Three Phases of Labor

Because the first stage of labor is the longest one, it is further subdivided into three phases: *early labor, active labor,* and *transition.* The different phases are used to describe the progress of cervical dilation and the differing qualities of the contractions. They serve only as general guidelines, however; bear in mind that labor is a process and an experience, not a precise and predictable science.

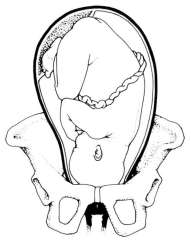
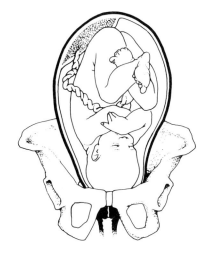

ANTERIOR POSITION   POSTERIOR POSITION

EARLY LABOR

During this phase, regular contractions occur every five to twenty minutes, last about thirty to forty-five seconds each, and are usually fairly mild. Women often compare these first contractions to the feeling of menstrual cramps or a low backache. An average early labor takes eight to nine hours, and during this time the cervix effaces to 100 percent and dilates to about three centimeters.

This may sound like a terribly long time to progress only a third of the way through labor, but you must remember that having a forty-five-second contraction every fifteen minutes is equivalent to three minutes of discomfort every hour. That leaves fifty-seven minutes for resting, reading, watching television, or taking a walk. The time passes very quickly if you go back to sleep or carry on with your normal activities. By the end of this phase, your contractions will probably last a full sixty seconds and occur every four or five minutes, and you'll be moving into active labor. This is the point at which many doctors want you to call them to tell them you are in labor—but this doesn't mean you are ready to go to the hospital or birth center.

Early labor varies for each woman. Many women realize they have gone through early labor only once they are past it and into active labor. They may not observe any regularity to the contractions until the intensity increases. Other women know immediately that they are in labor because the mucous plug dislodges or the amniotic sac breaks, followed by strong and frequent contractions.

Cervical dilation results directly from strong, regular uterine contractions. As long as your contractions are fairly mild and short, you should feel comfortable about staying home, even if this phase lasts a very long time. On the other hand, some labors can be very short. If your early contractions are painful, last a full minute, and quickly assume a pattern of three-minute intervals, you should forget about movies and warm baths and call your doctor or midwife right away. You may be in for what we call telescopic (shortened or condensed) labor. (For more on early labor, see chapter 8.)

ACTIVE LABOR

During active labor, contractions are three to four minutes apart and last about sixty seconds each. Because these contractions are stronger, longer, and closer together than the earlier ones, they dilate the cervix more quickly. Active labor lasts an average of three to four hours, and you will dilate to seven centimeters. As with all the other phases, a normal active labor can have many variations. You may dilate a respectable centimeter every hour, or you may move quickly to five centimeters and remain there for a few hours until progress resumes further, or you could race from three to eight centimeters in just one hour. (For more on active labor, see chapter 9.)

This is the phase when there is no doubt you are in labor. Your contractions are strong and you will have to work hard to stay on top of them. Unless you are having the baby at home, you should head for the hospital or birth center. There's no need to rush. Even if you're eight centimeters dilated, you probably still have about an hour or so of transition and then another one to two hours of pushing before the baby is born.

TRANSITION

Transition is the last phase of the first stage of labor, when your cervix dilates from eight to ten centimeters. It is the most difficult phase for many women because the contractions and rests are of roughly equal duration (60 to 90 seconds each) and because it comes when you are most tired. Contractions can also occur irregularly, sometimes stringing themselves together in double or triple form. This phase can also be accompanied by annoying symptoms—nausea, chills, shaking, irritability —making it the moment when most women declare, "Never again."

Transition usually does not last longer than an hour, however, and sometimes it consists of just a few contractions. (For more on transition, see chapter 9.)

Although most women find transition the most painful part of labor, the fact that the end is near makes it seem exciting as well. Once you are fully dilated, the first stage of labor is complete and you can begin to push.

THE SECOND STAGE OF LABOR

The second stage of labor begins when the cervix is fully dilated and ends with the birth of the baby. It lasts an average of one hour for a first labor, and 30 minutes or less for a subsequent delivery. During this stage, your contractions will return to a more civilized rhythm, lasting around sixty seconds each and spacing out to intervals of three or four minutes. Now instead of relaxing and breathing, you will actively push, helping your baby descend through your open cervix, into your vagina, and out into the world. You will push only during the contractions, and rest between them.

As you push, the baby will descend lower and lower into your vagina. Toward the end, the very top of the baby's head will be visible during each contraction, but it will recede when the contraction ends and the force of your pushing stops. When the top of the baby's head remains continually visible at the vagina, the baby is said to be crowning. Your doctor or midwife will decide if an episiotomy is necessary. After the head is born, the baby will turn once more, rotating back to the original side position, facing either your right or left hip. This movement is called the external rotation, and your baby will do this unaided (see illustration). Now his shoulders are lined up directly between your pubic bone and coccyx. Once the baby's shoulders are born, your doctor or midwife will literally catch the baby as the rest of his body emerges. The umbilical cord is cut, and the second stage of labor has ended. (For more on delivery, see chapter 10.)

THE THIRD STAGE OF LABOR

This final stage of labor is devoted solely to the expulsion of the placenta. It is relatively painless and short, usually lasting no more than thirty minutes. Now that the baby is born, the placenta is no longer needed.

Rotation and Descent of Baby

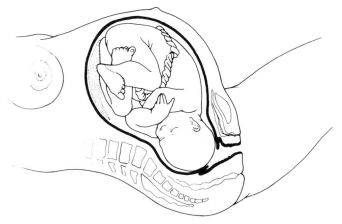

BEFORE FULL DILATION

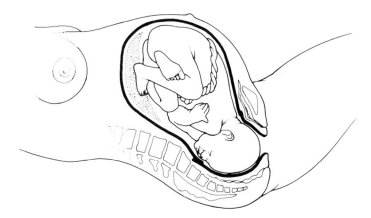

DESCENT INTO BIRTH CANAL

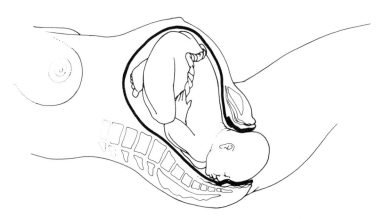

ROTATION OF THE HEAD COMPLETED

External Rotation

Uterine contractions continue, forcing the placenta to detach and closing off the placental site. The placenta will be expelled during a contraction, along with a show of blood.

The placenta is examined to make sure it is intact and complete. If any portion of it or the amniotic membranes remains in the uterus, it can cause hemorrhage. Nursing immediately after delivery encourages proper expulsion of the placenta because your natural oxytocin is released, creating efficient uterine contractions.

CHAPTER **5**

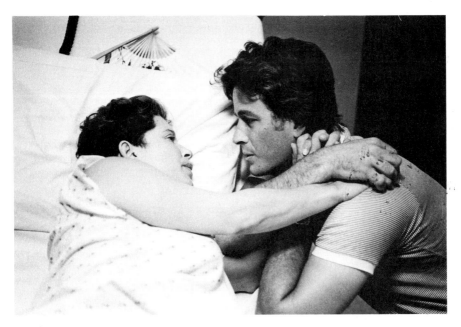

The Lamaze
Breathing

BREATHING FOR CHILDBIRTH

*A*ll physical activity, whether it be swimming, yoga, or weight lifting,
utilizes special breathing patterns. Since childbirth is very much a
physical event, it makes perfect sense that a specific breathing technique
would be helpful here, too. The Lamaze breathing patterns are not
magical rhythms to make the pain disappear. Nor are they techniques for
controlling labor. Rather, they are a coping mechanism that works on

many levels, both physical and psychological, to decrease the amount of pain you perceive. By coordinating your breathing with the contractions, you will work with labor instead of fighting it.

Contractions are often described as "waves" because they build, peak, and fade much like the real ones, and because they rise and fall, with periods of calm in between. If you've ever swum in the ocean (or watched others), you know there are two techniques for dealing with the waves. The first one is indecision. The wave approaches and you freeze, trying to choose whether to duck or run for shore. Suddenly it's too late, and you are dragged under by the force of the wave. When you come up for air, you're exhausted, out of breath, and a little shaken. Then there is only a short break before the next one comes, and then another, and another after that. It's frightening to contemplate, but this is probably analogous to the feelings our mothers experienced during labor, as they floundered through sensations that were incomprehensible and overwhelming.

The second technique for dealing with waves requires a little more finesse, but is much less taxing and a lot more enjoyable. By simply diving through the wave, you emerge easily into the safe, calm waters on the other side. You are not in control of the wave, but you are able to swim through it. You stay in the water for a while and dive through wave after wave. Each time it takes a concerted effort to dive in and come up on your feet. This technique is like using the Lamaze method—it requires concentration and timing, but the result can be exhilarating.

On a purely physical level, the Lamaze breathing keeps your body and baby well oxygenated. Working muscles produce waste products that, if allowed to accumulate, can cause soreness and cramping. This is the last thing you need on top of labor contractions. The oxygen you inhale will help to metabolize these waste products.

Breathing will also help you to relax. If you doubt this, try to hold your breath and relax your body at the same time. It is really an impossible task. Now breathe and let your body go limp. It's infinitely easier. Just by maintaining the flow of air you will experience a certain degree of relaxation.

From a psychological standpoint, the Lamaze breathing gives you something concrete to do and serves as a focus for your thoughts during contractions. Labor requires great passivity because you must step aside and allow your body to do what is necessary. This can be very difficult to accomplish, but by concentrating on your breathing, you can actively assist your body. As you breathe, the sensation of the contraction will

THE LAMAZE BREATHING

"I feel it is a very effective method. The pain is not as bad if you have a way of getting through it."

◆

"I wish I had practiced the breathing exercises until they were second nature. Looking back, I realize a person can't be too prepared."

◆

"It was well worth the time spent breathing and practicing. I knew what to expect and when to expect it, and the pain was minimized by the controlled breathing."

◆

"I had a hard time understanding how the way I breathed would help me deal with the pain. Afterward, I was amazed at how it really did help."

◆

"It was like someone teaching you how to ride a bike—it's funny until you find yourself on the bike for the first time."

◆

"I have successfully used Lamaze breathing in other painful situations, such as at the dentist's office. I used to be fainthearted, but Lamaze has helped me to overcome all fear of pain."

◆

"I'm amazed at the power of the human body. My contractions were very painful at times, but the relaxation and breathing techniques worked wonders."

decrease in intensity, in the same manner that background noises fade as you read an engrossing book. The pain of the contraction is there, but because it is not the object of your attention, you are less conscious of its presence. The Lamaze breathing will not decrease the amount of pain you have, but it will alter your perception of it.

The most natural response to a pain stimulus is to hold your breath and release it after the pain passes. The expression "It took my breath away" describes this common reaction. Another response is muscular tension, the tightening of the body in preparation for fight or flight. During active labor, when strong contractions occur every three minutes for several hours, you'll be exhausted if you fight each contraction in this manner. The ensuing fatigue will then decrease your ability to handle stress and will lower your pain threshold. One could say that the Lamaze method is really unnatural childbirth because breathing and relaxing in response to pain is a very unnatural thing to do. Learning the Lamaze method requires retraining and conscious effort.

During early labor, you will be reading, napping, taking walks, and continuing with your normal routine. Try to ignore your contractions for as long as you can. Your labor will seem very long if you drop everything at the first contraction and concentrate solely on these sensations. At some point, however, the sensation of your uterus will become the strongest stimulus, and all other distractions will fade.

You should start your first Lamaze breathing when you can no longer walk, talk, or just relax through the contractions, when other activities can no longer divert your attention.

While we can make generalizations, there's no telling when this will be or exactly what techniques you will want to use when. If your labor begins with strong, one-minute contractions from the very onset, you might start with the modified paced breathing. On the other hand, you may use the slow paced breathing throughout your entire labor and never need any of the other patterns. The relaxation techniques by themselves may be all you need for quite a long time, or they may work better for you if used in conjunction with a breathing pattern. You should experiment with what feels most comfortable for you and trust your instincts.

Many women are concerned about starting "the breathing" too soon and fear they will "run out" of techniques for the hard part. It's true that starting your breathing patterns too early can make your labor seem longer. However, if you delay beginning, tension can build and relaxation will suffer. You should start when you need to and not worry about how you will handle transition. There are always variations that can be devised if needed.

There is no such thing as doing the Lamaze breathing "wrong." If it feels right, it *is* right. There are no magic patterns or perfect numbers of breaths. You may want to learn a foolproof technique guaranteed to work, but this does not exist. Instead, you should consider the breathing patterns to be tools at your disposal to be used when needed.

TECHNIQUES COMMON TO ALL THE BREATHING PATTERNS

There are four breathing patterns: one for each of the three phases of labor and one for pushing. Though each one is different, there are certain components they all share.

The Cleansing Breath

The Lamaze breathing for a contraction always begins and ends with a deep sigh, called a cleansing breath. To do one, simply inhale deeply and then release it gently, slowly letting the air escape.

Cleansing breaths are helpful to both you and your partner. The first cleansing breath is a sign to your partner that your contraction has begun and he should begin timing; the second one tells him that the contraction is over. Conserving energy is important, and always having to say, "I have another one coming," or "Okay, that's it," wastes precious energy.

The cleansing breath is also your conditioned response to relax completely, stop whatever else you are doing, and get ready to do a breathing pattern. It replaces your natural response to tense your body and hold your breath. It's like a silent voice that says, "Get ready now, here's another one. You can do it." The final cleansing breath closes the door on each contraction, and the voice says, "It's over now, I'm doing all right. One less contraction to go."

Timing Within the Contractions

During each contraction your partner will time the passing seconds. He'll start timing as you take your cleansing breath and will say to you, "Fifteen seconds . . . thirty seconds . . . forty-five seconds . . . sixty seconds." He'll know the contraction is over when you take your second cleansing breath.

You should practice the timing for 60 seconds, even though actual contractions can vary in length from 30 to 120 seconds. A minute can seem like a very long time if you are in pain, and you'll be encouraged to hear that time is indeed passing. It is also reassuring just to hear your partner's voice and to feel his active assistance.

The timing will help you to handle each contraction more easily. Your contractions usually develop a rhythm, peaking at approximately the same point each time. If your peak occurs at twenty seconds, you'll learn that when your partner says, "Fifteen seconds," you must gear up for the hardest part. Then once the contraction eases, and you hear, "Thirty seconds," you know the worst is over and the rest is downhill.

The Focal Point

Another way to reduce your perception of pain is to concentrate your gaze on one point or image. Some women prefer an external focus: a tiny spot on the wall, a photograph of a beautiful place, or another child. Sometimes it's helpful to close your eyes and concentrate on an image (riding a wave or feeling the contraction as heat), a color, or a sound. You should be mindful, however, that closing your eyes may intensify the pain of the contraction; in order for this technique to be successful, you must maintain a strong inner focus. Practice with your eyes open and with them closed so that during labor you will be able to choose the method that works best for you. Again, there is no right or wrong approach.

Effleurage

One optional technique you may enjoy throughout labor is called effleurage. This is a French word, meaning stroking or light massage. If you bump your elbow, you automatically stroke it with your other hand. Rubbing a sore body part is a natural response, and an aching uterus is no exception. Even now it probably feels good to rub your belly, and there's no reason to discontinue this comforting motion once labor starts. You can rub a light circle all around your abdomen or just use a short stroke underneath your belly with one hand or with two. Better yet, ask your partner to massage your belly for you, letting him know the correct amount of pressure. If your belly is sensitive, you may prefer to exert firm pressure just above your pubic bone or have your partner massage your back, feet, or thighs instead of your abdomen. You can use talcum powder, cornstarch, or a little massage oil to prevent skin irritation.

In 1983 ASPO/Lamaze standardized the names for the breathing patterns for labor. This directive was in response to a need for a common professional language and a desire to eliminate regional differences in usage. These terms had originally been left to the discretion of individual teachers, but names such as *slow-chest, accelerated/decelerated,* and *pant-blow* have now been replaced by the terms *slow-paced, modified-paced,* and *patterned-paced.* In addition, the guidelines for performing the breathing patterns were made more flexible, allowing for greater individual variations on the part of both students and teachers.

Other comfort measures were updated as well. A greater emphasis was placed on teaching relaxation techniques, and effleurage, once confined to abdominal stroking, was expanded to include back or suprapubic pressure and leg, foot, and back massage. Though good Lamaze instructors had already incorporated many of these changes, they have now been officially endorsed.

THE LAMAZE BREATHING PATTERNS
Slow-Paced Breathing for Early Labor

The first breathing pattern is simple, slow, and very relaxing to do. Find your focal point. Take a deep cleansing breath in and out, and then breathe slowly and deeply for the duration of the minute contraction. Breathe in through your nose and out through your mouth. Relax your body completely, and let each exhalation help you to let go even more. At the end of the contraction, take another deep cleansing breath in and out.

During the contraction, your partner will time the quadrants of the minute, saying, "Fifteen seconds . . . thirty seconds . . . forty-five seconds . . . sixty seconds, the contraction is over." It will feel soothing to do the effleurage, or light belly massage.

If you count your breaths taken during the minute, you'll find that you probably take around six to nine (not counting the cleansing breaths), which is about half the pace of normal breathing. The reasoning behind this timing is that a more rapid rate will use too much energy and will fail to be relaxing, but if the pace is too slow, it won't be rhythmical enough to hold your attention.

Try to make the breaths in and out of almost equal length. If you have trouble, count slowly to yourself as you inhale, "One thousand, two thousand, three thousand," and repeat the numbers as you exhale. It is easy to breathe *out* very slowly, but it is difficult to breathe *in* slowly.

The timing is very individual. Singers and yoga enthusiasts are often most comfortable with five breaths per minute, and that is fine. The breathing should be calming, so establish a pace that is relaxing for you. The first few times you practice, your breathing will be slightly fast. The more you rehearse, however, the more confident you will be, and the slower and more soothing the breathing will become.

Feel free to breathe entirely through your nose, or in with your nose and out through your lips. Comfort is more important than style. If you have a cold or your nose is stuffed (a common condition called pregnancy rhinitis), you will have to breathe through your mouth. If you find your mouth gets too dry with this breathing, switch to all-nose breathing. Experiment a little and see what feels most natural to you.

Don't worry about whether you are doing abdominal or chest breathing. The style you intuitively select will be the right one. Remember, the purpose of the breathing is to relax you, not test your coordination.

You will continue this breathing pattern during the contractions only and use it for as long as it works for you. This may be for only two contractions or it may be for your entire labor.

Modified-Paced Breathing for Active Labor

As your labor progresses, your contractions will become stronger, longer, and closer together. You may feel more pain as the contractions intensify, and you may need a more active breathing pattern to keep up with your active labor. You may wonder now how you will know when to change to this breathing pattern, but this won't be a problem. In labor you will probably find you will change breathing patterns automatically.

Think about how your breathing adjusts naturally when you have to work harder than normal, how it changes as you walk up a flight of stairs or scrub a floor. Without conscious thought your breathing pace gets faster, and each individual breath becomes more shallow. Modified-paced breathing mimics these natural changes. You will accelerate the pace of your breathing as the contraction intensifies, and you will slow down as it fades.

Find your focal point and welcome the contraction with your cleansing breath. (Remember, by now it is a conditioned response to breathe and relax with each contraction.) Begin with slow breathing, then allow it to quicken as you reach the thirty-second mark. Once the peak of the contraction has passed, allow the breathing to slow down again. At the end of the contraction, take a deep cleansing breath and relax even more.

Your partner should still count off the quadrants of the minute and continue the belly, back, or foot massage. Feel free to inhale and exhale through either your nose or your mouth.

The modified-paced breathing is faster and more shallow than the slow-paced breathing for early labor. You will take about thirty breaths per minute now, but this figure is an approximation—you are free to set your own tempo. If this pattern of breathing seems difficult to grasp, try to breathe to a song. A slow rendition of "Love and Marriage" or the Beatles' "Yellow Submarine" are good ones, taking a breath in or out on each note. This is the pace for your fastest active-labor breathing done during the peak of the contraction.

To help you practice this breathing pattern, pretend you are going to walk up and down a flight of stairs. Your partner is at your side and you are ready to begin. Take your cleansing breath and focus mentally on the very top stair. Breathe slowly in and out, two or three times. You will hear your partner say, "Fifteen seconds," and you know you are about halfway up the stairs. It is harder work now, so allow the breathing to get faster and lighter as you climb those last few stairs. At the very top, you will hear, "Thirty seconds," and you know that the hardest part is over. Your breathing is still quick, but as you turn around and walk back down the stairs, it will return to the easy pace. When you reach the bottom step, take a deep cleansing breath and rest. The contraction is over.

It can be difficult to practice the active breathing without any real stimulus. You may feel the breathing seems too easy to be of any help when things get tough. To reassure yourself, you can conduct a small experiment by having your partner squeeze your upper arm, calf, or thigh to stimulate the sensation of a contraction. He should gradually increase the intensity of his squeeze so that his grip is tightest at the thirty-second mark; slowly, he should release his grip and end at sixty seconds.

Many women who try this exercise are amazed at how unconscious they are of the tight grip and how well the breathing works to decrease their perception of pain. It is also encouraging to try this simulation without doing the breathing, because then you are able to contrast the amount of discomfort with and without the breathing. Another experiment is to have your partner squeeze your arm or leg quickly and as hard as he did at the thirty-second mark. This demonstrates that pain is much more tolerable when it occurs gradually, as it does during normal labor.

Patterned-Paced Breathing for Transition

This technique requires the most energy and concentration, so use it only for the strongest contractions. The tempo is fast, light, shallow, and even throughout the entire contraction. This breathing is done entirely through the mouth, with lips and jaw slack and relaxed.

Because transition contractions peak quickly, you only have time for a quick cleansing breath. It is really more psychological than physical at this point—a mental "On your mark, get set, go" preparation for the contraction. The breathing for the contraction itself is done in one even rhythm, breathing in and out three times, then taking a fourth breath in and blowing it out through pursed lips, as if to blow out a match. The sequence goes like this: in/out, in/out, in/out, in/blow; in/out, in/out, in/out, in/blow; and so on. The breathing is so shallow and light that there should be no sound on any of the exhalations except for the blow, which is crisp and short, very staccato, and will act as an accent, not as a break or pause. At the end of the contraction, take one or two very slow cleansing breaths to unwind completely. Take advantage of whatever short rest you get between contractions.

This technique is the most difficult one, so at first, you should practice with a simulated contraction of thirty or forty-five seconds. As you become more confident, practice for ninety seconds. You will be tempted to make the sound of your breathing audible to your partner, but this is unnecessary. You may be aware of your exhalation but not of your inhalation. Don't worry about it—you are inhaling even if you can't hear it.

You may want your husband to rub your back or he can continue the effleurage. Your focus may be internal as you visualize your cervix opening those last three centimeters, or it may be external as you stare at a bit of color in a photograph. At this point, most women need direct eye contact with their partners, and this is the time when you will most likely breathe through the contractions together.

Your body works very hard during labor, and by transition you are tired. The last thing you want to do is struggle with your breathing. For this reason, you should practice the transition breathing until each breath is feather light and completely effortless.

Transition breathing lends itself to variations more easily than other types. This can be useful during labor, for varying the pattern can help force you to concentrate on your breathing. Practice the three breaths and the blow, but once you've got it down, you can experiment a little. Try two breaths and a blow, or five breaths and a blow. When the time comes, you can change your rhythm for each contraction if you like.

Another variation of transition breathing is called *pyramid breathing*. This pattern requires intense concentration, which some women find helpful.

Pyramid breathing consists of breathing in and out once, then breathing in and blowing out through pursed lips. The next time, you inhale/exhale twice and then inhale/blow; the third time you inhale/exhale three times and then inhale/blow, and so on until you reach five in-and-out breaths followed by an in-breath and a blow. It looks like this:

In/out, in/blow
In/out, in/out, in/blow
In/out, in/out, in/out, in/blow
In/out, in/out, in/out, in/out, in/blow
In/out, in/out, in/out, in/out, in/out, in/blow, and so on

If this variation seems very complicated to you, you are correct, it is. But many women like it for that very reason, so we present it as another option. Don't feel you have to learn it if you are too confused.

Breathing to Offset an Early Urge to Push

Usually, feeling the need to bear down (or have a bowel movement) is the signal that your cervix is completely dilated and you are ready to begin pushing. Sometimes, however, this urge is premature, occurring before you are fully dilated. Pushing now could cause your cervix to swell. So always wait for your doctor or midwife to examine you first.

If you are told you are not completely dilated, you must do some very active breathing to avoid pushing.

To resist this strong feeling, put your hands over your nose and mouth and blow out forcefully and quickly in multiple short exhalations for as long as the urge to push persists. Keep your hands over your face to prevent hyperventilation. When the urge subsides, you can remove your hands and return to your regular transition breathing. The desire to push may last for just a few seconds at the peak of the contraction or throughout the entire minute.

This breathing is an important technique, but one that will not make much sense to you until you need it. Practice it anyway so that it will be a familiar routine when the time comes.

Breathing for Pushing

During the pushing, or second stage of labor, you will bear down only during the contractions; in between, you will rest. The type of breathing you do for the contractions will depend on their length. If each contraction lasts a full sixty seconds, you will have time for an initial cleansing breath and then for three or possibly four pushes before it is over. If each one is shorter, you will skip the cleansing breath and begin to push immediately in order to take full advantage of the contraction's duration. Each push will take ten to fifteen seconds. There are two basic breathing techniques you can use during pushing: breathing in and then pushing as you continuously release your breath, or breathing in and then pushing while holding half a breath.

When you feel a contraction coming, you will take your cleansing breath in and out, then take another deep breath in and quickly blow some of it out. While holding the rest, you will completely relax your pelvic floor and bear down as your partner slowly counts, "One . . . two . . . three . . . four . . . five . . . six . . . seven . . . eight." Quickly, you will release the remaining air, take another breath in, let half of it out, hold the rest and push again, up to the count of between eight and ten. If the contraction is still there, you may even push a third or fourth time. After you release the rest of your last breath, you will relax your legs and finish with your cleansing breath. If at any time you feel any pressure in your neck or face, let a little more air out. Try to work your chest and upper abdominal muscles and relax the ones in your face and pelvis.

Another technique is to take your cleansing breath in and out once the

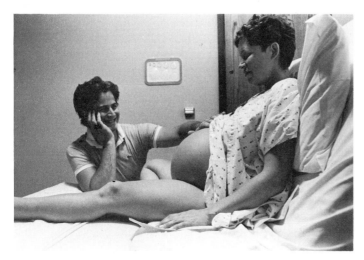

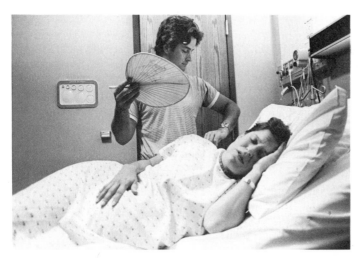

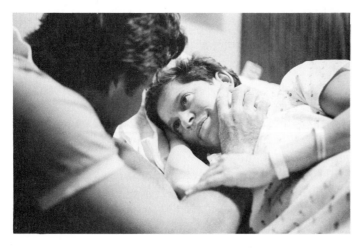

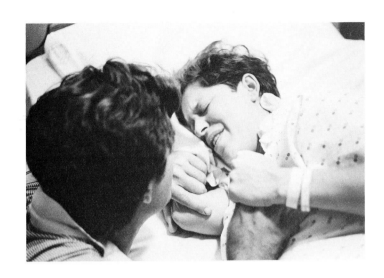

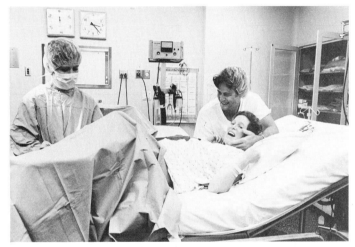

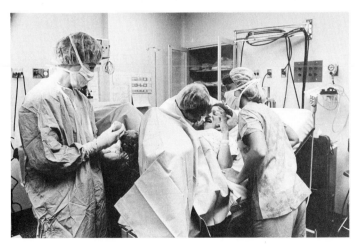

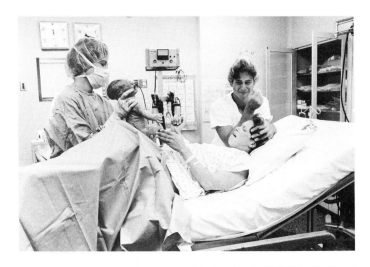

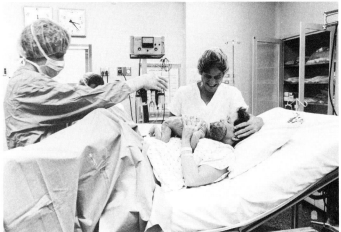

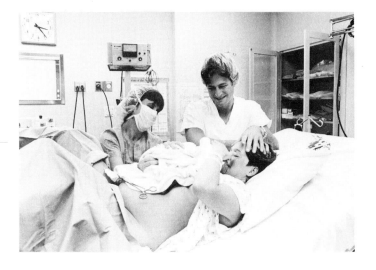

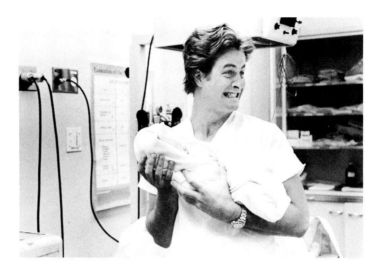

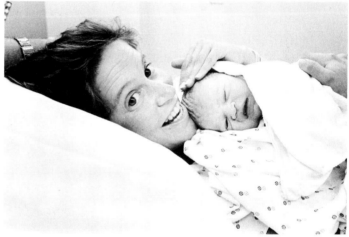

contraction begins, then to inhale again and continuously exhale as you push. This you will repeat three or four times, depending on the length of your contraction, and end with your cleansing breath.

There are many "right" ways to breathe as you push, and it will be an individual and instinctive choice when you will exhale and when you will hold your breath. It's possible you may not know how to push correctly, but it's unlikely you would breathe incorrectly. Don't focus on perfecting a specific breathing technique. Instead, practice different styles and keep in mind that when the time comes, your breathing will probably be an adaptation all your own.

Many women don't do any special breathing at all, simply following their natural desire to yelp, shout, or grunt as they push. If you're given the freedom to assume a comfortable, efficient position and you're not inhibited about vocalizing, this informal approach may work the best. The only breathing technique that should never be used is the Valsalva maneuver, which means pushing with a full held breath. It is commonly taught in the delivery room by nurses and doctors, but it is a dangerous and uncomfortable method. In *Nine Months, Nine Lessons,* childbirth educator Gail Brewer explains why: "This technique places severe strain on your already separated abdominal muscles, interferes with the return of blood to your heart by raising the pressure in your blood vessels to dangerous levels . . . and most significant for labor progress, causes the muscles of your pelvic floor to contract, not *release,* thus *inhibiting* your baby's descent."

To understand the effect of the Valsalva maneuver, take a deep breath in and hold it for about five seconds. You will begin to feel the pressure building in your face and neck. If you hold your breath and try to push at the same time, you will feel even greater pressure. Used during the delivery, this technique will exhaust you, making your face grow red with effort and the veins in your neck stand out. It can even cause capillaries in your face and eyes to break. In addition, the nurse may be exhorting you to "Push, push, push, hold your breath, don't let any air escape," while instructing you not to make any noise because that would be a waste of energy.

During this second stage, you will tune in to your partner's encouraging voice and push as you feel the need. You'll most enjoy giving birth if you can relax, breathing and pushing intuitively. Childbirth should be considered an art, not an athletic competition.

Learning how to push is important, but it's also inherently inadequate because giving birth requires on-the-job training. Practicing pushing without labor is like trying to swim without water. Prior to labor there is no urge to push and no way adequately to prepare for the effort it entails. Be reassured, however, that pushing is an instinctual act that every woman can perform, provided that she is allowed to choose her own position and that her pelvic muscles have not been deadened by anesthesia.

TIPS ON PRACTICING

Optimally, you should practice each breathing pattern at least five times every day with your partner and as often as possible by yourself. You can practice your cleansing breaths every time you feel the baby kick, so you begin to condition yourself to breathe in response to a stimulus. Do your slow breathing as you wait for a light to change or before you drop off to sleep at night; practice the active breathing during a television commercial or on a crowded bus; try the transition breathing as you go up a flight of stairs or ride your stationary bike.

When you practice the timing of the contraction, your partner can use a watch with a second hand or a stopwatch. Within a few weeks, however, he should develop the sense of the length of a minute and be able to do without the watch. This is preferable because during labor his attention should be on you, not on his watch.

Let your cleansing breath be the cue to your husband that your contraction has begun, rather than having him tell you when to start. This is what will happen during labor, so it is a way of establishing the correct habit.

Everyone has the tendency to speed up in the heat of performance. For example, a speech rehearsed at home in twenty minutes will take twelve minutes to deliver in front of an audience. A similar rush occurs during labor, so if there is doubt about the tempo of a breathing pattern, it is generally better to practice a little on the slow side, allowing yourself the leeway to speed up during labor.

Don't always practice in a peaceful environment where it's easiest to relax. Bright lights and loud noises can improve your powers of concentration and your breathing and relaxation skills.

Practice in different positions. Don't always settle yourself comfortably in bed, since you may not spend most of your labor there. You should become accustomed to breathing standing up, in the hands-and-knees position, sitting in a rocking chair and lying on your side. The breathing will feel slightly different in different postures, and since you can't predict what positions will feel best during labor, you should be prepared for all of them. This also holds true for when you practice pushing.

The breathing patterns should be rehearsed to the point where they are second nature. Practice until the rhythms are so familiar they are absolutely effortless to perform.

THE LAMAZE LABOR CHART

The following chart summarizes the information from chapters 4 and 5 on labor and Lamaze breathing. No two labors are identical, and there are many variations on labor and delivery. This is meant only as a general guide to the average labor. The chart can be used as a review once you have finished reading this book or as a summary you can refer to during labor.

	PURPOSE	CONTRACTIONS	AVERAGE LENGTH	WOMAN'S MOOD
Early Labor	100% effacement of the cervix and dilation to 3 centimeters	Regular contractions that last 30–45 seconds and occur every 5–20 minutes. Mild at first but gradually becoming stronger and more frequent.	8–9 hours	Excited Comfortable Confident Chatty Scared
Active Labor	Dilation of cervix 4–7 centimeters	Regular contractions 3–4 minutes apart, lasting for 60 seconds. Contractions are longer, stronger, and closer together.	3–4 hours	Become more internally focused Less verbal Busy concentrating on breathing and relaxing

THE LAMAZE LABOR CHART

BREATHING	PARTNER'S ROLE	WHAT TO DO
Slow Breathing: Relax, take a slow, deep cleansing breath. Continue to breathe slowly and rhythmically, in through the nose and out through the lips, 6–9 breaths per minute. Gently massage abdomen. Partner times quadrants to the minute, saying 15-, 30-, and 45-second marks. End with a deep cleansing breath.	Time contractions Emphasize relaxation Verbal reassurance	Rest, relax, conserve energy Read, nap, take walks, go to a movie Continue usual routine Eat lightly to keep up strength
Modified Breathing: Relax, take a deep cleansing breath. Take two slow breaths to about the 15-second mark and then accelerate breathing until the 45-second mark. Faster breathing is done either all through the nose or all through the mouth. As peak passes, decelerate breathing. End with deep cleansing breath.	Time contractions Check for relaxation Make comfortable Massage back if needed Protect concentration	Call doctor or midwife Finish packing suitcase and Lamaze bag Go to hospital or birth center Change position when needed

	PURPOSE	CONTRACTIONS	AVERAGE LENGTH	WOMAN'S MOOD
Transition	Dilation 8–10 centimeters	Contractions and rests of roughly equal duration, 60–90 seconds long. Contractions can be irregular, peaking twice or maintaining the peak for a number of seconds.	1 hour	Intense concentration Irritable Tired Loss of sense of humor
Pushing	Expulsion of the baby	Contractions become shorter and further apart. Usually return to pattern of active-labor contractions, 60 seconds long and 3–4 minutes apart	½–2 hours	Refreshed, having found second wind Intense concentration Excited Possibly irritable and confused Tired
Delivery of the Placenta	Expulsion of the placenta	Contractions continue but are brief and mild	10–30 minutes	Ecstatic! Exhausted!

BREATHING	PARTNER'S ROLE	WHAT TO DO
Patterned Breathing: Quick cleansing breath to start. Breathe through mouth, 3–4 breaths with short, staccato blow out through pursed lips as an accent. Breathing should be shallow, light, and rhythmical. Forceful blowing out with hands over nose and mouth for early urge to push. Cleansing breath to finish contraction.	Help relax between contractions Maintain her sense of perspective, assuring her it will end. Reassure, encourage Breathe together and maintain eye contact Set short-term goals, taking only one contraction at a time	Remember that this is the hardest part Change position Anything that makes you feel better
Breathing for Pushing: Deep cleansing breath to start. Take another breath in, let half of it out, then either hold breath or blow out slowly for a count of 8–10. Let out any air that is left, take another deep breath in, and repeat push as you hold breath or let out slowly. Maintain pelvic tilt and pelvic-floor relaxation.	Help with positioning so she is not flat on her back. Should sit, squat, or lie on side. Count from 1 to 10 for pushes Encourage	Push with each contraction Try different pushing positions

CHAPTER 6

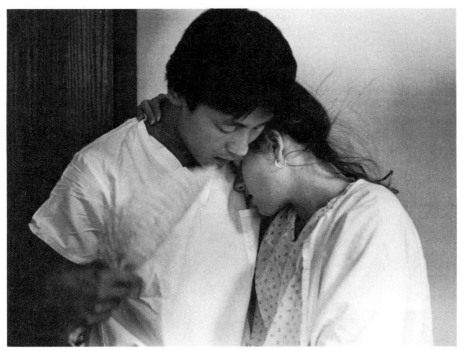

Exercise and Relaxation During Pregnancy

E xercise and relaxation may seem unrelated, but they are both physical disciplines that can improve self-awareness and body image. If practiced throughout pregnancy, both can give you an extra edge in labor. Relaxation is critical because it will permit your body to restore itself between contractions, while exercise will provide stamina.

Birth is more physical than you can imagine, and working with your body now will prepare you for the real work of labor. Before giving birth, if you can learn how to isolate muscle groups, how to breathe through strenuous activity, and how to work with physical sensations, you'll be very well prepared. We urge you to undertake the short exercise program that Diana has drawn up and to practice the relaxation techniques. We know they are good—and you may enjoy them so much that they'll become part of your postpartum routine.

EXERCISE

Ten years ago, women who exercised during pregnancy were a small minority. Doctors didn't recommend it, and women were concerned that exercise could in some way harm the baby. There were no books on the subject, and although pregnancy exercise classes were available (Diana's being one of them), they were few and far between. Most women stopped working out as soon as they realized they were pregnant and resumed only after the baby was born.

Today it's a whole new world for pregnant women who want to keep in shape. Pregnancy exercise classes are everywhere, as are books on the subject. Mothers-to-be are now concerned with not getting enough exercise, parents and peers expect them to work out, and obstetricians recommend exercise classes at the first checkup. The Lamaze movement is partially responsible for this change in attitudes because it has always recognized pregnancy as a healthy, vital state that permits normal activity. This shift has also occurred because women have spread the word about how invigorating and fun exercise regimens are and how terrific they felt after childbirth.

The Benefits of Exercise

Exercise will not shorten your labor, make it less painful, or enable you to wear your old jeans home from the hospital. It will not directly affect the amount of weight you gain, make your body thinner, or trigger labor. It will, however:

EXERCISE

"I never had a backache, I rarely was tired, I was strong, I never felt like a fat pregnant lady, I had an incredible amount of energy—and I attribute all this to my pregnancy exercise class."

♦

"Through getting in tune with my body, I got in tune with my baby. I felt so great about myself and life!"

♦

"What helped me to push was that I was in great shape and had done Kegels for nine months *religiously.* This helped me relax the sphincter muscles and surrounding ones to make way for a large baby."

♦

"Exercising throughout my pregnancy kept my physical and emotional energy up. I also felt in control of my body—although it did not look like mine when I looked in the mirror!"

♦

"I can't imagine not feeling good during pregnancy, and I think exercise has a lot to do with it. It kept me in touch with myself and gave me a wonderful time each day just to be with me and my unborn child."

♦

"I find pregnancy to be one of the hardest times during which to feel good about my body. I have aches and pains, seem to move at a snail's pace, and look enormous. Exercise not only tones my muscles but also elevates my spirits and helps to make the nine months a happy time in my life."

♦

continued

"Exercise made me feel that I was still in control of my body, that I was not getting completely out of shape. I became more aware of my breathing, and it was almost second nature for my delivery."

◆

"I enjoyed exercising with all the pregnant women because I could see others who were even fatter than I!"

- ◆ Help you feel healthier and have more energy
- ◆ Improve your circulation
- ◆ Alleviate many common complaints, such as leg cramps, lower back pain, and constipation
- ◆ Help maintain muscle tone so that you will carry the baby with more grace and return to your former shape more easily
- ◆ Teach you how to breathe and work at the same time, which will prepare you for natural childbirth
- ◆ Make you more aware of and confident about your body

It has never been scientifically proven that women with good physical fitness fare better in labor than those in poor shape, but many women who do exercise during pregnancy say that the preparation was at least as helpful as the Lamaze classes themselves. We believe an exercise regimen can only enhance your labor and delivery because fitness provides stamina for labor. This means you will hold up better during a long labor and have more energy for pushing at the end. Pain is felt more acutely if you are tired or run down, so the more stamina you have, the better you'll be able to cope. Being fit will also encourage greater comfort during birth because it will be easier to change positions during labor or to squat or stand while pushing. In many ways working out is similar to labor: It's hard work, it requires concentration, it helps if you breathe correctly, and it's not always enjoyable. But like labor, it feels wonderful when you're done.

We hope you've been exercising throughout pregnancy. If you haven't and are feeling well, you can begin today. It's not too late, and the following routine is a gentle one, geared to the last month of pregnancy. Just to be safe, check with your doctor or midwife before starting the exercises. Ask your husband to join you and you can make it part of your regular Lamaze practice. You can start with the exercises, review the breathing techniques, then wind down with the relaxation exercise at the end of this chapter. It should take about an hour, and you will feel very good when you're finished.

The Exercise Regimen

SITTING SIDE STRETCH

This exercise feels great. It also tones and stretches the waist and ribs, and helps to improve posture by strengthening the back muscles that support the spine.

To Start:
Sit tall with your spine long and straight, your shoulders relaxed and open, and your head centered on top of your spine.

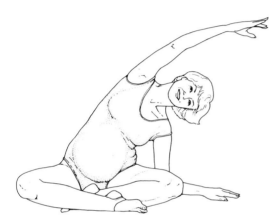

Exhale:
Stretch your right arm over your head and bend to the left. Relax your head to the side and let your left elbow drop toward the floor. Feel the stretch along your entire right side.

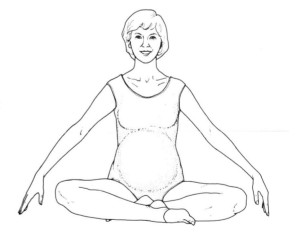

Inhale:
Try to maintain the length along your right side as you unroll to the center position.

Total:
Six times to each side, alternating sides each time.

FOOTWORK

Exercising the muscles in your legs improves the circulation. This exercise will be especially helpful if you are prone to leg cramps or if water retention is a problem.

To Start:
Sit tall with your legs straight out in front of you, hip width apart.

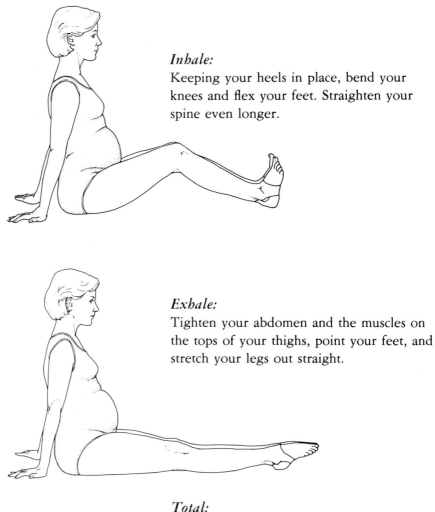

Inhale:
Keeping your heels in place, bend your knees and flex your feet. Straighten your spine even longer.

Exhale:
Tighten your abdomen and the muscles on the tops of your thighs, point your feet, and stretch your legs out straight.

Total:
Sixteen times

PELVIC TILT

This is a wonderful exercise because it strengthens the abdominal muscles while at the same time relaxing the lower back. Do it whenever your lower back feels achy or stiff.

To Start:
Lie on the floor with your knees bent, the soles of your feet on the floor about hip width apart.

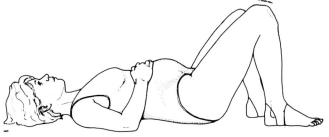

Inhale:
Allow the abdomen to rise and fill with air.

Exhale:
Tighten your abdominal muscles and think of giving your baby a hug. Feel your back flatten against the floor, your whole spine long and straight. Make sure you keep your buttocks completely relaxed.

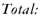

Total:
Eight times

LEG LIFTS

No exercise regimen would be complete without just a few leg lifts. The first part of this exercise works the inner thighs; the second part tones the outer thighs.

Part I:

Lie on your left side with both legs straight and your head on your bottom arm. Your body should be in one straight line.

Breathe normally throughout.

Stretch both legs even longer, then raise your right leg to hip height.

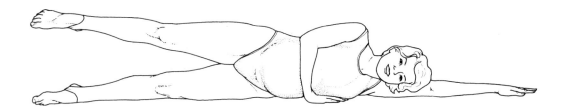

Leaving your top leg up, slowly raise and lower your left leg. This should be done in one smooth and even rhythm. Press your inner thighs together each time they meet.

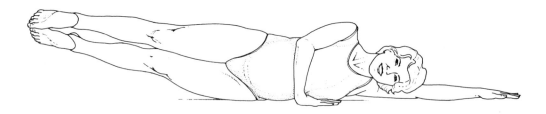

Total: ten times, then turn to your right side and repeat.

Part II:
Return to your left side and prop yourself
up on one arm. Bend your left leg, then
check to see that your body and right leg
form one straight line.

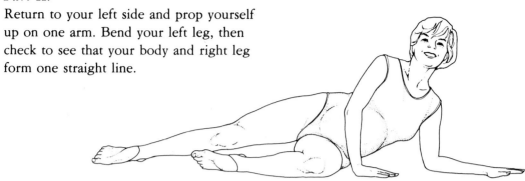

Lengthen your right leg, tighten your
buttocks, and slowly lift and lower the leg in
one smooth and even rhythm. Only lift your
leg three to five inches off the floor so that
you use your thigh muscles only and not
your hips or back.

Total: ten times, then turn to your right side
and repeat with the other leg.

UPPER-BODY CIRCLES

Tension often settles into the shoulders and upper body. Here's one way of relieving it. A warm bath and a good massage are also recommended.

To Start:
Sit tall.

Breathe normally throughout.

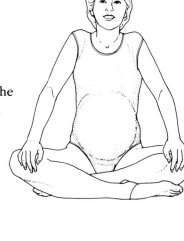

Shoulder Circles:
Circle your shoulders forward, up, all the way back and down to center. Reverse. Eight times to each direction.

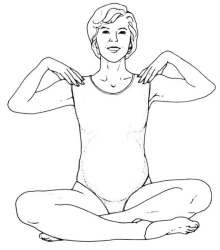

Elbow Circles:
Place your fingertips on your shoulders and circle your elbows forward, to the side, and behind you. Reverse direction. Eight times to each direction.

Head Circles:
Circle your head forward, to the side, around to the back, and to the other side. Drop your chin toward your chest and reverse direction. Four times each direction.

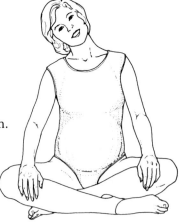

TWIST

Good posture is difficult to maintain as breast size increases. This exercise will help improve your posture, release tension in the upper back, and increase tone and flexibility in the waist and ribs.

To Start:
Sit with your legs crossed, your right hand on your left knee, your left hand by your buttocks.

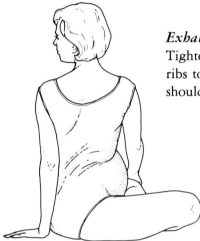

Exhale:
Tighten your belly muscles and twist your ribs to the left, looking over your left shoulder.

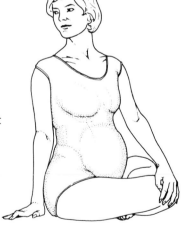

Inhale:
Change sides, your left hand on your right knee, and look over your right shoulder.

Total:
Six times to each side, alternating sides each time

BACK MASSAGE

This exercise strengthens your abdominal muscles and relaxes the ones in your lower back.

To Start:

Lie on your back with your knees bent and the soles of your feet on the floor, hip width apart.

Inhale:

Allow your abdomen to rise and fill with air.

Exhale:

Tighten and flatten your abdominal muscles and lift your hips off the floor. Do not tighten your buttocks or arch your lower back. Think of the tops of your thighs as the highest point, and your spine as a straight, diagonal line. Inhale.

Exhale:

Again, tighten your abdominal muscles and roll your spine, one vertebra at a time, back to the floor.

Total:

Six times

LEG STRETCH

This exercise stretches the hamstring muscles in the backs of your legs and helps you practice conscious breathing with the discomfort of a stretch. Never bounce or force yourself to go lower. Use your breathing and just think of lengthening your spine over your leg, not down to your knee.

To Start:
Sit with one leg straight in front of you and the other knee bent, foot to the inside of your other thigh. Relax your body over your straight leg.

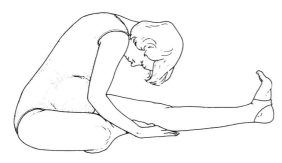

Inhale:
Slowly flex your extended foot. Feel the stretch along the back of your leg and along your spine, but keep your head and shoulders relaxed.

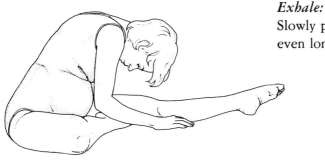

Exhale:
Slowly point your foot. Stretch your spine even longer over your leg.

Total:
Six times, then repeat to the other side

THE CAT

This exercise increases flexibility in the muscles along the spine and is wonderful for a tight or achy lower back.

To Start:
Support your weight on your hands and knees—hands directly under your shoulders, knees slightly apart and directly under your hips.

Exhale:
Tighten your abdominal muscles, do a pelvic tilt, and round your spine. Let your head relax and your chin drop to your chest.

Inhale:
Stretch your hips to your heels.

Exhale:
Return to the hands-and-knees position, the spine still rounded.

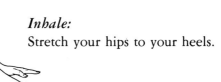

Inhale:

Slowly straighten the spine, feeling your back
lengthen as you stretch. Keep your belly
muscles working to support the baby, so that
your back doesn't arch.

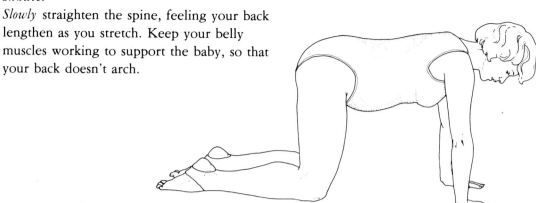

Total:

Six times

THE KEGEL EXERCISES

If you're only going to do one exercise while pregnant, let it be your Kegels. Named after a pioneering California doctor, Arnold Kegel, these simple exercises will increase sexual pleasure and help you recover from childbirth more quickly. If you've never done Kegels before, start now.

The Kegel exercises strengthen the pelvic floor muscle, which runs from the pubic bone to the coccyx and wraps in a figure eight around the urethra, the vagina and anus. This muscle can be thought of as a hammock, supporting the pelvic organs: rectum, vagina, uterus, and bladder. Good tone of the pelvic floor prevents urinary incontinence, strengthens orgasms, and maintains good support for the pelvic organs. And because healthy tissue is more elastic, it may prevent the need for an episiotomy.

During pregnancy, the baby's weight causes the pelvic floor to stretch and weaken (like a sagging hammock with an extra person in it). Years ago, urinary incontinence, uterine prolapse, and diminished sexual pleasure were considered the unavoidable results of childbearing. Today we know this isn't true, because the pelvic floor can retain strength and elasticity with a little exercise, just like any other muscle.

To work the pelvic floor muscle, try to stop and start the flow of urine as you sit on the toilet. It will be difficult to do this at first, but with practice, your skill will improve. You can also perform Kegels while making love, and both of you will be able to feel the pelvic floor muscle squeezing the penis.

Try to do the Kegels in groups of five, working up to about twenty groups a day. Even doing one hundred won't take more than ten minutes. Kegels are great because they can be done anywhere at any time; simply reminding yourself to do them is half the battle. The best way to remember is to condition yourself to perform them while you are doing some other activity, such as waiting for a traffic light, talking on the phone, or waiting on line.

Kegels are the single most important exercise you can perform during pregnancy and throughout your life.

The Benefits of Good Posture

Posture is always a matter of good health. Correct body alignment is important at all times in a woman's life, but particularly during pregnancy, when a constantly shifting center of gravity and added (but unequally distributed) weight can create lower-back ache, neck tension, and fatigue. If you want to look and feel well, improving and maintaining good postural habits is essential.

During pregnancy, the most common postural mistake is allowing the belly to relax forward while leaning back with the shoulders as a counterbalance. The result is weakened abdominal muscles and lordosis, an exaggerated curve of the lower spine. To correct this tendency, try to lengthen your spine and balance your head and shoulders over, not behind, your hips.

Good posture is achieved by strengthening the muscles that support the skeleton in alignment, not by tightening muscles here and there to make you look "straight." Proper posture doesn't mean walking like a pregnant soldier or being frozen in one position. Proper posture permits you to move like a dancer, with ease and grace.

Even if you've always had bad posture, you can correct it while pregnant. This is an excellent time to work on poor habits because improvements will be almost immediately apparent. Women commonly experience heightened body awareness during pregnancy, and this sensitivity makes it easier to remedy postural problems.

Here are three easy visualization exercises to help you improve your posture, concentrating on different areas of your body. At first, do them standing in front of a mirror so you'll be able to see as well as feel the changes. Then, once the exercises become familiar, practice them as often as you can, anywhere or anytime.

1. Stand tall and visualize the length of your spine, from your tailbone up to the top of your neck. Imagine your head as the last pearl on a string and each vertebra of your spine as one pearl on the strand. Concentrate on letting the pearls hang in one straight line.
2. Tighten your lower belly muscles and give your baby a hug. Allow your pelvis to tilt forward slightly, keeping your buttocks and knees completely relaxed. Imagine your tailbone directly between (not behind) your legs.
3. Shrug your shoulders up toward your ears as if you were a puppet and someone were pulling up the shoulder strings. Now imagine the strings being gently released and allow your shoulders to drop slowly. Feel your skull resting on top of the uppermost vertebra. Allow your neck to feel long and your chest and upper back to open.

RELAXATION

Most people acknowledge the fact that stress can have negative effects on physical well-being. The reverse, that relaxation can have positive effects, is equally true, though not as widely accepted. If stress can raise one's blood pressure, then relaxation can lower it; if stress can increase the pace of respiration, then relaxation can slow it down; if stress can upset the chemical balance within us, then relaxation can restore the balance. It seems to us that American culture in general resists the notion of relaxation as an important skill—perhaps because it's not an active pursuit or one with effects that can be measured. We look forward to the day when a housewife does not feel guilty requesting a few moments of peace and when an executive can sit at her desk with her eyes closed and not be considered strange.

The following relaxation techniques will be extremely helpful for you and your partner during pregnancy and labor, but please don't assume that once your baby is born, relaxation has served its purpose. Relaxation is a skill that will come in handy at other times as well, such as before a big presentation, driving in traffic, or not being able to get to sleep at night after an exhausting day. Both you and your husband will find it a useful tool. Continue to practice relaxation, both in times of stress and in times of peace. The applications are almost limitless.

Relaxation is a learned art, not an inherited talent. The ability to relax can be acquired with patience and practice, just like any other skill. Do not become discouraged if you find it difficult, for it is hard in the beginning. But the more you do it, the easier it gets, the better you are at it, and the more you will enjoy the feeling.

Included here are three different relaxation techniques: the progressive relaxation, the full relaxation, and the neuromuscular relaxation. Each exercise approaches the ability to relax from a slightly different angle, and each one will be helpful in its own way. The *progressive relaxation* is like an introduction. It is an easy way to discover how to release tension from the body and requires the least amount of assistance and knowledge from your partner. The *full relaxation* is more loosely structured and allows for greater imagination and creativity. It also enables you to experience a much deeper level of relaxation. It is based on relaxation through suggestion, and you will discover images or thoughts that will help you cope with your labor. The last technique, *neuromuscular relaxation,* is an active one, in which you learn to keep your body relaxed

RELAXATION

♦

"The Lamaze breathing was helpful, but what really worked for me was the image of the wave rising and falling."

♦

"I walked up and down the hall for almost the entire labor. When a contraction came, I would stop, hold on to my husband, and do the slow controlled breathing. I kept a mental image of how my muscles were working. I tried to stay relaxed and to let them do what they were supposed to do."

♦

"It was a very easy and fast labor. As long as I relaxed and stayed calm, it was fine, but if I even tensed my toes, the pain seemed to multiply."

♦

"I tried to relax my body completely and let the contractions simply wash over me—almost as if I could leave my body temporarily."

♦

"I think the only way I was able to deal with twelve hours of back labor was by relaxing completely during contractions. At first, I was startled and angry at the pain, but once I was able to really relax, it was not difficult. Between contractions I tried to make my body go completely limp and worked on removing any tension in my fingers and toes. I seemed almost unconscious. My doctor and all the nurses complimented me for adjusting so beautifully to a difficult labor."

even though one part is in a state of contraction. Obviously, this is the exercise that most directly relates to labor. Once you have mastered the progressive relaxation and established a number of images that help you to relax, this last exercise will be quite easy and fun to practice. You will truly feel prepared.

You can often squeeze in a few minutes between chores to practice a breathing pattern, but it is not a good idea to hurry through a relaxation. Though each technique takes only ten to fifteen minutes, you should set aside time when you and your partner are calm and when you won't feel rushed. The room should be comfortably warm and well ventilated, your clothes should be loose and unconfining, and your body should be well supported by pillows.

By practicing these techniques with your partner, you both learn what the feeling of relaxation is. You also learn about each other—where tensions are held, which strokes feel good, which words or images help deepen the feeling of letting go. You will also learn which touches and words to avoid, and this is equally important. You will become more sensitive to each other and you will learn to trust and appreciate each other in a different way. Without even being aware of it, you will condition yourself to relax to the sound of your partner's voice and the feel of his touch.

If your partner positively has neither the time nor the inclination to practice with you, you can do them by yourself or with a friend. It's preferable to have your partner involved, but it's not essential.

The Progressive Relaxation

This technique for relaxation is a very simple one. All you do is tense and then release each part of your body, one part at a time, slowly and thoughtfully. You can more easily sense the feeling of relaxation by first contracting muscles and then letting them go. By doing this exercise you will learn to be aware of each separate muscle group and to be able to distinguish between when these muscles are tensed and when they are relaxed.

Have your partner talk you through this tension/relaxation exercise. Then switch places and let him try it. You can practice this relaxation before rehearsing your breathing patterns or at another time altogether. After a week or two, you will be able to practice this technique by yourself (especially at night if you have trouble falling asleep). Time with your partner is limited, we know, so once this exercise is familiar, use your time together to concentrate on the neuromuscular and the full visualization relaxation techniques instead.

Begin by settling yourself comfortably in a semireclining position on your bed or couch. Arrange the pillows so that every limb is supported and there is no part of your body you have to hold up yourself. Have your partner read the following suggestions one at a time and check to see that you are complying. His voice should be calm and soothing, and he should give you enough time both to contract and to completely relax each muscle group. Encourage your partner to divide it into even smaller muscle groups if he likes and to feel free to use other images that come to mind.

Contract each body part for five or six seconds before releasing it. You will find that you will naturally want to hold your breath as you tighten each set of muscles, and you will begin to understand why the Lamaze method uses conscious breathing techniques. Try to breathe slowly and deeply all through this exercise—either your slow chest breathing or just your usual rhythm. Have your partner remind you to breath should you forget.

THE PROGRESSIVE RELAXATION EXERCISE
Take a deep cleansing breath in and let it out with a deep sigh. Close your eyes, take another deep sigh and breathe in and out, allowing yourself to exhale all your tensions with the breath. Let yourself fall into the pillows beneath you.

1. Tense your feet. Press your heels forward and spread your toes apart. Feel the muscular tension in the very tops of your feet.
   Now relax your feet. Let your toes hang loosely from your feet and let your feet hang from your ankles.
2. Tighten the muscles in your legs. Squeeze your inner thighs together and tighten the muscles on the tops of your thighs and around your knees. Breathe, even though there is tension in your legs.
   Slowly relax your legs completely and feel the tightness melt away. Allow your legs to open naturally and to be completely supported by the bed or floor.
3. Contract your pelvic floor muscles. Squeeze tightly as if you have to urinate desperately but the bathroom is occupied. Feel the pelvic hammock lift between your legs.
   Now relax these muscles completely as if to allow yourself the luxury of urinating.
4. Squeeze your buttocks tightly together and tense your abdomen as well. Feel the tension in your lower back and how difficult it is to keep breathing when you are working so hard. Tighten even a little bit more.

Slowly release your buttocks and belly completely and take a deep cleansing breath to help you relax even more.

5. Tighten the muscles in your chest. Feel how this stops your breathing.

    Relax these muscles and let the air escape. Allow your breathing to resume and sense your breastbone freely rising and falling with each breath.

6. Shrug your shoulders up to your ears as if you could wear them like earrings.

    Slowly let them fall back down to your collarbone, like sand smoothing out with a receding wave. Let them feel quite heavy.

7. Stiffen your arms like the sleeves of a wet blouse left outside on an icy day. Clench your fingers into tight fists.

    In your mind, bring the blouse indoors. Feel your arms soften to the warmth of the imaginary room and unfurl your fingers. Notice in passing how your fingers will remain slightly bent even when relaxed.

8. Lastly, tighten all the muscles in your face and neck. Pretend you are eating something very sour, like a lemon drop or a very sour pickle. Wrinkle your face in protest. Squeeze your eyes closed and deepen the lines in your forehead.

    Allow all tension to drain from your face and feel relief pass over it as if you just heard very good news. Let all the small muscles around your eyes relax and let your lower jaw hang loosely from your upper jaw. Smooth out all the wrinkles in your forehead and let your face grow smooth, calm, and free of expression.

Take a deep breath in, and let it out with a slow sigh. Feel your whole body relaxed and at peace.

The Full Relaxation

Saying to yourself or being told to "Just relax" is usually the very phrase that will make you tense. Contracting and then releasing muscles using the progressive relaxation just described is one helpful method to achieve muscular release. Another technique is to use specific mental images for relaxation. This is called visualization, guided relaxation, or relaxation through imagery. This technique is used for behavior modification, healing, and stress reduction through biofeedback. The premise is that the mind and body are integrated, one affecting the other in an on-going process.

Animals can respond only to a concrete sound or action—to the tone of a voice, the ringing of a bell, or the reward of a pat on the head or food in the dish. We, however, can respond to the abstract as well. The mere idea of something can create a physical response. Imagine you are eating a very sour lemon. Notice how saliva begins to form and how you can feel the tartness in the corners of your mouth. Or say to someone, "I'm going to give you an injection now," and instantly his breathing quickens, perspiration increases, and his heart begins to pound.

What visualization does is to use this ability physiologically to respond to an idea in a positive way. Now close your eyes and imagine yourself on a beautiful beach on a warm day. Feel the sand sift through your fingers, smell the fresh air, and listen to the rhythm of the waves lapping at the shore. Do you feel how your body responds without your having to think about "relaxing"?

Practicing this full relaxation is not a matter of becoming limp and going into a "trance." Nor is it a prelude to hypnosis. Rather, it is an opportunity to focus inwardly and to take the time to let the mind and body be one. We so often feel one way but act another, do one thing but think about something totally unrelated. We try to look interested even if we are bored, feign disinterest while keeping alert; we fold the laundry while thinking about what to make for dinner. The time spent doing the following full relaxation is simply a time to focus your thoughts and to do nothing—except allow yourself to relax. You can do this visualization yourself, but it's preferable to have the assistance of your partner.

Again begin by settling yourself comfortably on your bed, chair, or floor. You can be semireclining with pillows supporting your head, arms, and knees, or you can lie on your left side, with pillows between your knees or supporting your top leg. You and your partner should alternate guiding each other through this relaxation. Speak slowly and allow time for the images to be experienced. The relaxation can take ten minutes or it can take half an hour or more, depending on time and inclination. Images not mentioned here will occur to you or your husband as you speak, and you should feel free to incorporate them. Unspoken images will come to you as you relax, as well. This is fine. In fact, no two relaxations will ever be exactly the same. After each relaxation, discuss with your partner which images you liked the most. In the beginning you can use the images we've listed here. After a few days or weeks both of you will have developed your own repertoire, and you will be able to put this book aside and explore your own suggestions.

THE VISUALIZATION EXERCISE

Take a slow, deep breath in, then slowly let it go. Take another deep breath in, and this time feel your chest fill with air. Now slowly release the breath and allow your body to settle down even more comfortably onto the bed or floor underneath you. If you need to change your position, go right ahead. Often, changing the placement of your arms or legs will help you to relax even more. Sometimes, even noises around you can help you rather than distract you.

Concentrate your attention on your breathing and become aware of the rhythm of your inhalations and exhalations. Feel the breath deeply on the inside of your body. You can feel the rising and falling of your chest as you breathe in and out, and you can imagine your lungs deep inside your ribcage inflating and deflating like balloons. Now take another deep breath in, and this time as you exhale, see if you can release all tensions from your body out with the air. Breathe out all the tensions from your body, and from your mind, with your exhalation. . . . Let your legs relax heavily onto the floor or bed, let your head be supported by the pillows beneath it, and allow your shoulders to drop as all your cares melt away. You might even feel the bed or floor come up to support you firmly, allowing you to let go even more.

As you breathe, you will feel your chest rising and falling, like the waves at the ocean. The steady, ongoing rhythm of the inhalation and exhalation continues without your even having to think about it. It doesn't matter whether your breathing is slow or fast, deep or shallow. Just let it be. As you breathe in, you take the oxygen you need and release the carbon dioxide and other waste products you don't need. Breathe in what you need . . . release what you don't. Feel the amazing elasticity of your skin, expanding with each breath and then relaxing back with each exhalation.

During pregnancy, the hormone called relaxin causes the muscles and ligaments of the body to soften even more than usual, so that you may be aware of an even greater flexibility in your body right now and of your body's ability to make greater adjustments than at other times in your life. As you breathe, you might begin to be aware of your abdomen rising and falling along with your chest and to feel how your entire body responds to your breathing.

If you like, you might pretend that your body is like a bag of sand. The seams run along the sides of your body, the soles of your feet, in the back of your neck, down your spine, and anywhere else you would like to put them. But these seams are only loosely sewn, and each time you exhale, sand escapes out through these seams, and each time you inhale, air replaces the sand that you've lost. Exhale out the sand, and replace it with the air you inhale, until all the sand is gone, and your body feels light and full of air. [Pause to allow time for this image to be experienced.]

Imagine yourself in a favorite place. It can be the beach on a Caribbean island, a raft in a swimming pool with a cool drink in your hand, a warm bubble bath, a walk in a pine forest, or a cozy room with a fireplace on a cold winter's day. Smell the smells of your surroundings and hear the sounds. If you are at the seashore, you might hear the sound of the waves and the cries of the seagulls. You might feel the warmth of the sun and the coolness of the breeze and the texture of the sand sifting between your fingers. Perhaps you will smile as you enjoy the calm and peace of this place in your mind.

Now let just a color remain. It may be the blue of the sky, the whiteness of the sand, or perhaps no color at all. Allow the color to become the color of a very deep and plush carpet. Imagine yourself at the very top of a long staircase. As you walk down the stairs, you find that the carpet becomes deeper and softer. Step down to the first step and feel how yielding it is beneath your feet. Perhaps you are barefoot or perhaps you are wearing a pair of slippers. Now take your second step, and a third step, and at each step down the staircase you can feel yourself becoming even more deeply relaxed. Continue down the staircase, and now at the very bottom you are more relaxed than you have ever been before.

The relaxation is almost over now, but know that at any time you can return to this feeling of very deep calm. By closing your eyes and letting your thoughts wander to the images of the past few minutes, you can return to this feeling of total relaxation. Take a slow and deep breath in and allow yourself to feel the floor or bed beneath you, and to become aware of the room around you. Take another deep breath and feel the energy return to your arms and legs, along with a feeling of being refreshed and relaxed. On this last breath, slowly allow your eyes to open and return your thoughts to the here and now. Stretch your arms and legs, and very slowly come up to the sitting position.

The Neuromuscular Relaxation

The progressive relaxation introduced you to the feeling of muscular release; the visualization relaxation deepened these sensations and identified a number of mental images to help you. This third technique takes the relaxation one step further, teaching you how purposefully to tense one body part while consciously relaxing the rest of your body. Because the uterus will be contracting during labor while you try to maintain your mental and muscular relaxation, this exercise most directly relates to the skills you will need once labor begins. It is one thing to be able to relax while comfortably settled in bed thinking about warm beaches and cool breezes. It's another to maintain the relaxation while part of you is in pain.

Normally, pain is a message from your body to do something—remove your hand from the flame, take out the splinter, or fix a tooth. Ordinarily it is a stimulus telling us something is wrong. We tense our body instantly in preparation for action—a necessary and healthy response. Pain in labor, however, is an exception, the one time when pain is not a signal of distress and when muscular tension is an unhelpful response rather than a helpful one. If you contract your whole body each time a uterine contraction occurs, you will exhaust yourself after only a very short time. Only by letting the uterus work freely and actively by itself will you be able to free the cervix to open while at the same time conserving energy throughout the rest of your body.

The neuromuscular exercise is not exactly comparable to childbirth, for your partner will not be asking you to tense your arms or legs during labor. But it is valuable preparation nonetheless because you are conditioning yourself to relax your body in response to a muscular contraction (an arm or a leg now, the uterus later). In this exercise, your partner will ask you to contract an arm or leg and you will tighten that limb and relax the rest of your body at the same time. He will check your overall relaxation before telling you to release the tensed limb, and he will stroke it, a tactile aid to relaxation. You will learn to isolate and control separate muscle groups so that during labor one group can work while the others rest. You will also be conditioning yourself to let go of all muscular tension to the words *contract* and *relax,* to the sound of your partner's voice, and to the feel of his stroke on your body.

You will find that in the beginning it will be difficult to only contract one body part at a time. Your breathing will stop and your other limbs will want to tense also. You will understand why it is important to practice now to establish a new response and how your experiences from the previous relaxation exercises will help you.

The best position for practicing is one in which you are semireclining. Sit up in bed or on your couch with your legs at hip height. Prop pillows behind your head and shoulders and underneath your knees. Never put a pillow into the small of your back for support—it only increases the arch. Instead, add a second pillow under your knees.

This exercise really can't be done alone; you'll need your partner or a friend to help you. Have your partner read the following instructions and respond as best you can. When the exercise is completed, change places and have him be the one to try to stay relaxed. Besides being a helpful skill to know, it may also make him a more sympathetic partner.

THE NEUROMUSCULAR EXERCISE

1. To begin, relax your body completely. Allow your limbs to be heavy, totally relaxed, and easily manipulated. Breathe deeply and slowly and focus on a mental image from the full relaxation to help you let go even more.

   Partner: Check each of your wife's limbs to see that it is completely relaxed. If you pick up her arm at the wrist, it should feel very heavy. Feel how easily the elbow bends and how you can even swing the arm gently and easily in the shoulder socket. If you place the elbow on the floor and let go, her hand should drop to the floor with no resistance. Now check her other arm, then make sure her legs are relaxed. Put one hand under her knee and the other under her heel. Check to see if her leg feels heavy and if you can easily bend her knee (but keep her heel on the floor). Stroke your hand along the inside and outside of her thigh and help her to relax to your touch. Then check her other leg. Use a soothing tone of voice, and reassure her that she need not help you to lift her arm or leg. Be patient. It will take time before she can trust you to gently manipulate her arms and legs while keeping them relaxed.

2. Contract your right arm.

   Partner: Your wife should stiffen her right arm and hold it straight out, inches off the floor. Remind her to breathe and give her a moment to relax the rest of her body. Now check to make sure her legs and left arm remain relaxed. If she finds this difficult, remind her she is only just beginning to learn and that very few people do this perfectly the first few times.

3. Relax your right arm.

Partner: Stroke her arm as she relaxes it completely. Make sure all muscular tension is gone.

4. Contract your left leg.

Partner: Your wife should flex her foot, toes to the ceiling, and tighten the muscles in her thigh. She should not try to lift her leg off the floor or bed. Make sure her left leg is completely stiff. Now check her right leg and both arms to see if they are still relaxed, and make sure she is not holding her breath.

5. Relax your left leg.

Partner: Stroke her leg from her thigh all the way down to her toes and see if you can bend her leg easily at the hip and knee joints. Tell her what a great job she is doing.

6. Contract your right arm and right leg.

Partner: This is more difficult, so give her a moment to figure out which is right and which is left and to relax her left arm and leg completely. Check her right side to see if these are contracted, then check her left arm and leg to see if these limbs are relaxed.

7. Relax your right arm and leg.

Partner: Stroke first her arm and then her leg and check to see that she has released all muscular tension.

8. Practice this tension/release exercise with both arms contracted, then with both legs; with the right arm and leg contracted, and then with the left arm and leg tensed. For the greatest degree of difficulty, have her contract opposite arms and legs. Finish each practice session with a cleansing breath and with her whole body completely relaxed.

THE LAMAZE RELAXATION CHART

	PURPOSE	HOW TO PRACTICE	PARTNER'S ROLE
Progressive Relaxation	Easy way to release tension from body and learn to tell when muscles are tense or relaxed. During labor, relaxing between contractions allows the body to replenish and sustain itself.	Tense and release each part of your body, one section at a time, starting with your toes and ending with the muscles of your head and neck.	Verbal instructions and image suggestions. Reminders to keep breathing slowly and deeply.

Full Relaxation	Deeper level of relaxation through imagery; allows for greater creativity and visualization. During labor, this technique will promote relaxation and the inward focusing of attention by means of suggestion and imagery.	Assume a comfortable position and use mental imagery, such as waves, a beach scene, a bubble bath, a certain color or texture, to promote deeper relaxation.	Verbal exchange of relaxation images.
Neuromuscular Relaxation	Learning to keep your body relaxed even though one part is in a state of contraction. During labor, you will need to keep your mind and body (particularly the pelvic floor) relaxed, even though the uterus will be working hard.	Alternately tense and release different limbs while keeping the rest of your body relaxed. Start with an arm or leg and work up to various combinations (both arms, both legs, right arm and leg, and so on).	Verbal instructions and encouragement; stroking, checking for full relaxation of limbs.

CHAPTER 7

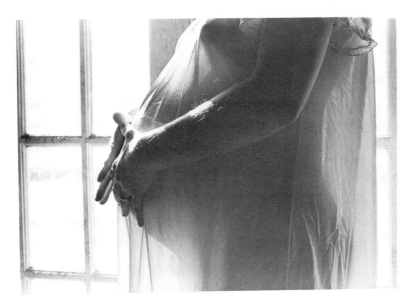

The Last Month

*T*he last month of pregnancy is not the best—you're swollen and tired of feeling fat, but not sure you're really ready to be a mother. You may be having difficulty sleeping because of your size, the baby's activity, leg cramps, and the constant need to go to the bathroom. The ninth month is when many women lose their good humor about being pregnant and when the anxiety about having a healthy baby reaches a peak. If you're late—and more than 40 percent of first-time mothers are— many of these feelings are intensified. If this is your second or third child, you will be worried about the effect the new baby is going to have on your family life.

If you haven't already been driven crazy during your pregnancy by people telling you what to do, it will surely happen in these final weeks. Some will advise you to buy your entire layette now. Others will instruct you to prepare and freeze lots of nourishing meals so you won't have to cook later. If you are working, many people will tell you to stop immediately. If you have already stopped, at least one person will ask when you're going back, even though you've only been home three days. This also seems to be the most likely time to hear horror stories about fifty-hour labors and emergency cesarean sections.

The last month can be trying, but fortunately, all this ends when labor begins. Be patient, remind yourself that pregnancy does not last forever, and do what pleases you most. In our opinion, this final month is a perfect time for ignoring most of that well-intentioned advice and, if you feel well enough, for you and your husband to have fun—go to the movies, out to dinner, visit friends, in short, many of the things you won't be as inclined to do as parents of an infant.

As we've said before, a good doctor or midwife is essential for a good birth experience. But if you're exhausted, even the most skillful practitioner can't help you find the energy to make it through a long labor. If you go to the hospital worn out from unpacking boxes in your new apartment or from completing one more project at work, all your childbirth preparation will be for naught. You must be as well rested as possible to maximize your chances of having natural childbirth.

IF YOU WORK

It is difficult to strike a balance between pregnancy and the demands of a job. How long to work is a favorite topic of self-appointed pregnancy experts. Some will warn you not to work beyond your fifth month, while others will counsel you to stay on the job until your water breaks. Your pregnancy may make your co-workers uncomfortable, so their opinions are not always in your best interest. And in the words of one of our friends, "They treat you like a bomb that is about to explode." The decision about how long to continue working is between you and your doctor or midwife; you shouldn't let yourself be pressured by anyone else.

There are lots of considerations to weigh when deciding how long to remain at work. Professional women commonly underestimate their

THE LAST MONTH

♦

"It's an extremely difficult time emotionally. There's a good deal of soul-searching."

♦

"I did a lot of nesting—getting everything cleaned and organized in the apartment."

♦

"There's greater anxiety about the pain of labor now, but I feel my mind is open. I can't wait for the arrival of the baby."

♦

"It's been the best month of all because I've learned so much, feel the best I've felt since the pregnancy began, and finally feel comfortable and knowledgeable about my pregnancy. Everything is in place at home, and we are looking forward to the baby."

♦

"The whole process of being pregnant seems to be one of physical and emotional realization that there really is a baby in there. And in the last month, I find myself learning that I must focus on the baby as a separate being who will no longer be a part of me."

♦

"Even though I've only been in the last month of pregnancy for two days, it seems like the longest month."

♦

"For the first time I started feeling uncomfortable and bulky."

♦

continued

"The ninth month becomes a contest of patience. No more sleep, no more peace. It's such a countdown, but you're really ready."

♦

"As they say, the ninth month is a trimester unto itself. Hungrier, heavier, slower than I ever imagined myself to be. All my funny symptoms showed up—swollen feet, tingling hands, quirky appetite and fatigue. The afternoon nap became a necessity."

♦

"I'm looking forward to the birth while at the same time fearing it. Anxious about the baby's health, and so forth, and need lots of support."

need for some time off before giving birth. The transition to motherhood can be more difficult for these women, because in addition to adjusting to the baby, they must also suddenly get used to being home. We think you should plan to leave work at least two or three weeks before your due date so that you can rest and prepare yourself and your home for the baby. If this is absolutely impossible, at least consider working part-time in the final weeks. Perhaps you could work at home instead of going to your office every day, or modify your schedule so that you don't have to commute during the rush hours.

In determining when to leave your job, the most important factor should be your health. If you are well and your work is not exhausting (every woman is tired during the last trimester), you could stay until your ninth month if you want. A critical consideration should be the effect of your commute. If you have to stand on a packed bus or drive more than an hour, you shouldn't continue this grueling pace until the very end if you don't have to. ·

Women are just as competent as men and we should be able to do anything we want, but there are differences between the two sexes, and being nine months pregnant is one of them. When you are pregnant, your body is working hard, and everything is exaggerated—you're sleepier, hungrier, warmer, queasier, heavier, and you worry more. The vast majority of women experience these changes, and it's pointless to deny them. It's regrettable that the current superwoman movement makes pregnant women feel guilty if they don't work until the first contraction.

Midwife Elizabeth Davis has observed that women who work until they deliver almost always have overdue babies. In her book, *A Guide to Midwifery*, she says, "An invariable part of preparing for parenting is surrendering to the pregnancy and experiencing it with enjoyment. If a woman has worked all along, she will take a couple of weeks to get ready regardless of due date." Women frequently claim they'll be bored if they don't work until the last minute, but by clinging to their jobs they may be trying to avoid the scary and inevitable change to motherhood. Perhaps you feel reluctant to surrender your work identity, even for a short time, or you may be afraid the office will self-destruct without you, but try to keep your priorities in place. Having a healthy baby should be your most important task right now.

If You're Not Working Outside Your Home

If you are pregnant with your first child and are at home, you are in an ideal position to stay rested and fit. Don't let yourself feel pressured to keep busy. Set aside leisure time and take advantage of it. Things will never be like this again.

If you are not employed but do have other children, you do have a full-time job; it just doesn't pay anything. You need to slow down during this last month, too, but it may be difficult. In some ways it is still more socially acceptable to say, "I had a hard day at the office, leave me alone," than to state, "I'm exhausted, I need some time for myself." You deserve special consideration even if you aren't bringing home a paycheck. You are tired, you are pregnant, and you need your rest.

TASKS FOR THE LAST WEEKS

This can be a perfect time to do many of the things you won't have time for once your baby is born—reading, shopping, cooking, seeing friends,

CHOOSING A PEDIATRICIAN

◆

Right now is the time to choose your child's pediatrician. Although you may be tired, in a month or so you'll be lugging around a bigger baby, a stroller, and a bulging diaper bag, and even the smallest outing will seem like an enormous affair. It's reassuring to begin labor knowing you have already selected your baby's doctor, and should your infant need special attention after birth, you'll be able to call on someone you already know and trust.

Before the interview, try to determine what kind of doctor you would like. Is it someone who will tell you what to do, or someone who will give you the choices and let you decide? A doctor whose only concern is the baby, or someone who views the family as a unit?

Getting recommendations should be easy. You can start with your obstetrician or midwife and then ask your family doctor, your friends with children, or your Lamaze teacher. The pediatrician does not have to be affiliated with the hospital where you deliver. Some hospitals will extend privileges to allow your pediatrician to perform the newborn exam. If not, the staff pediatrician will care for your baby, and your doctor can see you and your newborn in his office later.

We suggest you screen prospective pediatricians by going to the office for an informal chat. This meeting should give you a fairly good idea of whether you can work together.

To help you evaluate the doctor, we've composed twelve questions concerning different areas of pediatric practice. Many doctors give a standard talk to new parents regarding child rearing, feeding, discipline, and office procedures. This will answer some of your questions and give you a sense of the doctor's personality. Ideally, your child's doctor should be someone who can sympathize with the normal anxieties of caring for a new baby and who says, in effect, "I'm here to help you."

THE PEDIATRICIAN'S QUESTIONNAIRE

1. **What is the doctor's hospital affiliation?**

It's very important that a doctor be affiliated with a good hospital, or else have arrangements to connect you with one with special facilities. For day-to-day concerns your

continued

local pediatrician may be fine, but if your child becomes seriously ill, you may want a doctor affiliated with a top hospital noted for its pediatric care.

2. Is this a solo or a group practice?

The solo pediatrician is becoming extinct. There are many different group arrangements, however, and sometimes your baby can see the same doctor for every visit, even though it's a group practice.

3. What are the office hours?

See if there are evening or weekend office hours, which are helpful for working parents and for emergencies.

4. Will the doctor make house calls?

5. What is the fee schedule?

6. How do you like the office?

You'll want a location that isn't too far away and that has convenient parking. Check also to see if you like the atmosphere of the waiting room and of the doctor's office. See if there are toys and books available and if the waiting room is childproofed.

7. Are special provisions made for sick children?

Sometimes sick children are segregated in the waiting room or are asked to come in through a separate entrance. A special location or special hours for normal checkups is ideal.

8. How are phone calls handled?

Find out if the doctor has a special call-in time each day, and if not, how phone calls are handled. Are there nurses who can answer common questions over the phone?

9. How long do office visits usually last?

You do not want to be whisked in and out of the office in five minutes, nor see the doctor for two minutes and then the nurses for twenty. Nor do you want to wait for hours with a small child before seeing the doctor. If the waiting room is generally crowded, it could mean that appointments are not being handled efficiently—although one child with a medical emergency can throw off the most careful scheduling.

continued

10. What is the doctor's philosophy?

You will want to be in agreement on such topics as child rearing, breast-feeding, discipline, working mothers, and the like. Find out the doctor's attitude on scheduled-versus-demand feedings, when to introduce solid foods, and other points you care about. If you are a vegetarian and your doctor thinks this constitutes child abuse, keep looking. If you want to nurse and the doctor is a mother herself, ask if she breast-fed her baby.

11. Is the doctor willing to talk about behavioral and social issues as well as medical ones?

Caring for a baby is more than just keeping him healthy, and an experienced doctor should be able to talk with you about the whole context of child rearing.

12. Are you comfortable with this doctor?

If you can discuss things freely, if he or she really seems to enjoy children, if you feel at ease and are not afraid to call the doctor with your questions—even in the middle of the night—these are good signs. You need a doctor whose presence is reassuring, whose attitude is not scary or abrasive to you, and whom you can trust.

sleeping, or enjoying hobbies. One important thing you should do before the baby arrives is find a pediatrician.

Now is also the optimum time to hire household help for the postpartum period if you can afford it. This is another instance in which the superwoman image conflicts with reality. Most women truly believe they'll have plenty of time for cleaning, cooking, running errands, sending birth announcements and thank-you notes, and showing off the baby, who will be blissfully sleeping all the while.

We've never heard anyone say that taking care of a new baby is easy. In fact, most women say it's the hardest job they've ever had. Once the baby arrives, you'll be grateful for any help you receive, even if it's only a teenager who will dust or wash dishes for a few dollars an hour. Almost every woman who filled out our questionnaire expressed gratitude for the help she received after giving birth. The few women who did not have any assistance at all complained more about fatigue and were generally less enthusiastic about this time of their lives.

If we still haven't convinced you to take it easy before giving birth, consider that you are doing this for the good of your child. The last trimester of pregnancy is the time babies gain most of their weight, and it's essential that you have the energy to prepare and enjoy meals. Even if your husband makes you a beautiful dinner, you're not going to feel like eating it if you're exhausted.

Nesting

During the ninth month, you'll probably hear some jokes about the nesting syndrome, which is the preparation couples make to prepare their home (nest) for the baby. This is a basic, practical urge, but it can be carried to comic extremes. Men and women usually express this instinct differently and with varying intensity. Your husband, for example, may finally get around to building those bookshelves in the den, while you may become preoccupied with the neatness of your hall closet. Often this behavior peaks just prior to labor with a sudden desire to scrub the bathroom tile or buy out the baby department.

Whatever strange ideas you have about cleanliness and order, keep in mind two things: (a) Babies don't know or care if their room is ready or not; and (b) your number-one priority right now should be to stay well rested and ready for labor. There's no point in sanding woodwork if that means you'll be too tired to practice your Lamaze techniques or that you could possibly go into labor desperate for a good night's sleep.

Hints for Better Sleeping

One of the biggest complaints women have in their last month is that they have great difficulty getting to sleep and remaining in that state. Anxiety, an inability to get comfortable, leg cramps, and a frequent need to urinate all contribute to something less than a restful night.

There's very little you can do about your many nocturnal trips to the bathroom, except to limit the amount you drink in the late evening. In the final weeks of pregnancy, the baby's head engages, putting extra pressure on the bladder and creating a need for more frequent elimination. A positive thinker might believe this wakefulness is good preparation for the many night feedings that lie ahead, but most women consider it simply annoying.

One difficulty in waking up frequently is that you can't always get back to sleep right away. For maximum comfort, we suggest arranging pillows under your stomach and legs to support your weight more evenly and ease the pull on your back (see drawing). You might use several small pillows or a regular-sized bed pillow. The only problem with pillow propping is that when you turn over, you may be required to wake up fully just to rearrange the pillows.

Sleep Positions

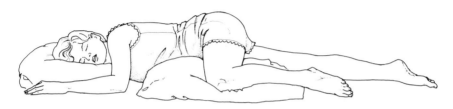

FOR STOMACH SLEEPERS

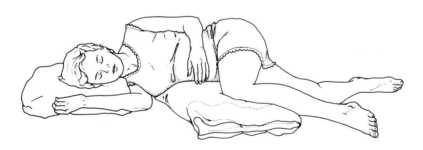

FOR BELLY SUPPORT

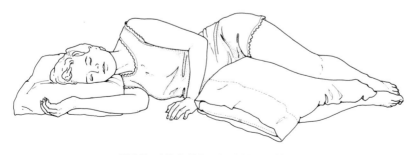

FOR ADDED COMFORT

To help you get to sleep, we suggest warm milk or cocoa, wine if that makes you sleepy, a warm bath, or the progressive relaxation exercises in chapter 6. Try not to go to bed on a full stomach; you'll sleep better if you've had a few hours to digest dinner. If your back is hurting or leg cramps are bothersome, do some stretching right before bed or, better still, do an exercise routine (see chapter 6) during the day.

Traveling for the Last Time

This final month may be your last opportunity for quite a while to enjoy a romantic interlude with your husband or a last-minute family visit. The advisability of travel depends on how much traveling is involved and how anxious you are about leaving home. It's not worth trekking to the beach if you will spend every minute waiting to feel the twinge of a contraction. But the same trip can be relaxing if you know that you'll have ample time to return home if labor begins. Perhaps all you need is the name of a local obstetrician and the route to the nearest hospital "just in case."

You shouldn't be worried about taking short trips. Although some babies are born in cabs, this usually happens to fourth- or fifth-time mothers. Most women take eight or nine hours to reach the first three centimeters of dilation during their first pregnancy. Doctors generally advise not traveling if you're past your due date or if there has been any cervical progress in terms of effacement or dilation. Obviously, it wouldn't be prudent to go away if you have a history of premature labor, are carrying twins, or have high blood pressure.

If you want to fly anywhere during your ninth month, you should check with your doctor or midwife first. Then call all the airlines that service your route because their policies vary greatly. For example, one domestic airline allows you to travel unrestricted until seven days before your due date, yet another requires a doctor's letter for travel in the first two weeks of the ninth month—and after that point, you're not permitted on board. Some airlines reserve the right to refuse a passenger who merely appears too close to her due date. At no time during pregnancy should you fly in small planes with unpressurized cabins.

Going anywhere by car is obviously a lot simpler, and the only precaution you should take is to get out and move about once in a while to avoid leg cramps. If you're not driving, you might consider stretching out full-length in the backseat so that you can keep your feet up and change position more easily.

You should have been wearing your seatbelt all these months. Some women think they can harm their babies by using the belt, but this isn't true. If your car has a lap belt instead of the more up-to-date shoulder strap, you should adjust the belt snugly and as far below the uterine bulge as possible (see drawing). Although it may seem odd to tighten the belt, this will decrease forward motion and injury if you are in an accident.

Whether you should continue to drive until the day you deliver seems to be an open question. Some doctors want women to stop driving as the due date approaches, others are so casual about driving that the subject never comes up. Obviously city women have an advantage here because they can take public transportation, whereas rural women may have no choice because they can't go anywhere without getting in a car. A good general rule may be to let someone else do the driving when possible.

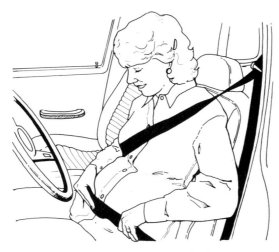

Wearing a Seatbelt

Packing Your Lamaze Bag

Your suitcase will contain whatever you will want for your hospital stay (see next section). Your Lamaze bag will hold the items you may need for labor. You will probably only use one or two of the things in the bag, but since you can never predict which ones they will be, go ahead and take it all.

Item	Use
Books, cards, radio	To pass the time in early labor
Object for a focal point	For concentration and attention
Lip gloss	Dry lips
Washcloth	Refresh face
Cornstarch, baby powder, or lotion	For effleurage or backrubs
Large safety pins	To preserve dignity in hospital gown
Lollipops	Energy and dry mouth
Food and drink for partner	To assure his continuous energy and presence
Pillows, small ones and bed-sized	Hospitals never have enough
Socks	Cold feet
Freezer or cold pack, hot-water bottle	Back labor
Tennis balls or rolling pin	To provide counterpressure for backache
Mirror	To help you push in the labor room
Camera, film	To remember the happiness forever
Champagne	To celebrate
Change and necessary phone numbers	To announce the good news

Packing Your Suitcase

It's possible to just walk into the hospital or birth center and deliver your baby without lugging along a suitcase, particularly if your partner can go home later and bring back whatever necessities you lack. Most women are happier, however, knowing that their own clothes, makeup, and toothbrush are close at hand. The following is a list of items to consider:

Nightgowns
Bathrobe
Slippers
Underpants
Nursing bras, nursing pads
Toothbrush, toothpaste
Shampoo, conditioner, brush, comb, and any other toilet articles you
   might want
Makeup, manicure kit
A few dollars for miscellaneous items
Radio or tape recorder
Travel clock or watch
Scented soap, other luxuries
Address book, telephone numbers, stationery, announcements
Notebook and pen for questions (and answers)
Reading material
Loose clothes to wear home
An outfit for the baby to wear home

Most women spend less time in their own nightgowns and new bathrobes than they expected because of the risk of bloodstains. Generally it's easiest to relax in your hospital gown and then add a pretty bathrobe for visitors.

Hospitals may not provide everything you will need—a local anesthetic spray, for example, for episiotomy stitches, or self-sticking sanitary napkins if you've had a cesarean. Don't wait for the nurses to offer you things, since they may never indicate what is available; ask for what you want. Sometimes you may have to ask your doctor to leave orders for you.

Check out local parking lots, eating places, and public transportation in advance. The less energy you or your partner have to spend on frantic searches during or after delivery the better.

Be on the lookout for items of sentimental value that you can collect, such as the daily newspaper, a copy of your newborn's footprints, or your ID bracelets. Some hospitals have a routine for taking pictures of babies; if this interests you, find out how it works.

Checkups During the Last Month

The type of checkups you will be having during your last month of pregnancy will depend on the manner of practice of your doctor or midwife. First-time mothers are generally seen once a week at this point and then twice a week if they go past their due dates. Some doctors routinely perform internal exams throughout pregnancy, others do them only in the final month.

From your examinations, the doctor or midwife should be able to determine the position of the baby. If the baby's breech, there are certain measures you may want to take (see the section on breech in this chapter). If the baby's posterior, however, there's very little you can do except hope that he turns, although the chances of this happening decrease as you get nearer to your due date. It's very likely any cervical effacement and dilation will be noted as well as the baby's station. And your urine, blood pressure, and weight will be checked as they have been during previous visits.

Now is the time when many doctors and midwives really begin to talk about labor, addressing such topics as when you should call them, how to recognize early labor, and when to go to the hospital. These last visits are a good time to clear up any questions you may have about hospital policies or your doctor's particular practice. Often during the final Lamaze classes important issues can be identified that you haven't yet thought about or discussed. If your partner hasn't accompanied you to any office visits, you should insist that he do so now. You'll both feel more comfortable during labor if he's at least met the doctor or midwife once.

IF YOUR BABY IS BREECH

By now, most babies will have assumed the vertex position (head down), but a few, approximately 3 to 4 percent, are breech, which means they present buttocks, legs, or feet first. If your baby is in a breech presentation when you go into labor, you're likely to have a cesarean, especially if this is your first birth. Fifteen years ago, breech babies were routinely delivered vaginally. Today 75 percent of all breech babies are delivered by cesarean because of the increased safety of the operation. Studies have also shown improved infant outcome with cesarean delivery.

There is no known cause for the vast majority of breeches. A small percentage are related to multiple births; a uterus stretched out from many pregnancies; excessive amniotic fluid; an abnormal position of the placenta, such as placenta previa; and congenital and uterine abnormalities. Women who have had a previous breech birth have an increased chance of having one again, although no one is quite sure why.

Types of Breech Presentation

There are three basic variations of the breech position (see illustrations):

- *Frank breech.* This is the most common breech presentation, and it is considered the safest to deliver vaginally. The baby's legs are straight up and pressed against his or her chest.
- *Incomplete breech* (also known as single or double footling). In this position one or both of the baby's legs may drop down into the vagina. This category also includes a baby who comes out knee first.
- *Complete breech.* The baby has his legs crossed almost tailor fashion.

Breech Positions

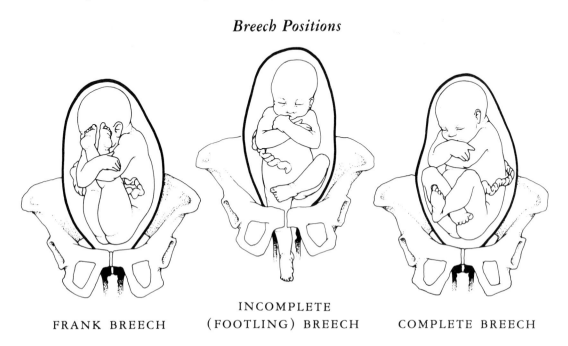

FRANK BREECH   INCOMPLETE (FOOTLING) BREECH   COMPLETE BREECH

The Risks of Breech Birth

Breech births carry a greatly increased risk for the baby. The mortality rate is four to five times higher than for vertex vaginal deliveries, and breech babies have a much greater incidence of neurological impairment. This is because it is possible for the baby's body to slip through an incompletely dilated cervix, but not his head. Doctors and midwives are most fearful of this occurrence, particularly if a woman is having her first child and there is uncertainty about the size of her pelvis.

In his excellent book *The Pregnancy Book for Today's Woman,* Dr. Howard Shapiro describes a doctor's worst fear: "There is no obstetrical situation which is more frantic and desperately tragic than the inability to successfully and atraumatically deliver the head of a baby in the breech position. Time is crucial in these circumstances since a delay of four or more minutes is likely to result in permanent brain damage due to lack of oxygen received by the fetus. At this stage, the point of no return has been reached, because it is too late to perform a cesarean section." If there is any delay in the after-coming head, most doctors will assist the delivery with Piper forceps, an instrument that is especially designed for this purpose.

Breech deliveries also have a greater chance of cord prolapse, a dangerous condition in which the baby's oxygen supply can be compromised. A University of Michigan Hospital study found a 5 percent incidence of prolapsed cord with complete breech, a 15.7 percent with double footling, and 14.5 with single footling. There was no incidence of prolapsed cord in 345 women with frank breech presentations.

Ways to Turn a Breech Baby

If your baby is breech, there is a good likelihood he will turn by himself, which would enable you to avoid a cesarean. There are techniques, however, to coax the baby into the normal vertex position.

EXTERNAL VERSION

External version is one method of turning a breech baby, although it is not performed or even recommended by every doctor or midwife. During this procedure the baby is externally manipulated into the normal vertex position. Two doctors who perform them routinely are: Dr. Thomas Kerenyi, clinical professor of obstetrics at Mount Sinai Medical

School in New York and former chief of perinatology at Mount Sinai Medical Center; and Dr. Daniel Clement, director of maternal fetal medicine at Saint Luke's Roosevelt Hospital Center, also in New York, and assistant professor of obstetrics and gynecology at Columbia University.

Both doctors have had great success with external versions for their own patients as well as for women whose doctors or midwives don't do them. Dr. Clement feels the technique got a bad name during the 1960s when case reports appeared describing placental and cord accidents. In attempting to perform a version, the location of the placenta was unknown, and X rays were the only way to confirm the baby's position.

As Dr. Kerenyi sees it, obstetrics today has become either "straightforward natural childbirth or cesarean section. There is still something to be said for the obstetrical maneuvers in between, which can make a big difference." External version is one such technique. He feels the optimum time to attempt the version is around the thirty-fourth week of pregnancy because the amount of amniotic fluid decreases as pregnancy progresses. Roughly 20 percent of all babies are breech at thirty-four weeks, but at forty weeks, only 3 to 4 percent are still in that position. Dr. Kerenyi believes that if left alone, most babies will eventually turn themselves around and that he is simply giving nature a helping hand. Dr. Clement likes to do his version a bit later, around the thirty-fifth or thirty-sixth week, so that in case a problem arises and delivery is warranted, the baby will be more mature. (He's being extremely cautious, since he has never induced labor or created a placenta problem by performing a version.)

Versions are done wherever there is an ultrasound machine—either at the doctor's office or at a hospital. The sonogram will show the baby's precise position, the placenta and frequently the umbilical cord. If the sonogram reveals fibroids (benign growths), a bicornate (double) uterus, a very large placenta attached to the anterior (front) wall of the uterus, or an abnormality with the fetus, the version will not be performed because it would either be unsafe or it wouldn't be likely to work. If conditions are favorable, and most of the time they are, the baby will be firmly prodded to perform an in-utero somersault. This may feel uncomfortable, but undue force should never be used, and there should never be pain.

Often a second ultrasound will be done midway through the procedure to ascertain the baby's new position. The fetal heartbeat will also

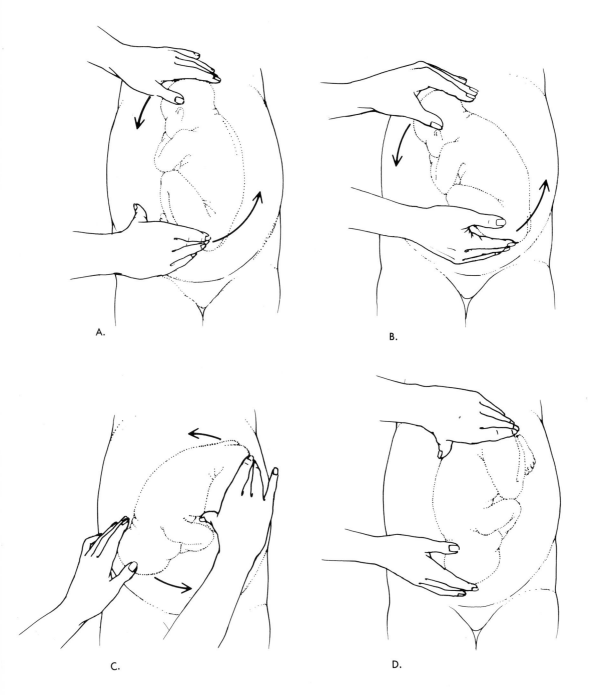

A.

B.

C.

D.

MANIPULATION OF FETUS
DURING EXTERNAL VERSION

EXTERNAL VERSION

♦

"I knew at thirty-five weeks that the baby was breech. I had done some reading about breeches and therefore I was prepared to discuss a version with my doctor when he confirmed the baby's position. I knew what the risks were, but given my doctor's expertise, I felt fairly comfortable about consenting to the procedure. My husband went with me to that appointment and he encouraged me to try the version.

"The whole thing really went off without a hitch. There was no pain, and I can't even say there was any discomfort. Other doctors in the group came in to observe what was going on, and my doctor did a running explanation as he turned the baby. First, he looked at the baby on the ultrasound and then he moved him. I had one Braxton-Hicks contraction, and he stopped and then brought the picture up on the ultrasound again before proceeding.

"It was very reassuring to see all of Benjamin's parts on the ultrasound. My husband is extremely scientific, and this was better than going to a movie—he found it fascinating.

"After the baby was turned, I felt incredible pressure in the pelvic region because his head was now in the proper place. For the first twenty-four hours, I was really nervous about him turning back and I tried to sleep in a semiupright position. But after a few days, I felt confident he was going to remain vertex, and he did."

---

be checked several times. If at any time the uterus starts to contract or the baby seems to resist, he is simply eased back into the original position. Approximately one-third of all babies will resume the breech position within the next day or so; the other two-thirds will remain vertex.

If your baby is breech, ask your doctor or midwife about having an external version. If you are advised against the procedure but want to pursue it, you can call the ultrasound department of your local hospital for a referral.

EXERCISE

Another way to turn a breech baby before delivery is through exercise. You should lie in a position that places the hips higher than the head for fifteen minutes every two hours or as often as possible for five days. This can be accomplished by lying on the floor on your back with your knees bent and putting a few pillows under your hips. Or you can get on your hands and knees with arms bent on the floor and your hips in the air. You can also use a tilted board or ironing board to get the same effect. Although this can be a bit tedious, it seems to work and it's definitely worth trying.

RELAXATION

Feelings of fear and anxiety are common during the last month of pregnancy, and there is a belief among obstetricians and holistic practitioners alike that this tension can affect the baby's presentation. Actively working through these fears and/or simply experiencing total muscular relaxation is another method to try to turn your infant.

Dr. Neil Nathan of the University of Minnesota School of Medicine reported in the professional journal *Ob.Gyn.News* that he used relaxation techniques for thirty-four women, all past thirty-seven weeks gestation and all with babies in the breech position. Studies indicate that only about 5 percent of breech babies will usually turn past the thirty-sixth week, but his success rate was 40 percent.

Dr. Lewis Mehl, a practitioner with the Holistic Psychotherapy and Medical Group in Berkeley, California, has been using relaxation techniques for turning breech presentations since 1977. He sees about two women each month and his success rate is roughly 90 percent. He takes an interdisciplinary approach, using one or more techniques, including visualization, biofeedback, hypnosis, and individual counseling.

AN ORIENTAL REMEDY

There's also no harm in trying a remedy for turning breech babies used by practitioners of shiatsu, Japanese pressure-point massage. First, you must locate a point known as Spleen #6 (see drawing), which is on the inside of the leg in the depression behind the shinbone, just above the knob of the ankle. Then, place a small ball bearing or grain of brown rice over this point and hold it in place with clear plastic tape. You can change the tape whenever necessary. If this doesn't work, you can exert some hard pressure to the point, but only when you are a week or so

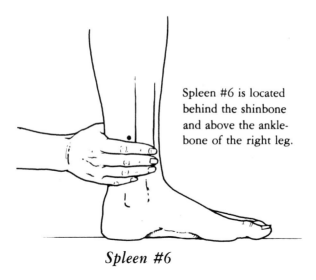

Spleen #6 is located behind the shinbone and above the ankle-bone of the right leg.

Spleen #6

away from your due date. It is believed that Spleen #6 is extremely sensitive and that, if manipulated, it can trigger labor.

WHEN TO ATTEMPT A VAGINAL DELIVERY

If the baby doesn't turn head down, you may not need a cesarean if you meet a certain set of criteria. Most obstetricians evaluate the following conditions before attempting a vaginal delivery:

- *The baby's position.* If the baby is in the frank breech position, there is much less chance of prolapsed cord than if the baby is in the other two breech positions.
- *The mother's previous birth experience.* If the woman has given birth before, her pelvis is known to be adequate in size.
- *The baby's weight.* Breech presentation is most common among premature babies, but vaginal delivery is considered unsafe for babies under five and a half pounds because tiny infants are less able to compensate for minor injuries. A large breech baby, over eight pounds, is more difficult to deliver vaginally.
- *The baby's due date.* The baby's estimated age should be between thirty-six and forty-two weeks.
- *The baby's condition.* There can be no evidence of fetal distress.
- *The progress of labor.* A normal labor is important, since Pitocin should not be used.

- *The doctor's experience.* Today most young doctors have never even seen a breech birth and wouldn't consider a vaginal delivery.
- *Emergency backup.* You will need an operating room available in case a cesarean is necessary.

As an additional precaution, some obstetricians recommend having a flat-plate X ray taken. This would show the position of the baby's head; if the chin is lifted (military position), the cord could be wrapped around the baby's neck. In this instance, normal delivery would be unsafe.

IF YOU PASS YOUR DUE DATE

As we said at the beginning of this chapter, there is an excellent possibility that if this is your first pregnancy, the baby will be late. More than 40 percent of all first babies arrive after their due dates, and only about 5 percent of all babies are born on the day they are expected. Being late should never be considered a medical emergency, unless there is a sudden decrease in fetal movement. Your due date is merely an estimate, and having a baby on time actually means he can arrive anytime within a twenty-eight-day range—that is, two weeks before and two weeks after your due date. (Your doctor may refer to your due date as your EDC, meaning estimated date of confinement, but we prefer EDD, or estimated date of delivery).

Also try to keep in mind that the calculation of your due date is subject to error because doctors use a standard approach that doesn't account for individual variations. Your due date is figured by taking the first day of your last menstrual period, counting back three months, and then adding seven days. This method is precise if you satisfy three standards: (a) you know exactly when your last period began; (b) you ovulated and conceived two weeks later, and (c) you have a twenty-eight-day cycle. Obviously, there are not many women who can meet all three criteria, and therefore there are not many pregnancies that can have an exact due date. Most couples cling to their due date because it's neat and tidy and makes scheduling easier. But babies arrive when it's right for them, not you, and this inability to plan is probably good preparation for parenthood.

Although you shouldn't be overly concerned about your due date, you will want your calculations about the baby's arrival to be as accurate as possible. This precision is critical because some doctors talk of induction as soon as your due date has passed. You certainly don't want to set yourself up for an induction by giving your doctor incorrect information. Unless you've had a sonogram between your eighth and twelfth week of pregnancy, it's very difficult to figure your baby's age precisely. Sonograms performed between the eighth and twelfth week have an accuracy range of plus or minus five days. Between twelve and sixteen weeks, clear readings are difficult to obtain because of the curled position of the fetus. Between twenty-six and thirty-two weeks, the accuracy range is plus or minus eleven days. After that point, the test is not useful for determining gestational age.

Postmaturity

Induction should be considered only if the baby is truly postmature, not just a little late. A baby in this condition cannot remain in the womb any longer, because his food and oxygen supply is being compromised by an aging placenta. The placenta is considered to be a timed organ, and at approximately forty-two weeks it can begin to atrophy, causing a post-term baby to lose weight or suffer distress during labor. A postmature baby appears wizened, skinny, and dry-skinned. This condition is relatively uncommon, however, occurring in less than 5 percent of all pregnancies.

Many doctors are quick to induce as soon as a pregnancy reaches forty-two weeks. This is because studies have found postmaturity to be a leading cause of death among babies born to first-time mothers. This fear may be easing today, however, because sophisticated testing permits the baby's health to be more accurately gauged than in the past. A 1985 review of literature on postmaturity, published in the *Journal of Nurse Midwifery,* states that, "The routine induction carries a greater risk than a prolonged pregnancy. . . . The majority of literature states that the routine induction of labor at 42 weeks does not improve perinatal outcomes." Many practitioners believe that true postmaturity is rare and that what is more commonly seen after forty-two weeks is a miscalculation of the due date. There are many inductions performed in the name of postmaturity, but there are many fewer babies delivered who are truly postmature.

If you are late, your doctor or midwife may ask you to have a few tests to check the condition of the fetal-placental unit.

TESTS FOR POSTMATURITY

Fetal-Movement Counting

One simple but accurate test of fetal well-being is fetal-movement counting. Activity is usually a sign of health, and counting fetal movements can be a reassuring check on the baby. Normally, babies who are older than thirty-two weeks move an average of 282 times a day, although all these motions are not felt by the mother. In general, a count of at least 10 movements in a twelve-hour period would signify that everything is fine with the baby. If at any time there are less than that number of movements or you detect a sudden drop in your baby's level of activity, call your doctor or midwife.

The Nonstress Test (NST)

One reliable check on your baby's condition is the nonstress test (NST), which monitors the fetal heartbeat in response to the baby's movement. The NST has largely replaced estriol testing (measuring estrogen levels in blood or urine). Formerly thought to be an indicator of placental well-being, estriol testing is now considered to be inaccurate.

Prior to the NST, you may be asked to eat or you may be given orange juice to drink during the test in an attempt to increase the baby's blood sugar and level of activity. You will be hooked up to a fetal monitor and instructed to notify the doctor each time you feel the baby move. A good, reactive pattern is one in which the fetal heartbeat accelerates with movement, increasing by fifteen-beats-per-minute for about thirty seconds. This should occur two to three times within a twenty- to thirty-minute period. With the NST, a reaction is good. You will probably be told everything seems fine and to go home. A nonreaction could mean fetal distress —or a sleeping baby. Some obstetricians will ask you to have a nonstress test as soon as your due date has passed. This practice is questionable because it inflates medical costs and subjects expectant couples to unnecessary anxiety. We are against the nonstress test being given routinely or without reasonable medical cause. If there is a question about your baby's age, or if you are more than five days past your due date, it can be a useful diagnostic tool. In addition to suspected cases of postmaturity, the nonstress test is recommended if there has been decreased fetal movement, in high-risk women with hypertension, diabetes, or a history of stillborns.

The Stress Test (ST)

If your baby has not demonstrated a reactive pattern in response to the NST, your doctor will probably want to do an immediate stress test (ST), also known as the contraction stress test (CST). During this procedure, the baby's response to uterine contractions is recorded. You may have an intravenous that will feed you Pitocin, or you will be asked to stimulate your nipples. Because contractions can be stimulated by either Pitocin or nipple stimulation, the test is now known as a contraction stress test. Again, you'll be attached to a fetal monitor, recording the baby's heartbeat. There is some controversy about whether a nonreactive nonstress test should be immediately followed by a stress test. In a 1982 study, Rayburn, Motley, and Zuspan recommended waiting a few hours and then repeating the nonstress test instead of immediately giving the more invasive procedure. They found that approximately two-thirds of all nonreactive nonstress tests later became normal or were followed by a normal stress test. They suggest that a nonreactive pattern is often caused by a sleeping baby, who will perform quite well once he wakes up.

If you do have to undergo a stress test, your doctor will be watching for a slowing down of the fetal heart rate during contractions. In this case, a negative reaction—nothing happens to the heart rate during a contraction—is good news. If deceleration patterns appear, it could mean that the placenta is aging or that there is a problem with the position of the umbilical cord. If the fetal heart pattern is alarming, your doctor may want to take emergency measures. If you are receiving Pitocin for the ST, the obstetrician may increase the dosage to induce labor. In extreme cases, an immediate cesarean would be performed.

If you have a stress test and the results are negative—that is, all seems well—be reassured and then get up and go home. Don't let yourself be talked into an induction. It may seem very convenient to just stay in the hospital and let your doctor begin or continue the Pitocin until labor really gets going. It may also seem particularly tempting if your favorite doctor in the group has performed the stress test and will be on call that weekend, or if you're simply tired of being pregnant. You must remember, however, that induction represents a major intervention in an otherwise normal pregnancy. Induced labors can be difficult (see chapter 8) and greatly decrease your chances for natural childbirth.

The Tenth Month

Most first-time mothers get pretty anxious once their due date has passed. At this point, you're probably fairly uncomfortable and you're ready for this endless pregnancy to be over. You're also probably very eager to meet the person you've been lugging around for nine months. The phone calls about your status increase daily, and it seems each time you leave your house, you bump into someone who says, "You're still here?"

It's very easy to get undone about this situation and consequently not sleep very well or enjoy the unexpected freedom. Women who are at home on maternity leave are bound to be upset because this waiting period is cutting into the time they will have later on with the baby. It is hard to use your days constructively because the longer you go past your due date, the more frequently you will be having examinations and nonstress tests. It seems that all you do is answer the phone and go for checkups.

You may not be feeling too well physically either, because you're so keyed up about experiencing the first signs of labor. Any new symptoms, whether it be a stuffed nose or a mild headache, are embellished in your mind with the hope that they'll really turn into something. You may be feeling fine, but you'll mope around in a sort of vague malaise, hoping for something to materialize.

The best advice we can give you is to relax and try to get in touch with how you really feel about having this baby. Midwife Elizabeth Davis believes that "normal healthy women will, nine times out of ten, have their physical factors in readiness at term unless psychology has created chronic tension or inhibition." She has described some typical situations that contribute to going past the due date and beyond: (a) a woman who's having her last baby and is thoroughly nostalgic about it; (b) a woman who is having her first baby and is frightened of the responsibilities of parenting; (c) both parents being uncertain about their changing roles and this vacillation prolonging the pregnancy; and (d) a woman who has felt obligated or otherwise compelled to work right up to her due date and now may be taking some time to savor the experience.

Becoming a mother for the first time can be a bold and frightening step. You'll be giving up a lot of freedom in exchange for great responsibility. If you're past your due date and fairly anxious, you may want to talk to friends who've had children or your Lamaze teacher about your feelings. Sharing your anxiety can't hurt, and you may gain some insight into your situation. To relax, try the visualizations in chapter 6 and do something you enjoy in your last few days as a free agent.

NATURAL WAYS TO GET LABOR GOING

Anyone who has been ten months pregnant—or even a few days late—will forgive you for wondering if there isn't some way to get things moving. Following is a list of natural alternatives that might help trigger labor:

- *Castor oil.* This is an old trick used to induce labor, especially if the membranes have already ruptured. It may taste awful, but it usually works, though no one knows exactly why. Take two tablespoons of castor oil orally, followed by one tablespoon half an hour later. It will make you go to the bathroom, so make sure you drink plenty of fluids so you don't get dehydrated.
- *Lovemaking.* Ina May Gaskin, the author of *Spiritual Midwifery,* is a great believer in erotic activity as a means of inducing labor.
- *Nipple stimulation.* This method can be used to stimulate contractions for a stress test, an induction, or during labor. It's common knowledge that breast-feeding causes the uterus to contract; nipple stimulation prior to or during labor is simply an application of this phenomenon.

  Dr. Benjamin Chayen, assistant professor of the Division of Fetal Maternal Medicine at the Thomas Jefferson Medical College in Philadelphia, has conducted a great deal of research on nipple stimulation and has used it successfully in many different instances. He presented some of his results at the ASPO/Lamaze annual conference in October 1985, and we spoke to him about his work. One of his most interesting findings is that nipple massage activates the production of the hormone prolactin, not oxytocin (as commonly believed), to create uterine contractions.

  In one particular study, sixty-two high-risk women were induced, thirty with electric breast pumps and thirty-two with Pitocin. Nipple stimulation was as successful as Pitocin for inducing labor and in fact took much less time to establish strong, regular contractions, thereby shortening the early phase of labor. Another difference was the cesarean-section rate of the two groups: 43.7 percent of the women whose labors were induced with Pitocin were delivered by cesarean section (mostly for failure to progress), while only 26.6 percent of the nipple-stimulation group gave birth surgically. Dr. Chayen speculates that prolactin is more effective because it is a natural hormone, while Pitocin is "a totally artificial" way to induce labor.
- *Shiatsu massage.* Shiatsu practitioners claim they can induce labor by

pressing Spleen #6, a special point just above the anklebone (see the illustration on page 159). Even if your labor is induced with Pitocin, pressing on this point may help establish a regular pattern of contractions.

We do not want you to have a medically induced labor if it is not essential. We believe that too many inductions are performed, but this phenomenon is not created solely by a small group of trigger-happy obstetricians. It's a complex medical problem, fueled by women putting tremendous pressure on their doctors to "do something" once a due date has come and gone. It's also encouraged by doctors protecting themselves from litigation by ordering unnecessary tests, which should be reassuring but often only further increase a mother's anxiety.

Being late is the one issue that really tests both a doctor's and a mother's confidence in the natural scheme of things. This last month may be one of the longest in your life, but there's no reason to try to hurry things along without good cause. The more patient you are and the more you trust in the natural workings of your body, the better chance you have of enjoying a healthy baby and an uncomplicated birth.

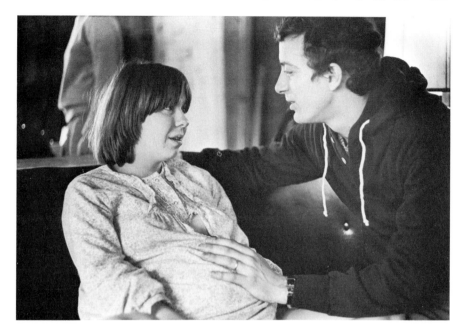

CHAPTER 8

Labor Begins

EARLY LABOR

*E*arly labor is exciting and scary. It's thrilling because you've waited so long to see your baby, and that moment is now close at hand. As you feel labor beginning, you are filled with a sense of wonder about your body, which is performing in a new and powerful way. But early

EARLY LABOR

♦

"This is it! Why didn't I rest more and eat more before this started? I had cleaned the entire house and gone to bed one hour before labor started. I went to the hospital and had to lie flat on my back for the fetal monitor to work. Thought I was near delivery—but was only two centimeters dilated! Progressed very slowly until they let me sit up."

♦

"The only surprises were good ones. I missed out entirely on the first phase of labor. My doctor had said, 'Call me when the pains are five minutes apart,' but they were never five minutes apart. They started between two and four minutes apart, and that was it. I kept thinking that at any time they would get further apart so I could call my doctor! I got to the hospital at noon and delivered at 3:30 P.M."

♦

"In the beginning I had contractions that were very erratic. There would be a span of twenty minutes and then two contractions next to each other. Since my contractions weren't regular, we assumed it was false labor. It wasn't."

♦

"I was scared and nervous, but very excited and happy. I felt my first labor pains low in my pelvis. I talked and joked during contractions."

♦

"The beginning phase was extremely mild. In fact, I thought I was suffering from indigestion until my water broke."

♦

"Woke up at 3:00 A.M. with diarrhea and happily discovered I was in labor. Contractions slowly got stronger and closer together. I was comfortable, had breakfast and lunch, even went shopping."

continued

♦

"I don't know what I was thinking, but I was totally surprised! My first contractions were mild, close together, and very irregular. I stayed up all night timing contractions and wondering whether I should call the doctor or not."

♦

"Had no idea the contractions could be so painful so early, knowing they're only to get worse. Back labor was already starting."

♦

"I was awakened at 6:30 A.M. by the rupture of my membranes. I knew this was it. I was very excited and happy that we would have our baby soon."

♦

"I had felt crampy all day but didn't know I was in labor until the doctor, at my regular clinic visit, told me I was four centimeters dilated."

♦

"I had felt crummy all day, so when it started that evening, I thought I was getting the flu. I was a month away from my due date and almost positive it wasn't time for the baby."

♦

"It was just little twinges—no more than a mild stomachache."

♦

"I had taken castor oil at lunch to hopefully start labor. At around 3:00 P.M. I had cramps, but I didn't realize I was in labor until my 'show,' around 6:00 P.M."

♦

"I had been three centimeters dilated for two weeks. Labor began with stomach cramps. Within two and a half hours the contractions were five minutes apart."

continued

"My water broke at home, and my pains went immediately from ten minutes apart to three minutes apart. When I got to the hospital, I had only dilated to three centimeters; forty-five minutes later, I had dilated to nine centimeters."

♦

"When I lost the mucous plug, I announced to my husband that the process had started. Shared grin, handshake, congratulations, and joint feeling of 'here we go,' not just for the process but for the beginning of parenting."

♦

"The moment when my water broke was remarkable. I'll never forget that feeling of inevitability and 'There's no turning back now.'"

labor is also frightening, because you've never felt a contraction before and you don't know what lies ahead.

How Labor Begins

Sometimes it's only in retrospect that you realize when labor actually began. If your water breaks and you have regular contractions, you can be pretty sure this is the real thing. But for most women, labor starts as discomfort in the lower abdomen or as a tightening of the uterus, a feeling similar to a Braxton-Hicks contraction. It can also be heralded by mild backache or cramps in the upper thighs. All of these signs may be confused with the common discomforts of late pregnancy, making it difficult to determine if you really are in labor. It is often only in retrospect that you will be able to pinpoint when labor began.

True early labor can start in an erratic manner, but usually a pattern is established. As we described in chapter 4, your initial contractions may last thirty to forty-five seconds and occur anywhere from five to twenty minutes apart. To determine the correct frequency of your contractions, you must time from the beginning of one to the beginning of the next. For example, contractions are four minutes apart when you have a one-minute contraction and a three-minute rest.

These first contractions are generally mild, and women frequently compare them to menstrual cramps. As time passes, the rhythm will change, and the contractions will become longer, stronger, and closer together. When this occurs, you will know that labor is really progressing. For a first pregnancy, an average early labor lasts eight or nine hours. During this time, the cervix will efface completely and dilate to about three centimeters.

While you're at home, it's hard to tell what phase you're in and how quickly your cervix is dilating. Obviously, you can't examine yourself, but you can get some idea based on the contractions. If they are mild, ten minutes apart and lasting only thirty seconds, you can be pretty sure there is not much progress being made. On the other hand, if your contractions are at least sixty seconds in length, are occurring at least every five minutes, and are strong enough to require Lamaze breathing, there will be some effacement or dilation. Of course, there are exceptions to this pattern, but in general progress can be gauged by the strength, length, and frequency of your contractions.

Variations of Early Labor

The patterns of early labor are more diverse than the patterns that occur later on. Most labors begin as we've just described. There are, however, a few common varieties of early labor and they are easily recognizable because they're so distinctive. They are

- *Telescopic labor.* This labor begins with intense, frequent contractions that produce full dilation within a few hours. It's the kind of labor that seems easy in retrospect because it's so short. But telescopic labor is often difficult because even these early contractions require your utmost concentration. There's no chance to warm up to labor and no idea at the time that it will be over quickly.
- *Prodromal labor.* This technically means false labor, but it can also mean just a long warm-up phase, perhaps as long as eighteen hours. This type of labor can be spent at home because discomfort is minimal. Contractions are generally mild and widely spaced. Although

prodromal labor isn't usually painful, its length and vagueness can wear you out.

 • *Strong early labor.* This variation begins with a bang—with strong contractions, five minutes apart—and the contractions remain strong and frequent for hours, for the labor is of normal length. For this type of labor, you need stamina because you will be doing a lot of breathing for a long time. It's a tough labor, but like all other kinds, it, too, is finite.

Starting the Lamaze Breathing

You should begin the slow chest breathing when your contractions are strong enough to demand your full attention. You don't have to start your breathing if other distractions work, but if the breathing relaxes you, by all means don't be afraid of starting too early. For some women, early labor is the hardest part. If you begin with strong contractions or with immediate back labor, the pain can be startling. This might happen in the middle of the night, and you may feel tired, lonely, and unable to handle what's ahead. Even if your partner is wide awake and support- ive, it can be hard not to dwell on the pain and fantasize about what you'll do if it gets worse.

Try not to fall prey to these doubts. Just allow your body to take over and work automatically as the contractions intensify. If you surrender and let labor happen, you will find unknown resources for coping. One axiom to remember is, "Take one contraction at a time." Fantasizing about future pain will only undermine your present efforts. During each contraction, concentrate exclusively on your breathing, and when the contraction has ended, don't think, just rest.

You will find that Lamaze breathing increases in effectiveness as labor progresses. This is because, like anything else, breathing becomes easier with practice. Also, you get to know your contractions and you learn what to anticipate. You become more proficient and relaxed because breathing becomes an automatic response that doesn't require thought.

False Labor

A precursor and component of false labor are Braxton-Hicks contrac- tions. These are commonly referred to as warm-up contractions, and are usually painless. Most women describe them as a tightening, almost like the feeling in your arm when your blood pressure is taken. During the contraction, the uterine muscle becomes very hard. Braxton-Hicks can occur all throughout pregnancy but are more strongly felt as the due date approaches. The terms *Braxton-Hicks* and *false labor* are often used interchangeably.

Labor is only considered real if you are having contractions that produce continual effacement and dilation of the cervix. You may be having contractions, but if they are not creating significant cervical change, you are experiencing false labor. Approximately 25 percent of all women will experience a bout of false labor before real early labor begins. This can be maddening because the contractions can keep you awake and you can get tired, but no closer to delivery. There's very little good about false labor except that the contractions do flex and strengthen the uterine muscle and they provide an opportunity to practice your breathing.

We dislike the phrase *false labor,* since it is a negative term that implies the body is somehow inefficient, but it is the commonly accepted name. The correct medical term, as we mentioned earler, is *prodromal labor,* meaning pre- or practice labor.

There are at least two typical patterns of false labor. One is found among women whose babies are large but not engaged. They experience twinges as the baby drops into the pelvis, and these pains can be mistaken for labor. Usually at this point there is some effacement, but not much at the cervical opening. The best remedy for this situation is a hot bath and some relaxation exercises.

Another sort of false labor is more like the real thing because there are actual contractions, which cause some pulling discomfort. These spasmlike contractions tend to be irregular in length, which suggests that uterine movement is poorly synchronized. Women with this type of false labor should have a stiff drink to try to relax the uterus sufficiently to stop the inefficient contractions.

It's often hard to determine when false labor ends and the real thing begins. False labor is often lumped together with real labor to produce the childbirth horror stories we've all heard. "I was in labor for thirty-six hours." "I had contractions for forty-eight hours." "My mother was in labor for three days." In most cases, women experience a long bout of false labor and then a normal amount of real labor. For example, a thirty-six-hour labor might be broken down into twenty-four hours of warm-up contractions and twelve hours of the real thing. You may think this is just a matter of semantics because contractions are contractions whether or not they produce dilation. We know that, but in defining false labor, we are attempting to temper some of the more harrowing birth stories you've been told.

False labor can be truly annoying. You may leave for the hospital, only to be sent home. You may have contractions for a whole day and then go to your doctor's office to find you haven't even dilated one centimeter. You will probably be bored, tired, and quite uncomfortable. The pain of false labor may wear you down and cast doubts on your ability to have natural childbirth.

The advice we have is to rest and then rest some more. Try not to become discouraged; labor will happen. Take hot baths (if your water hasn't broken), drink wine, and turn off the phone. Do your utmost to nap or sleep through the night. Eat easily digested foods and drink plenty of juices and water. Think about how wonderful it will be when it's all over.

What to Do During Early Labor

You should call your doctor or midwife when you know you are in labor. This is a matter of courtesy as well as reassurance. Most doctors and midwives want to know what's happening and prefer to schedule professional and personal engagements accordingly. Some women are inclined to call their doctors as soon as they feel the first contraction. This isn't necessary, but if you need to touch base, that's fine. If it's the middle of the night, why not let your doctor or midwife get some sleep and call in the morning? As a general rule, doctors or midwives want to hear from you when contractions have been five minutes apart for at least an hour or ten minutes apart for two hours.

For further reassurance, you might also call your Lamaze teacher. She can answer your questions and suggest ways to make you more comfortable. If you're feeling scared, she can also just talk to you. You shouldn't feel strange about asking your instructor for help. Her job isn't limited to instruction of the Lamaze method; she is there to offer support to women in labor.

If contractions begin during the day, you may want to go to the office for an examination. If you've made even slight progress, you may want to go to the hospital or birth center, believing that you'll be more comfortable there. If you're less than four centimeters dilated, feeling well, and have no special problems, we think you should return home. The best time to be admitted is when you are in active labor, five to six centimeters dilated. Medication is usually withheld until labor is well established, so there's no reason to leave home just to get pain relief.

Of course, if you are classified as high-risk, early labor at home is not recommended. Or if you are experiencing any unusual symptoms, such as bleeding or acute pain, don't hesitate to go to the hospital. If this is not the case, stay home.

A hospital is no place to be in early labor. Home is more enjoyable because there you can listen to music, watch television, eat and drink what you want, and use the bathroom in privacy. You can also talk on the phone, assume any comfortable position, and exercise total control over your environment. Your sense of time will also be different, depending on whether you're home or in the hospital. Three hours spent at home feels a lot different from three hours spent in a labor room. There's nothing inherently dangerous about spending early labor at home.

It's an unusual woman whose labor is so short that she barely has enough time to get to the delivery room. In general, the longer you stay at home, the more control you have over your whole labor. If you arrive at the hospital too soon—before labor is clearly established—you may be sent away. Once you are admitted, your labor will be charted, which means you have punched a time clock. If your labor fails to progress satisfactorily, certain measures will be taken. To get labor moving, your doctor may rupture your membranes or administer Pitocin to strengthen your contractions. You may also be hooked up to a fetal monitor, which in turn may hamper your mobility. All of these interventions work against your chances of having natural childbirth.

While at home, there are four important things to keep in mind as you labor:

+ *Rest.* If you wake up in the middle of the night with some mild contractions, try to go back to sleep. Even if your water has broken, you should go back to bed after changing the sheets. You may sleep fitfully, waking up for contractions, but you are still getting more rest than if you were reading or watching television. If labor begins while you are at work or out of the house, return home and put your feet up. The most important thing to do during early labor is rest; it's essential that you conserve energy for the hard part.

- *Eat.* You must keep up your strength. A lot of people believe women in labor are not able to digest food, but recent research has shown this to be untrue. You know that going all day without food makes you feel weak and light-headed, so it seems unwise to approach a rigorous activity such as childbirth without nourishment. Obviously we're not recommending that you eat an eight-course Chinese dinner, but you can eat light foods that are easily absorbed, are low in roughage, do not form a ball or clot in the stomach (such as milk or soft bread), and do not rest in the stomach for extended periods of time (such as fats). This would include toast, honey, plain cookies, applesauce, broth, and fruit. It's also important to keep well hydrated, so drink lots of fluids: herbal or decaffeinated tea, juices, and water. Even if you don't feel hungry, you should make yourself eat something. Some women do throw up during labor, but this is not the result of having eaten earlier. Don't avoid eating just because this might happen to you. It's important to keep your strength up.

- *Drink.* This is the one moment during pregnancy when you should be encouraged to have a stiff drink. If you're experiencing false labor, alcohol can relax the uterus and stop contractions. Even if you're not having false labor, a drink will help relax you, and that's good. After months of abstention, you may feel odd about drinking, but a few ounces of liquor will not harm your baby, who is fully formed and hours from being born. It's preferable to relax with a drink at home instead of with some Demerol at the hospital.

- *Shower or bathe.* Warm water is always relaxing, and a shower is often helpful when labor gets stalled. (If your membranes have ruptured, you should not bathe because of the possibility of infection.) A French surgeon, Michel Odent, has recently been attracting a great deal of publicity with his birth clinic in Pithiviers. Dr. Odent has found that a bath helps women to become more instinctive and relaxed, making labor go more smoothly.

Although most doctors have at last adopted a more flexible attitude about "prepping" a woman for labor, some still require an enema and a trim of the pubic hair. You can do both these things while in early labor at home, thus avoiding any disruption in your concentration at the hospital.

Many women don't need an enema because they experience diarrhea just before or during early labor. Others don't want one because it can be a dehumanizing and uncomfortable procedure under the best of circumstances. If you are constipated, however, or worried about having a bowel movement on the delivery table, you can buy a small or child's-sized enema at the drugstore and use it before going to the hospital. Be sure to drink lots of liquids afterward because enemas are dehydrating. As for pubic shaves, they have proved to be useless in preventing infection, so there's no reason you must have one. Some doctors are concerned, however, about hair becoming caught in the stitches of an episiotomy repair. Trimming your pubic hair can be done at home, preferably by your partner.

We know early labor is exciting, but you should not call your family and friends to announce it has begun. The difficulty with sharing this news is that progress reports will then be expected, and this task will distract you and your partner from the job at hand. It's also possible that you may be experiencing false labor, and then you'll feel obliged to call everyone back and apologize for raising their hopes.

As we've mentioned, if your labor is progressing normally, you should avoid going to the hospital too early. See chapter 9 for a discussion of the best time to go.

BACK LABOR

Women frequently describe back labor as the most difficult part of their birth experiences. Back labor is caused by the baby resting in a posterior position, which means the back of his head is pressing against your sacrum (see the illustration on page 181). With each contraction, the baby's hard bone jabs against your hard bone, and you experience a knifelike pain in the back. True back labor is reported to occur in about 25 percent of all births, but the incidence in the responses to our questionnaire was higher, more like 30 or 40 percent. Some women experience intermittent back pain during labor, but it's not the continuous ache of real back labor.

A baby born in a posterior position emerges looking at the ceiling. Most babies (97 percent), however, are born in an anterior position, which means they come out facing the floor. If your baby assumes a posterior presentation, it is likely he will turn around during labor or as

BACK LABOR

◆

"The pain did not radiate, it did not throb, it was just There. My husband used a roller on my back, which helped a great deal—as did being on all fours."

◆

"Back labor feels like the baby doesn't have any room and decides to come through your back."

◆

"Counterpressure from my husband helped, and the knowledge that I would either die or deliver eventually."

◆

"We put three tennis balls in a sock and my husband rubbed those along my lower central back. No matter how hard he pushed, I wanted the pressure to be harder. I needed someone on the order of Arnold Schwarzenegger to *stand* on my back."

◆

"I felt as if my back were being crushed by a truck. Massaging helped."

◆

"Walking was the only thing I could do. I couldn't sit or lie down. I would press my tailbone against the wall."

◆

"I used a Tupperware rolling pin and filled it with ice to numb the area."

◆

"It was terrible. I could not get comfortable, counterpressure did not help, and my husband wouldn't let me have an epidural. We really worked on our breathing, and that got me through it."

continued

"My entire spinal column ached, and I was not *allowed* to deal with it. Once I turned on my side when no one was watching and was infinitely more comfortable. As soon as the labor nurse discovered my transgression, she scolded me like a child and insisted I stay on my back, and in pain."

♦

"Very painful. Almost no position offered comfort, although toward the end being on my hands and knees was best."

♦

"Back labor felt as if my lower back were tied in a knot. I realized then how important being able to relax was."

♦

"The only way I was slightly comfortable was sitting in a hot shower with the water hitting my lower back."

♦

"Elephants could have napped on my back and I wouldn't have felt them at all. The pressure was extremely intense. When the baby was finally delivered, I was so relieved about my back that I forgot to ask if it was a boy or a girl."

you push. But until this happens, you will feel a sharp pain in your back each time the uterus contracts. True back labor may last for an hour or two or for the entire labor. The pain often radiates around to the front, making your stomach and back feel like one big sore spot.

The problem with back labor is that you don't have any moments that are pain-free because you must cope with a backache while recouping from contractions. Women who have experienced back labor say there are no discreet contractions, just greater or lesser degrees of pain. In addition, back labor can mean a longer labor because the baby's head tends to enter the pelvis slightly deflexed, causing slow dilation due to an asymmetrical fit against the cervix.

Coping with Back Labor

Lamaze breathing is not as effective for back labor as it is for normal labor, because back labor is doubly painful and therefore twice as wearing. Back labor has been the undoing of many women who planned on natural childbirth. Remember, however, that even if your baby begins labor in the posterior position, it's very likely he will turn around. Getting through back labor takes a slightly different approach and a greater commitment to relaxation. The ability to relax between contractions is critical because tension will only exacerbate the back pain. You'll also be working harder during contractions because there's more pain to breathe through, and you'll really need the rest periods.

There are three good techniques for pain relief you should try along with your Lamaze breathing. They are

- *Hot or cold.* Hot means a heating pad or hot-water bottle, and cold is a cold pack. To compare effectiveness, you can start with one and switch to the other. You should also play around with the positioning of the pad or pack, since the pain can shift, making it difficult to hit just the right spot. Whether you prefer hot or cold is a matter of taste and of climate.
- *Change of position.* The worst thing you can do for back labor is to lie flat on your back. In that position, the entire weight of the baby's head is pressed against your spine. Instead, any position that gets the baby off your back is good. Try resting on your hands and knees, standing, lying on your side, or sitting while leaning forward over a table or a pile of pillows. You can also experiment with sitting on a hard surface, such as the toilet or a wooden chair—or, in the hospital, a metal instrument tray. Anyone with a bad back will tell you that a soft surface can be torture.
- *Counterpressure.* People instinctively press on something that hurts. If you stub a toe, your first impulse is to rub it, so it's no surprise that you have the same reaction to a shooting pain in your back. To apply counterpressure, your partner can use his fist, tennis balls, a rolling pin, or a folded-up towel. Don't worry about rubbing as hard as you need to—it can't hurt the baby, and it will only feel good.

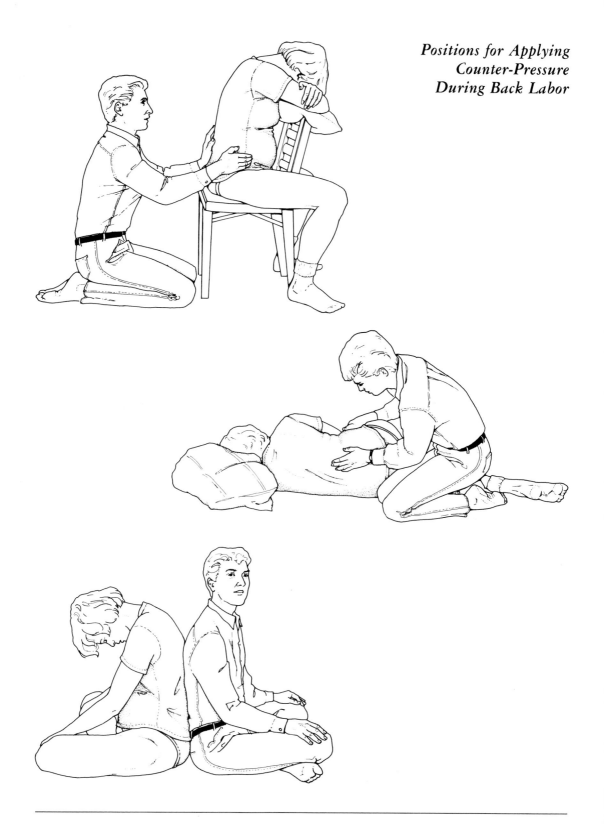

*Positions for Applying
Counter-Pressure
During Back Labor*

You have to experiment to find a comfortable and effective amount of counterpressure.

The Partner's Role

Back labor is a situation that can make or break your partner. It's a very demanding sort of labor because there's a need for constant experimentation with breathing patterns and alternative methods for pain relief. Often, as soon as one position or pressure point will work, the pain shifts and you'll be forced to find a different strategy. Your partner will be completely involved if you have back labor, working very hard to provide physical support and a careful balance of encouragement and sympathy.

PREMATURE RUPTURE OF THE MEMBRANES

There is great disagreement even among obstetricians about what to do if your water breaks before labor has started—a condition known as premature rupture of the membranes, or PROM. The controversy about treatment centers on the risk of infection to the mother and her baby if labor and delivery do not take place within a prescribed number of hours. The dispute also touches on the risk-benefit ratio of many standard hospital practices, such as internal exams, Pitocin stimulation of labor, and fetal monitoring.

Some doctors and midwives believe that if the membranes rupture, there is very little that should be done except to wait for labor to begin. Until that happens, good hydration and impeccable standards of hygiene are essential. This means no oral-genital contact, no tub baths, and drinking lots of liquids to offset the lost amniotic fluid, which is continually being replenished. It also means periodic temperature checks to monitor for possible infection. All of these measures can be performed at home, and if you are lucky, labor will begin soon—80 percent of all women go into labor within twenty-four hours of rupture of the membranes.

Other doctors, however, believe that women with ruptured membranes should be hospitalized immediately and given Pitocin to bring on contractions. These obstetricians usually set a strict twenty-four-hour limit for labor and delivery—that is, your baby must be born within twenty-four hours of your water breaking. If labor doesn't progress sufficiently to meet this standard, a cesarean will be performed. The reason stated for this urgency is a fear of maternal or fetal infection. Some doctors will extend the deadline for delivery to forty-eight hours and may allow you to wait awhile at home, particularly if your water breaks during the night.

We believe in treating premature rupture of the membranes as conservatively as possible. This means staying at home until labor is well established and being alert for signs of infection. If your water breaks, you should insist that your doctor give nature a reasonable chance to take its course. A recent study has shown that the risk of infection following PROM increases dramatically after the initial vaginal examination and incrementally after each subsequent exam. This is because the ruptured membranes have created an open passage into a formerly sterile uterine environment, and with each check on cervical progress, normal vaginal bacteria is pushed toward the uterus. Obviously, you will not receive an internal exam at home, and by remaining there, you minimize the risk of this kind of infection.

Statistics indicate that cesareans are three times as likely following an induced labor, compared with a labor that begins normally. If you go to the hospital after your water breaks but before you experience contractions, you will be given Pitocin to induce labor. If you stay home with PROM and take good precautions, chances are excellent that you will have a normal natural delivery.

There are three instances, however, when there can be no debate about going immediately to the hospital with ruptured membranes:

♦ *If the amniotic fluid is stained with brown or greenish matter,* it can mean fetal distress. The dark material is meconium, the baby's first bowel movement. This does not mean that your baby is in imminent danger; he may have experienced a temporary distress, or he could be in a breech position (breech babies frequently pass meconium because there is great pressure on their presenting part, the buttocks). If the amniotic fluid is colored with meconium, you shouldn't be unduly worried because recent studies have shown that most babies in this situation are not compromised. The fear, however, is that the baby could aspirate the meconium, impeding breathing at birth or increasing the chances of respiratory infection. However, if there is evidence of meconium, your doctor or midwife will want to monitor the baby carefully throughout labor.

♦ *If your water breaks and the baby is not yet engaged,* you should go to the hospital immediately. This situation can be dangerous because you could experience cord prolapse. If cord prolapse does occur, you must assume a knee-chest position with your hips in the air. This condition necessitates a rapid trip to the hospital and an emergency cesarean.

♦ *If the baby is in an unusual position,* such as breech or transverse, a prolapsed cord is again a possibility. Sometimes it's difficult to know if your membranes have really ruptured because there may be just a trickle of water. It could be urine that is being involuntarily released on account of the constant pressure of the baby's head on your bladder. If in doubt, you can call your doctor or midwife and describe your experience or go to the office and be checked there.

PROM occurs in about 10 percent of all women at term, making it a common labor variation. This is certainly one topic you'll want to discuss with your doctor or midwife before your due date so that you'll know what to do if your water breaks. Usually, membranes will rupture between eight centimeters dilation and the delivery of the baby. If your membranes rupture and labor doesn't begin, try stimulating labor contractions by using the measures listed on page 165 and/or by walking around at home. (Do not engage in lovemaking after your water has broken.) Sometimes one of these methods will work and sometimes a combination will do the trick. Sometimes nothing will help, but at least you will have done all you can.

INDUCED LABOR

No one knows how many inductions are performed each year in the United States, because they are done in a variety of ways and for a variety of reasons. Inductions can be done manually in two ways: by breaking the amniotic sac with a plastic hook (an amniotomy) or by stripping the membranes during an internal examination (separating the amniotic sac from the lower uterine wall, usually done with a fingertip). They can also be done chemically, by administering Pitocin. This drug mimics the effects of the body's natural hormone, oxytocin.

Of course, your membranes can rupture naturally before labor begins, but you should never allow your doctor to break your water before labor is well established. If this happens, you become a good candidate for induction by Pitocin or for a cesarean, because once the amniotic sac is broken, you and the baby are susceptible to infection. If your doctor ruptured your membranes prematurely and labor failed to begin, he'd probably insist on putting you on Pitocin. If that failed to establish labor, you'd likely have a cesarean, either because you'd contracted an infection or chances were good that you would.

INDUCED LABOR

♦

"I was looking forward to being induced—I knew that by the end of the day I'd have a baby in my arms. Now that it has happened, I think maybe I should have gone against the doctor's orders and let it happen naturally."

♦

"My water broke and I never went into labor. After eighteen hours I was induced with Pitocin. I was totally unprepared for labor to begin with contractions three minutes apart, and my contractions were peaking twice. I totally lost control! The breathing was absolutely useless."

♦

"After two hours on Pitocin I had an epidural. The pains were too much for me."

♦

"I was opposed to it even when I got it. However, I was grateful when I saw my daughter five hours later."

♦

"I had an induced labor, and on a scale of one to ten, the labor pain for me was a thirty-six. There was no gradual buildup of contractions, and I never got those 'rest periods' they tell you about in class. Total labor and delivery time was three hours and forty-five minutes. This is too much like a record attempt in a sport at which I am not well trained."

♦

"I've had two normal deliveries, so I have a basis for comparison. Induction is much more painful. I can't even begin to describe the pain. I had back and stomach labor."

Pitocin induction should never be performed because you're a few days late or because you want to deliver on a certain date. In 1977 the Food and Drug Administration (FDA) recommended that doctors refrain from performing elective inductions due to the risks associated with this procedure. This action more or less halted the practice of timing of a baby's birth with a husband's business trip, an anniversary, or a doctor's vacation, although there are some practitioners who will still induce for these reasons.

The risks of Pitocin induction are greater for the baby than the mother. They include:

+ *Respiratory-distress syndrome.* If labor is induced before the baby is fully developed and his lungs are still immature, respiratory problems commonly develop. Without sophisticated testing, it's impossible for a doctor to assess the baby's maturity accurately and therefore know when an induction would be absolutely safe.
+ *Fetal distress during labor.* If the dosage of Pitocin is too high, it produces contractions that last too long and prevent the uterus from relaxing between them. The result of this overstimulated labor is that the baby's oxygen supply can be compromised, causing possible asphyxia and brain damage.
+ *Neonatal jaundice.* The reasons for this are unclear. The incidence of jaundice is increased with smaller or premature babies.

Women consistently report that contractions produced by Pitocin are sharper and more painful than natural ones and therefore harder to handle. An induced labor also starts abruptly, allowing a shorter warmup period and less time to get used to the feel of labor. By the time you've gotten the knack of how to breathe and relax with early contractions, you are headed into active labor.

There is no question that the use of Pitocin increases a woman's need for medication; there are numerous studies which have proved this relationship. Obviously, an induced labor is to be avoided whenever possible. There are, however, instances in which inductions are justified. They include:

+ If a woman has toxemia, diabetes, hypertension, or kidney disease
+ If the baby is truly postmature
+ If a positive contraction stress test shows fetal heart decelerations
+ If a woman's membranes have been ruptured for more than twenty-four hours and labor has not yet begun

If your labor must be induced, you will go to the hospital where you will be hooked up to an intravenous line with an attached Pitocin drip. Your labor must be continuously monitored by either an internal or an external fetal monitor (the internal is more common because it is more accurate). This is one instance in which your doctor should be actively overseeing your labor, actually spending a good deal of time in your room checking the monitor and regulating dosage.

The dosage you receive should be administered by an infusion pump, calibrated in increments of miliunits per minute. It's difficult to state an ideal dosage of Pitocin because women react very differently. One woman may experience good strong contractions with two milliunits per minute, whereas another might have no results at all with twenty. Your doctor will probably start with a small dosage and gradually increase it by two milliunits every fifteen minutes until you have regular contractions, roughly three minutes apart.

Whatever amount you are given, you should never experience continuous contractions. This would be caused by too high a dose, and if this occurs, your doctor should be notified immediately. The drip should be turned off. If the uterus is unable to relax sufficiently between contractions, your baby may not be able to get the necessary replenishment of oxygen. Also, an overdose of Pitocin puts you at risk for placental separation because the uterus is contracting so hard that the placenta can become detached. Women who have had several children or previous uterine surgery also risk uterine rupture if they receive an overdose of Pitocin.

Sometimes an initial dose of Pitocin may be all you need to trigger your body's own production of oxytocin. If labor is going well, you should request that the drip be turned off to see if you can maintain the contractions on your own. If this doesn't happen, the Pitocin can be hooked back up again.

An induced labor doesn't figure into many women's fantasies about birth, but under certain circumstances, it is necessary. It may not be the easiest way to begin, but it doesn't necessarily have to ruin your experience. When properly handled, it can even save you from a cesarean, and that's no small thing today. You can still have a good birth experience, even if one of its components was Pitocin.

We know all of this sounds unappealing, but there's some consolation in the fact that induced labors are usually shorter than normal ones. Your labor may be pretty intense, but you will see your baby in a little while.

CHAPTER 9

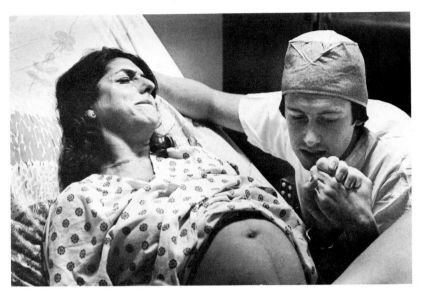

Active Labor and Transition

ACTIVE LABOR

When you are in active labor, you will know it. Yes, there are some women who feel vague pains and then leave for the hospital to discover they are eight centimeters dilated, but they are truly exceptional. For most women, active labor is powerful, recognizable, and compelling.

As we described in chapter 4, active labor generally occurs between four and seven centimeters of dilation and produces contractions that are stronger, longer, more frequent, and more regular than those experienced during early labor. For a first pregnancy, the average length of this phase is three to four hours, although it can last as long as ten hours and still be considered normal. Contractions are generally one minute long, with rests of two to three minutes between each one.

Active labor will require your undivided attention, and you'll no longer be able to walk, talk, or to be distracted through a contraction. Women in active labor have a tendency to become inwardly focused and they are less observant of their surroundings than they were in early labor. The repetitive alternation of breathing and relaxing becomes mesmerizing, and everything fades as you focus on each contraction. Relaxation by itself may no longer be enough to help you cope with the pain, but the combination of conscious relaxation and rhythmic breathing will enable you to ride the wave of each contraction. Suddenly it will become clear how the Lamaze technique works and why you have been practicing.

GETTING TO THE HOSPITAL OR BIRTH CENTER*

This is the time that both you and your partner will begin thinking about leaving for the hospital. As we've said before, most couples arrive there too soon rather than too late. As long as you are comfortable, stay put. Trust that you will know when you'll want the security of medical support. If you're perplexed about whether it's time, it's probably not. If you need a more concrete guideline, consider going to the hospital when contractions have been about four minutes apart for at least an hour.

As we keep stressing, you should try to remain at home as long as you are physically and emotionally comfortable. It's really discouraging to get to the hospital and discover you've dilated to only one centimeter. Sometimes a laboring woman will feel fine at home, but her partner will be entertaining fantasies about having to deliver the baby. If this happens to you, reassure him that everything's fine and attempt to channel this nervous energy into something constructive, like going to

*Most of the information in this chapter applies to hospital birth rather than birth-center birth.

PAIN

♦

"My labor was extremely painful. I felt as if my insides were being torn out of me."

♦

"I could easily have twenty children! I've had worse pain from soccer and gymnastic injuries."

♦

"I tried to convince myself that I was feeling pressure, and by power of suggestion, I felt a little more comfortable."

♦

"I even loved the pain, because I knew it was getting me closer."

♦

"The pain was constant, with peaks and valleys but no real break between contractions. I was totally unprepared for the intensity of the pain; nothing I had read and no one I had talked to had really prepared me for it."

♦

"The pain was not outrageous to me. It's only pain I don't understand that I can't bear."

♦

"Not pain, but severe discomfort. I felt like my uterus was going to pick me up and throw me out the window!"

♦

"I'm sensitive to pain, but there was no pain that I couldn't bear for the length of time it lasted."

continued

PAIN

♦

"The best way for me to describe the feeling is *isolation.* Your coach, nurse, doctor can help, but when you get right down to it, labor is something *you* have to cope with. No one else can take the pain for a few minutes and give you a break."

♦

"It was worse than I expected, but not so bad I wouldn't do it again."

♦

"I kept thinking I wanted to freeze this moment as I was feeling intense, intense pain. I was aware of a sort of anthropologic connection with all women through history—centuries and millennia of childbirthing pain."

♦

"I had a very easy, short labor, and the most painful thing was waiting."

♦

"My mother always told me that you would forget all the pain when you saw your child. Well, I still remember, but I'd do it again in a minute."

♦

"Very painful, but it seemed as if I were in a daze. I could hear everyone around me and knew they were there, but I wasn't really aware of them. It felt as if I were standing on the outside of myself, watching everything that was going on."

♦

"It was very uncomfortable, but I never felt like screaming the way women do in movies! I had a positive attitude, and my husband's presence was terrific. Prayer helped, too."

♦

continued

"I can honestly say my labor was not painful. It was wonderful! I enjoyed every minute of it, and as soon as the baby was born, I was sorry it was over. My sisters hated their deliveries and they say I'm crazy because I liked mine so much."

◆

"I thought labor was the most painful thing that I've ever been put through in my life. I told my husband that being hit by a semitrailer would have hurt less, because you would at least be unconscious."

◆

"It wasn't painful for me except when my daughter's head was crowning. I felt I was being stretched more than possible, and it burned."

◆

"I quickly realized I could not escape the pain and let it come over me, each contraction, yielding to it and emerging out the other side. It could not be fought."

the store or walking the dog. (One couple we know had a real disagreement about when to leave. The husband prevailed because he headed for the door, saying, "I don't know about you, but I'm going to the hospital.")

Sometimes women feel frightened and confused as active labor takes off. This is the phase when contractions become quite painful and when the novelty of being in labor has worn off. You'll know you have hit active labor when you ask yourself what you'll do if the pain gets worse. Early labor can be fun; active labor is not. It has been described as a "time of shifting gears, a time of giving in and letting go." Women often require much guidance at this point. The person who will provide that is your partner. He will breathe with you, time contractions, massage your back, fetch things to drink, answer the phone, call the doctor or midwife, and be there just to comfort you.

We presume that your suitcase and Lamaze bag are packed (see chapter 7), but there will be some last-minute things, such as a toothbrush, chilled champagne, food, and a cold pack, to be thrown in. You should also bring along anything that is proving useful to you at home, such as a hot-water bottle, pillows, or a picture used as a focal point. Your partner can call the doctor or midwife to say you will be leaving soon. Actually, this exit can be one of the longest you've ever experienced, because you will have to stop each time you have a contraction.

The best way to get to the hospital is to have someone drive both of you. If your partner doesn't have to watch the road, he can help with your breathing or massage your back. This also means you will not have to wait alone while he parks the car. Obviously, it's not always possible to find someone to chauffeur you in the middle of the night, but in big cities, you may be able to take a cab. Calling a taxi service is easier than trying to hail a cab.

If your partner is driving, don't allow him to run all the red lights. Each bump will intensify the pain, and the ride can seem excruciatingly long. You will be convinced you are further along in your labor than you are. If this is your first labor, the chances of your having the baby en route are negligible. Try to get comfortable with some pillows in the backseat or recline the passenger's seat if that's possible.

GETTING TO THE HOSPITAL

♦

"When we were going to the hospital, I was still doing first-phase breathing because I needed my husband to do the second-phase breathing, and he had to drive. So he just kept one hand on the wheel and the other on my belly and talked me through."

AT THE HOSPITAL

There are two possibilities once you arrive at the hospital: Should you park the car with your partner, or should he drop you at the door and then take care of the car? We advocate going to the parking lot with him, if you can stand it. If not, he should drop you at the entrance, and you should wait right there until he arrives. In any case, you should stay together, so you can go through the preliminary hospital routines as a team.

Most hospitals insist that you stop by the admitting department on your way to the obstetrics ward, even if you have preregistered. If you're too uncomfortable to wait while forms are filled out, it can be done later, either by your partner returning to the office or by a clerk coming up to the labor room. The admissions office can be a boobytrap in the normal hospital process, because laboring women and their partners often get separated there. This won't happen to you if you are adamant about staying together. Unfortunately, you may have to be adamant.

Once you arrive on the obstetrics floor, you will be shown to a labor room, and there a nurse will go through the standard admissions procedure. This usually includes a temperature check, a blood pressure reading, a urine sample, a short medical history, and a few questions about the progress of labor and what you've had to eat or drink. You will be given a hospital gown to wear, and the nurse will check the baby's heartbeat by hooking you up to an external fetal monitor or by listening with a stethoscope. You shouldn't be concerned about any of this; it's all routine fare for laboring women and none of it means there's anything wrong with you or your baby. (You can be detached from the fetal monitor as soon as a pattern has been established.)

If you are having your baby at a teaching hospital and your doctor's not already there, a resident will probably be the one to do the first internal exam. This is to make sure you're really in labor and it is standard procedure, but if you are a private patient, you don't have to permit it. We don't think there's anything inherently wrong with a resident doing one cervical check for purposes of admission, especially if you want to know your progress. If contractions have stopped or if you're less than one centimeter dilated, you'll probably be sent home, in which case there's no sense in having your doctor leave the office.

If you are in active labor, however, your doctor or midwife should be at the hospital within the hour, and any further checks should be performed by him. There's only one instance in which you should refuse a preliminary exam by a resident, and that's if your water has broken. The risk of infection increases greatly after the first vaginal exam, and since your doctor will want to perform his own exam when he arrives, it's prudent to wait.

We object to a resident making repeated checks because he is watching your labor on behalf of your doctor, who is someplace else. We also object to repeated vaginal exams by a variety of people for purposes of instruction. At a teaching hospital, you will meet residents, interns, medical students, and student nurses. They are all learning how to practice medicine and they'll practice on you, if you let them.

Theoretically, unless your life is at stake, no one except your doctor is permitted to touch you without your explicit permission. We're not advising that you refuse the assistance of a resident, we're just saying you should know your rights and assert them when necessary. If your concentration is being shattered or your breathing interrupted by hospital staff, your partner should nicely but firmly ask them to leave. No one but your doctor and a labor nurse has to be in your room. A laboring woman is under no obligation to be a good sport for the benefit of medical education.

The Pubic Shave, Enema, and Intravenous

While we're on the subject of assertiveness, we should mention that there may be other moments during the admission process when you must speak up about what you want. Unfortunately, some hospitals will still try to give you a pubic shave, an enema, and an intravenous. As we've said before, the only hospital procedures you must undergo are the ones you and your doctor have decided upon. All doctors practice differently, and this difference is reflected in the orders left for their patients. For example, the nurses know that Dr. Smith's patients get an IV at five centimeters, whereas Dr. Jones's don't have one unless they are dehydrated.

All parts of the prep are unnecessary, but the pubic shave has got to be the most useless of all. It's an annoying and dehumanizing procedure which causes great discomfort a few weeks later when the hair begins to grow back. A pubic shave was once thought to decrease the chance of infection, but several studies have disproved this theory. One study even found the risk of infection to be greater with a shave because of the incidence of razor nicks. *The Practical Manual of Obstetrical Care,* edited by Frederick Zuspan and Edward Quilligan, states: "There is no evidence that shaving the perineum alters the incidence of postpartum infection or breakdown of the episiotomy." If your doctor demands the shave be done, ask him for a copy of the study which encourages this archaic practice.

We were amazed at how many of the women who filled out our questionnaire had pubic shaves. Women who didn't get full shaves received a miniprep, in which just the area between the vagina and rectum (the episiotomy site) was shaved. This is an improvement over a total clip, but still unnecessary.

Enemas don't appeal to us, but many women want them so that they won't have to worry about having a bowel movement during delivery. There is, however, no medical justification for requiring an enema. *The Practical Manual on Obstetrical Care* says, "There is no evidence that an enema stimulates labor, despite the widely held belief. Unless the rectum is greatly distended with hard or impacted tissues, the discomfort imposed by this procedure is not warranted."

In many cases, women experience a slight diarrhea during early labor, making an enema doubly unnecessary. You shouldn't really worry about defecating while pushing because if it does happen, it's no big deal and it's something everyone has seen before.

Using some gentle persuasion, you should be able to avoid the pubic shave and enema, but it may be a bit more difficult to negotiate regarding the use of an IV. Some doctors don't hook you up immediately to an IV, but they will want one in place once active labor begins. If your doctor insists on this intervention for you, he will probably cite the two following reasons:

+ It keeps a vein open in case of emergency. If you should hemorrhage or go into shock after delivery, your veins can collapse, making it more difficult to insert an IV and necessary medication.
+ It will keep you hydrated. Most hospitals don't allow food or drink during labor (although they will allow a woman to suck on ice chips), and that tends to make women dehydrated and fatigued, particularly those with long labors. This is why the IV consists of a solution of dextrose and water.

Using an IV to prevent dehydration seems almost contradictory. If you were just allowed to drink, you wouldn't get dehydrated. The rationale for prohibiting the intake of liquids during labor is that if an emergency arose and general anesthesia had to be given, there would be a risk of asphyxiation from vomiting, since it is true that drinking fluids increases the likelihood of vomiting under anesthesia. But even if you fast for two days, there's a chance you could vomit, aspirate stomach secretions, and die. This is, in fact, the more dangerous situation because stomach contents after fasting are so acidic, chemical irritation and infection can occur. This is known as Mendelson's syndrome and is the leading cause of anesthetic deaths in obstetrics and the fourth leading cause of all obstetrical deaths. We're not suggesting you eat full meals during labor, just that you be allowed to prevent dehydration by drinking liquids. It seems excessively conservative to withhold liquids from all women when only a tiny percentage would require general anesthesia, especially since this prohibition does not totally eliminate risk.

You may feel reassured to have an IV in place, but most women find it immobilizing, uncomfortable, and even painful. It causes a subtle psychological change in the way you feel and the way you're treated by the hospital staff. You go from being a healthy woman in labor to being a patient on an IV. It takes a lot of motivation to get out of bed and drag the thing behind you on a rolling pole. An IV actually makes it too handy to administer medication. It promotes intervention just because it's there. It takes so little effort to give you a dose of something with the IV all set up.

In lieu of a routine IV, we prefer a wait-and-see attitude. An IV can always be put in if you become dehydrated. If your doctor is particularly insistent, he may have had a patient who actually did go into shock. Although rationally he knows there is little chance this will happen to you, he may not be willing to capitulate on this issue. As a compromise, you might suggest the Heparin lock. This is a plastic catheter that is inserted in a vein and then attached to a two-way valve. The tube is taped to your wrist and leaves you virtually unencumbered, but prepared for a complication, since medication can be given through the valve.

If you absolutely must have an intravenous or a Heparin lock, make sure that it's put in a comfortable spot. The inside of the forearm is the preferred location. The top of the hand should only be used as a backup, since it is a more sensitive area. If you're in a teaching hospital, a resident is most likely to insert your IV. There is no reason to want your doctor to do this, because a resident gets lots of practice and should be quite adept.

Fetal Monitoring

The fetal monitor is a machine that shows the baby's heartbeat, your contractions, and the relationship between the two. Until the beginning of the 1970s, the heartbeat was listened to (auscultated) with a fetoscope, but today electronic fetal monitors have replaced the human ear.

There are two types of monitors: external (noninvasive) and internal (invasive). Both look like large boxes with dials, similar to a stereo receiver, and they are wheeled about on metal stands about as high as your bed. To use the *external monitor,* two straps will be placed around your stomach; they are connected by two wires to the monitor. Some gel will be rubbed on your abdomen to provide contact for the electronic leads. The upper strap will record your contractions, and the lower holds an ultrasonic transducer to detect the baby's heart rate. Both your contractions and the fetal heartbeat will be recorded on graph paper, which runs through the monitor. Some machines have a microphone, amplifying the baby's heartbeat; it can be turned off if it's too distracting. There will also be a small flashing light on the machine and sometimes a flashing digital number, providing a computation of the baby's heartbeats per minute (normally in the range of 120 to 160 beats per minute).

With the *internal monitor* the lower strap is replaced with a long wire that is attached directly to the baby's scalp by a clip or screw electrode. In order to insert a fetal-scalp monitor, the cervix must be dilated at least two centimeters and the amniotic sac must be broken. The internal fetal-heart monitor is considered more accurate than the external, and it is often used when Pitocin or an epidural is given. Sometimes a second catheter is inserted into the uterine cavity to measure the contractions, and this replaces the external upper strap.

The purpose of a fetal monitor is to determine how well the baby's supply of oxygen is being maintained during labor. Decreased blood flow can occur if the mother is lying flat on her back, if there are problems with the umbilical cord or the placenta, or if the dosage of Pitocin is too strong. Often the patterns revealed by the monitor will indicate the particular problem. The three types of patterns are:

+ *Type I.* This pattern is a reverse image of the contraction. The fetal heart rate is at its slowest when the uterine contraction is at its strongest. This is a physiologic phenomenon, and a reassuring sign of fetal well-being.
+ *Type II.* These patterns are called late decelerations and are of an

abnormal nature. Here the fetal heart rate begins to drop (even slightly) close to the end of the uterine contraction. This occurs because the baby's oxygen supply is diminished, possibly because of poor placental transfer. The baby doesn't have enough of a reserve for the forty to sixty seconds during the contraction while the blood supply is diminished. This could be dangerous, and the baby's condition will be assessed, if possible, with a fetal-scalp sample.

♦ *Type III.* These are varied decelerations that occur due to intermittent interruptions in the supply of oxygen and nutrients to the baby. It may occur during a contraction if there is a cord wrapped once or twice around the baby's neck, when downward pressure during the contraction causes a brief interruption or a diminished supply of oxygen. There will be a sudden drop in the fetal heart rate (to about 80 beats per minute), it will stay there during the contraction, and then it will recover once the contraction is over. A deceleration can also occur between contractions if there is a compression of the cord between the baby's body and limbs and the amniotic sac. If this happens, the mother's position will be changed, she will be given more fluids (usually intravenously) and oxygen through a mask. A fetal-scalp sample may be taken, too.

With both Type II and Type III patterns, the baby's condition will determine the course of events. If fetal-scalp samples show sufficient oxygen, nothing more will be done. If this is not the case, the baby will need to be delivered quickly, either by forceps or by cesarean section.

One last element, especially of concern for high-risk patients, is the beat-to-beat variability of the fetal heart rate in general. This can be measured only by internal fetal monitoring. Normal circumstances indicate a fetal heart rate that varies from five to ten beats from the baseline. A rhythm that shows no variability could mean fetal distress.

A baby's heartbeat is normally in the range of 120 to 160 beats per minute. In addition to the late and varied deceleration patterns, distress can also be indicated when the heartbeat goes above the normal rate (tachycardia) or below (bradycardia).

Monitors are controversial. Proponents of the machine attribute lower infant mortality rates to their widespread use. Opponents refute this and link the use of monitors to the escalating cesarean rate. Doctors claim that monitors now constitute accepted medical practice and consider it foolhardy from a legal standpoint to do without them. Many couples don't like the idea of interventions during labor, yet they are afraid not to utilize the monitor, afraid that fetal distress could go undetected.

A fetal monitor is not without risks. It's a gadget subject to malfunction and the error of human interpretation. Studies have shown cesarean rates to rise dramatically immediately after monitors were introduced in a hospital, but once people learned how to use the machines, the rates dropped. Sometimes a monitor can give out many "false abnormal" readings that show fetal distress but are really machine malfunctions. Other common operational problems include: the electrode falling off, causing the baby's heartbeat to disappear; the monitor picking up the mother's slower heartbeat instead of the baby's; the baby moving out of range; and the monitor picking up indiscriminate tracings from the mother's movement or vibrations in the room, which interfere with an accurate reading of the baby's heartbeat.

No one doubts the benefits of monitoring for high-risk women—such as those with kidney disease, a history of stillborns, or high or low blood pressure—but the benefits for low-risk women have not been proved. In 1979 Dr. Stephen Thacker, of the Centers for Disease Control, and Dr. David Banta, of the federal Office of Technology Assessment, reviewed the literature on fetal monitoring. Their conclusion was that there is no evidence to show that monitoring is of any benefit in low-risk labors and that it carries substantial risks, including a greater chance of cesarean section. They noted that the monitor lacks the precision to distinguish normal from abnormal heart rates. This can result in unnecessary cesareans as well as cases of real fetal distress going undetected.

The external fetal monitor works best when you're lying down. No woman in labor wants to be immobilized, and the supine position can be excruciating, especially with back labor. Yet many women who filled out our questionnaires reported being forced to lie in this position. If you have complete freedom of movement, you'll feel more comfortable and therefore be less likely to need medication. Also, if you can sit up or walk, the force of gravity will aid your contractions and you will be less likely to require Pitocin. We have also heard complaints that nurses tend to focus on the fetal monitor rather than on the woman herself. When nurses listened to the baby's heartbeat by fetoscope, there was certainly more physical contact and perhaps more attention. Sometimes, it almost seems that the monitor has taken over the labor and everyone, including the woman herself, is focused on the machine.

We were surprised, however, to discover in reading the responses to our questionnaires that there were many couples who really liked the fetal monitor. The one great advantage, cited again and again, was that it was comforting to hear the baby's heartbeat throughout labor and know that everything was all right. The women also liked having their partners announce the points when a contraction was beginning, peaking, and fading. This can be a big help with the breathing, and it certainly permits a woman and her partner to work as a team. The disadvantage of this technique is that you both begin to rely on the machine rather than on your feelings to determine the strength of contractions and the progress of your labor.

There's nothing inherently wrong with fetal monitoring; it just shouldn't become the focus of your labor and it shouldn't prevent you from assuming a comfortable position. We suggest that you have the external monitor on intermittently, perhaps for five or ten minutes out of every thirty or forty minutes. If the heartbeat is fine, there's no reason you shouldn't be able to walk around or arrange yourself comfortably in a chair or bed.

You have less mobility if an internal monitor is used. This is because it is not done routinely, but is usually required by a specific condition, such as administration of Pitocin or anesthesia, demonstration of fetal distress, or maternal diabetes. The internal monitor carries a risk of infection—about 10 percent—for the mother, and most people become quite squeamish when they learn the electrode is attached to their baby's scalp. It's more accurate than the external monitor, however, and your doctor may dismiss the idea of a cesarean if the internal monitor doesn't reveal a difficulty. Contrary to popular belief, the use of the internal monitor does not prevent mobility. The electrode can be detached from the wires leading to the machine and then taped to the woman's inner thigh if she wants to walk around.

If There Are Signs of Fetal Distress

If the external monitor shows signs of fetal distress and all possibility of a mechanical problem has been eliminated (they've already tried changing machines), there are three things that are done:

- You will be asked to lie on your side. If one side doesn't work, you will try the other. The fetal distress could be caused by cord compression or by reduced blood flow to the uterus because of your position.

- You will be given some oxygen. This will give the baby a little boost and often brings the heart rate back to its normal pattern.
- If you are getting Pitocin, it will be turned off, so that the uterus can rest more completely between contractions.

If the heartbeat stabilizes, nothing further need be done. If, however, the baby's heart rate is still showing distress, you will probably be switched to an internal fetal monitor.

Fetal-Scalp Sampling

If the distress is still present, a fetal-scalp sampling may be done. In this procedure, a small sample of blood is taken from the baby's head, and its pH is tested. This reading will indicate how much oxygen the baby is receiving and whether it is safe to proceed with labor. The normal pH of fetal scalp blood is above 7.25; readings between 7.25 and 7.20 suggest that hypoxia (oxygen deprivation) may be occurring; and a reading of below 7.20 indicates that hypoxia is definitely present. If the scalp sampling determines the baby is in real distress, a cesarean or quick forceps delivery will be done.

LABORING AT THE HOSPITAL

It can take an hour or more, what with all the tests and comings and goings, to get settled in your labor room. Once this occurs, your contractions may intensify or they may peter out. Both responses are normal reactions to a new environment. In either case, the thing to do is to close the door, cover up the clock, and focus on each contraction, one at a time. Your state of mind will depend a great deal on how much progress you've achieved. If you're barely one centimeter, natural childbirth may be the furthest thing from your mind, but if you've managed to dilate to five centimeters, you'll probably feel quite positive. Whatever your situation, now is the moment to dig in and get serious about having your baby.

If your contractions have slowed down or stopped, you should get out of bed and walk around. Don't lie in bed waiting for labor to pick up. If you have an intravenous, ask that it be attached to a pole and drag the pole around with you. As we said earlier, if your doctor wants you on a fetal monitor, try to use it intermittently, so that you can walk around.

ACTIVE LABOR

♦

"I had to concentrate and wanted to be left alone. I didn't even want the bed to be jarred. I felt exhausted and wondered how long I could last."

♦

"Contractions came hard and fast and were very regular. It took a lot of determination and concentration to get through my breathing patterns. I didn't move or talk or want to be touched."

♦

"I was permitted to take a long shower about halfway through my labor, which helped a great deal to relax me and give me a second wind. I hadn't slept for about thirty-six hours."

♦

"I was sent to the hospital by my doctor, who didn't show up himself for twelve hours. I was unable to sleep in the hospital, with the IV, fetal monitor, and noise. We were tired and angry."

♦

"It was difficult for me to separate active-phase and transition because I went from four to ten centimeters in less than two hours."

♦

"The initial excitement wore off, I was tired and tried to nap between contractions. The monitor and periodic checks by the nurse were uncomfortable. I was awed by the strength of the contractions and I realized I had to focus on the breathing and relax as much as possible."

♦

"Even though this labor was relatively short, I think some of my distress came from the feeling of not having control over what was happening. I felt my body

continued

was a machine going through these contractions and I could not stop it or help it."

♦

"I imagined a roller-coaster ride during contractions: up, up, peak, down, down."

♦

"Both my husband and I were elated when the nurse checked me and said I was eight centimeters dilated. Not thirty minutes before, I had been 4 centimeters."

If labor has stalled, walking is a most effective way of bringing on contractions.

Some labors are harder to get moving than others. If your contractions are still not as regular as they were at home, you might try some nipple stimulation. This method is commonly used by midwives and is now gaining acceptance among obstetricians. Your partner can massage your breasts or you can do this yourself. You should also attempt to just relax, because sometimes the tension of being in a hospital can stall labor. Do some deep-breathing exercises and ask your partner to give you a massage. If there's a shower available, take one. This is an excellent way to release inhibitions and just unwind.

Sometimes contractions of similar intensity can seem more painful in the hospital than at home. This occurs because you may feel less in control, or because a hospital can be a frightening place. If your contractions suddenly seem much bigger and harder to handle, try to forestall panic. Attempt to make yourself oblivious to the new surroundings and adjust your breathing to whatever feels good. Your partner can sponge you with cool water, feed you ice chips, fix the bed, or do whatever you find comforting.

The Presence of Your Doctor or Midwife

If a midwife is delivering your baby, she will probably be at your side soon after you arrive at the hospital or birth center. If you have a doctor, he ordinarily comes to the hospital after you have been admitted. Where he will spend your labor is another matter, and it's a subject you should have discussed with him during an office visit. Women have very different expectations of where their doctor should be until it is time to catch the baby, ranging from being somewhere in the hospital to hovering at bedside, doing Lamaze breathing with her.

It's impossible to dictate correct behavior in this circumstance because so much depends on what you want and what kind of labor you have. If you're dilating slowly but normally and it's the middle of the night, there doesn't seem to be any harm in your doctor catching a few winks in the lounge. But on the other hand, if you're having telescopic labor and are sure you're dying, your doctor shouldn't be having a snack in the cafeteria. Some women want to be left alone with their partners during labor, others want as much medical supervision as possible. Ideally, you should be able to tell your doctor how available you want him to be.

The Plateau Phenomenon

Sometimes at around five centimeters of dilation, progress seems to slow down or stop. This hesitance, which we call a plateau, can occur in active labor or even in transition. A common scenario is strong contractions and dilation to five centimeters. Two hours later, contractions have maintained their intensity, but dilation remains at five centimeters. An hour later, no further progress has been made, and two hours after that, dilation still rests at five centimeters.

This phenomenon is known as *failure to progress* and it has to be one of the most discouraging patterns of labor. A 1980 study done by the National Institute of Health on the great increase in cesareans cited failure to progress as the single most important contributor to the rising cesarean rate. Failure to progress is frequently confused with cephalopelvic disproportion, but that condition is believed to occur in only about 2 percent of all deliveries. Sometimes a doctor will perform a cesarean because of failure to progress and then say as a kind of after-

P L A T E A U

•

"By 2:00 P.M. I was six centimeters dilated. I went into the office, and the doctor sent me to the hospital. Things slowed down when I got there."

•

"I stayed at two fingers dilated for almost ten hours and then jumped to ten. After that it was only another hour and a half until my daughter was born."

•

"I was three centimeters dilated and two weeks late when I was finally induced. After hours and hours of being on and off the Pitocin, I was still only 3 centimeters dilated. At one point I said, 'I can't take this much longer.' My doctor had examined me forty-five minutes earlier and then had gone off the floor, but I insisted that the resident examine me. He did and said, 'Oops! Just a rim left!' Then I felt the need to go to the bathroom (a classic symptom, I was later told), and suddenly I was fully dilated and ready to start pushing."

•

"Contractions slowed down once I got to the hospital. After two hours, my doctor suggested taking some castor oil but thought it would be easier to send my husband to the drugstore for it than dealing with the hospital staff. I guess the reality of the castor oil hit me, because by the time my husband got back, my contractions were booming."

thought, "Oh, your pelvis was too small anyhow." However, most failure to progress is simply that, a stalling or failure of labor, and has nothing to do with the size of your pelvis.

Generally, a plateau is a physical manifestation of a psychological occurrence. It usually comes at a time when there is no turning back, when everything must be surrendered to the labor, when the hard work is about to begin. During this kind of plateau, women and their partners often insist on frequent cervical checks, but this is misguided, because lack of progress gets everyone discouraged. Also, the exams can be uncomfortable, adding new discomfort when you are already becoming tired and less tolerant. In addition, if the water has broken, examinations will increase the chance of infection.

In this situation, cervical checks are requested because women want to know how much longer it will take and how much longer it will hurt. This thinking is not going to help dilation; labor takes as long as it takes, and that's all there is to it. You shouldn't be looking for external verification of internal feelings. What you should be doing is trying to let go. When labor stalls, you must do what your intuition tells you feels right. This may mean removing the monitor and going for a walk, having a snack, taking a shower, calling a friend, yelling out or having a good cry. Surprisingly, loss of control can help, because tears produce a tremendous release of tension, which will allow labor to proceed.

Last spring we attended a Lamaze workshop that was taught by veteran instructor Anne Rose. She recounted attending the labor of a friend, who was having her first child. This woman was admitted to the hospital with little dilation, but once there, labor began to progress slowly, up until the point of four centimeters. Then everything stopped for several hours. The doctor had left the room, talking about Pitocin, when this woman's husband noticed that her rear end was peeking through the gap of her hospital gown. Impulsively, he leaned over and kissed it, saying, "You've always had the greatest behind." Well, that gesture seemed to be the equivalent of a megadose of Pitocin, because contractions increased in intensity, and about fifteen minutes later the woman had the urge to push. Anne then ran out to get the doctor to do a cervical exam. He almost refused because he couldn't believe dilation could occur so quickly. He was wrong, and the baby was born within the hour.

Anne's explanation for what happened was that even though her friend was fully prepared and totally committed to having her baby, there was a part of her that was unable to let go. That one quick kiss made her feel confident and comfortable enough to let things proceed. Although this story is a little unusual, there often can be one tactic or one moment in a labor that can make a big difference. The difficult part is figuring out what works for you. Our best advice is to do what feels right to you at that particular moment.

TRANSITION

This is the part everyone dreads, and we'd be dishonest if we didn't tell you it can be bad. Fortunately transition is the shortest phase of labor, lasting about an hour and consisting of roughly ten to twenty contractions. It's the most difficult stage of labor because it comes at the end (8 to 10 centimeters) when you're the most tired. It's also the stage when you are the most tuned in to your body, feeling every breath, every movement as the cervix opens to its fullest extent. In some ways it's horrible, in some ways it's great.

The difficult part about transition is that when your contractions are the most intense, they will lose their wavelike pattern and predictability. It's not unusual to have a double or triple contraction or a very short rest period between contractions.

Not everyone experiences this, however, and for some the pace of labor continues unaltered. Transition can also include its own special sort of symptoms, which may make you feel pretty sick on top of it all. There are six classic symptoms of transition. Although you won't have all of them, it's good to know what they are. These feelings can be scary, but you should understand they are a normal part of labor, signaling that you're very close to having your baby.

- *Irritability.* Some women can be grouchy all throughout labor, but often a sudden ferociousness makes it very clear that transition has begun. This feeling is most frequently directed to the person closest to you, your partner, and neither one of you should feel sensitive afterward. Many women we know have been nasty to their husbands during transition, but the men have never taken it personally. Women in transition commonly say things like, "I'm never having another baby," or "I've had it, let's go home," or "Don't tell me what to do, I'm the one in labor, not you." You may develop an extreme skin sensitivity and announce that you don't want to be touched. This doesn't mean you're not relaxing properly, it just means you're in transition.
- *Nausea.* This is a very common symptom of transition and one of the worst. The best thing is to just let go and throw up, because you'll feel better afterward. Letting go is what you need to do, and throwing up often leads directly to full dilation. Every labor room is equipped with kidney-shaped basins you can use.
- *Chills.* Your body is exhibiting a classic shock reaction when you get

♦

"All I knew was that it would eventually be over if I could just hang in there. After all, you certainly can't stop and say, 'Excuse me, I'd like to leave now.' "

♦

"While in labor I kept thinking that anyone who does this twice should be committed. But sitting here two days later with the baby, I'd do it again."

♦

"It was the most painful going through transition while in the bathroom after an enema, without a coach."

♦

"I kept trying to figure out if I could kill myself without hurting the baby."

♦

"My grandmother told me I would enter 'the valley of the shadow of death' and then suddenly return. She was exactly right . . . but it was completely worth it."

♦

"I thought to myself, 'This can't go on forever.' It seemed like many hours. My husband thought the time flew by—but I felt as if the clock had stopped!"

♦

"During transition, I wanted the whole pharmacy in my veins. But later I was glad I was able to be awake to see our baby being born."

♦

"It took a lot of determination and concentration to get through my breathing patterns. I didn't move or talk or want to be touched at all."

the shakes. Your feet feel like they're freezing, and your arms and legs start twitching uncontrollably. This can happen during transition as well as after the delivery. Have your partner get your socks from your Lamaze bag and ask the nurse for an extra blanket.

+ *Bloody show.* This is different from the loss of the mucous plug that heralded the beginning of labor. As the cervix stretches, tiny capillaries can break, producing bright red bleeding. Don't be alarmed, just be excited that labor is finally ending.

+ *Backache.* Even though the baby is not posterior, backache is common during transition. Your partner should try all the tricks for dealing with back labor—massaging, exerting counterpressure, or applying hot or cold packs. You may consider a stabbing backache to be the final straw, but don't despair—it will be gone in a few contractions.

+ *Desire for medication.* This is often the time when, despite a prior commitment to natural childbirth, you're ready for the entire pharmacy. Although it's the most common time to ask for medication, it is also the worst in terms of both the progress of your labor and its effects on your baby (see chapter 11). Bear in mind that this is the shortest phase of labor and that in just a few more minutes you will be able to start pushing.

In addition to all the things we have just described, you may also feel an urge to push. As the baby descends, pressure is exerted against the broad ligaments of the spine, triggering a reflex urge to bear down. This shows great progress, but don't push until you are examined. If dilation is not yet complete, pressure from early pushing will cause the cervix to swell, decreasing dilation. Often, you will spend the latter part of transition blowing to offset the strong desire to push. (To review this breathing pattern, see page 95.) This can be very frustrating, because you're dealing with the most difficult part of your labor while trying to prevent yourself from doing what feels right.

Loss of perspective is a sure sign of transition. At this point, women frequently ask for a cesarean so that they can be put out of their misery. They feel as if they have been in labor forever and can't make a connection between what's happening to their bodies and the coming of the baby. Labor is regarded as a sadomasochistic conspiracy among their partner, doctor or midwife (no one is sacred), and the hospital staff. This is the time when every woman knows she can't take any more pain. It's often hard to convince someone in transition that it won't get worse, because that argument defies her experience of labor. But in almost every case, contractions do subside in frequency and intensity during the expulsion phase.

Transition is the time when some women are ready to throw in the towel. Others, however, take a perverse pleasure in this phase and enjoy it, knowing they are so close to the end.

CHAPTER **10**

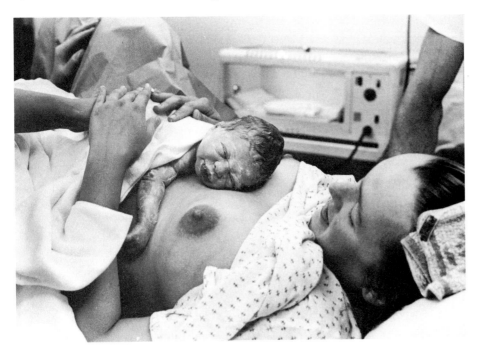

Birth

PUSHING

*M*any women regard pushing as the hardest, but most rewarding work they've ever done. Transition ends at last when the doctor or midwife says, "Okay, you're fully dilated. You can push now." This stage is a completely different experience from labor, and making the change from relaxation and conscious breathing to vigorous activity is often difficult.

Even if you have a strong urge to push, you will be surprised by the immense effort involved and the amount of energy needed. For some women, pushing is instinctive and delightful. For others it can

PUSHING

♦

"Felt great when it was okay to push! There was an excitement and a relaxation going into the delivery room where 'it' was finally going to happen."

♦

"I hated everyone who kept telling me to push! push! I *did,* but they kept yelling for me to do it again and again. I couldn't wait for it to be over."

♦

"I pushed on all fours for a while and then moved to the bed. All fours was easier. Grunting really helped. The lower and deeper the grunt, the better the push. All I could think of was getting that baby out so that my perineum would stop burning and stinging."

♦

"My doctor instructed me to 'push as if you're having a bowel movement.' I could never make sense of using those muscles and I think it could be better explained."

♦

"I felt as though I were the most powerful person in the world."

♦

"I did not enjoy pushing. It did not feel good to me as many films, books, parents have described it. It was really hard work, though not painful. I cried. I was tired. I specifically remember saying, 'I want to go home! I can't do this!' But I did it beautifully."

♦

"The undeniable fact is that it is up to you *alone* to get the baby out, and every ounce of your being comes together to do it."

♦

continued

♦

"It's like you're emptying out all the pain."

♦

"Squatting helped a lot. Also completely relaxing my muscles in that area. The more I could relax and not worry about what I looked or sounded like, the easier it was."

♦

"Between pushes I looked into the mirror and saw my baby's head crowning. It was then that I knew he was really here."

♦

"Our Lamaze teacher told us, 'Bulge your Kegel, push down and out.' The doctor said I pushed great."

♦

"It's like holding your breath and trying to move a brick wall."

♦

"I had two hours of pushing, which was very hard, but my husband would practically push with me, and that made it easier. He would get so excited when he could see the baby's head coming closer and closer that I got excited too!"

♦

"My doctor was very gentle and encouraging. He said, 'Make up your mind,' and that did it."

♦

"All of a sudden you don't have to concentrate on relaxing anymore. It felt good just to tense up and push!"

♦

continued

♦

"I found that if I waited for the first fifteen seconds of the contraction to pass and then pushed, it didn't hurt as much. I found my contractions had a peak near the end when I could push extra hard. If I followed my natural desire about when and how hard to push, it went easier."

♦

"Once I used the right muscles to push, my son was born after two pushes."

♦

"I never got the 'urge' that other women have told me happened to them. Pushing hurt, and I wasn't entirely sure I wanted to have the baby if I had to keep doing it—but the doctor jokingly told me that I'd be pregnant 'forever' if I didn't start to push."

♦

"One nurse held her finger by the vaginal opening and said to push against it, and this really helped."

♦

"I never want to hear the word *push* again!"

♦

"No matter what you learn in Lamaze, you don't really know until you give birth —especially the pushing. I didn't get the hang of pushing until the very end, and by then I was so tired I wasn't doing as well as I wanted."

♦

"Contractions began to slow down once I had to push, and it took me three hours with a Pitocin IV."

♦

continued

"A countdown to motherhood . . . painful, but a good pain that was going to end in something perfect."

♦

"I felt as though my baby had taken over; it knew what to do, and the pushing was involuntary."

♦

"It felt great! I remember burning and feeling like I would burst open, but, oh!, I wanted to push that baby out. I would watch his head crown and see lots of black hair. That was the greatest sight in the world."

♦

"It was great feeling the baby come sliding out and knowing that I did it totally naturally. It was a real sense of accomplishment for me."

♦

"The actual moment of birth was the best! The real discomfort was over; I even experienced an orgasm as her head was delivered."

be painful and exhausting, and not at all the relief they were expecting. It all depends on the position and size of the baby, the length of labor, whether you've had anesthesia, your feelings about birth, and the amount of support you have. The less of an urge you have, the more difficult pushing is; the greater your urge to push, the easier it is to do.

There's no correlation between the length of labor and the amount of time it takes to push out the baby. You can have a long first stage and a short second stage, or vice versa. There's also no correlation between the stages in terms of ease. In short, you just have to be prepared for whatever kind of labor or delivery you might get. The first-time mother spends an average of fifty-seven minutes pushing out her baby; the second-time mother averages eighteen minutes.

Often there is fear accompanying this stage, and naturally that can inhibit effective pushing. For those who are ambivalent about motherhood, this is the last chance to hold back. For most women, however, the fear is on account of the physical act of expulsion. There is a horror of being ripped apart, of being stretched so badly that you'll never be the same. Every woman is bothered by this fantastic notion to some extent, because it seems impossible that a seven-pound baby could emerge from a normal-sized vagina. Pregnancy seems unreal enough, but the fact that babies are born this way defies comprehension. The experience has been likened to having built a boat in the basement and then wondering how you will get it out.

To overcome this feeling, you must suspend your disbelief the way you did when you were three months pregnant and saw a woman who was ready to deliver. At that time you said with conviction, "I'll never get that big," but of course, you did. The emergence of the baby from the womb is perhaps the most amazing part of childbirth, and even women who have just watched themselves giving birth have a hard time believing what has just happened.

Once transition is over, contractions continue, but they occur less frequently, and they don't last as long—more like the pace of active labor. Your contractions may have piggybacked, but now they will probably space out again to three to four minutes apart. You may feel like pushing or you may have no urge at all. Either way, you will be instructed to bear down during these contractions. Now that the task of softening and opening your cervix is completed, you must work with the contractions to help the baby descend. You will push hard during each contraction, and when it stops, so will you. Although the physical effort is great, the rest periods will permit you to recoup your energy for the next contraction.

Sometimes contractions become much weaker or disappear altogether, even though you're being given permission to push. Usually they resume again in another twenty minutes or so, and this break can give you a second wind. This can be just a natural lull between stages, and nothing need be done right away. You might close your eyes for a few minutes or take a walk to encourage contractions to begin again. Many doctors or midwives, however, would want to give you Pitocin in an effort to get things going. We would advise patience as long as the baby's heartbeat remains strong. This pause isn't harmful. If it happens to you, don't worry about holding up the show. You should be the center of attention, and your rhythms should determine the pace.

The second stage of labor lasts long enough to permit ample time to find a comfortable position and figure out how to push effectively.

The Physical Process

Babies must negotiate an almost ninety-degree angle as they travel from the uterus to the vagina. Go back to the illustration on page 84 and study the pathway your baby takes. Study how the vagina and uterus form an almost ninety-degree angle. As you push, think to yourself "down and forward" while slightly rounding your pelvis. Don't push toward the rectum—it's the wrong direction. Instead, push vaginally as if you were doing the opposite of a Kegel exercise.

As you push, the baby gently stretches and opens the elastic walls of your vagina. During each contraction, the force of the uterus and your expulsive efforts will combine to cause the baby to descend. At the end of each contraction the pressure will stop and your baby will retract a bit. This gentle back-and-forth motion of two steps forward and one step back eases your vagina open and your baby toward birth.

Positions for Pushing

Unless you use a birthing room, you will do almost all of your pushing in the labor room and then move to the delivery room when the baby's head crowns. If you are in the birthing room, you remain where you are. Either way, you have great flexibility in finding comfortable positions for pushing. Try to get away from equating the postures for pushing with the position for delivery. They can be quite different. For example, you might squat for most of the time and then sit to give birth, or stand for some of the time and then lie on your side for the final pushes. Don't be afraid to try a somewhat unorthodox position if that's what feels right. You can always switch back to a more conventional position for the actual delivery.

There's no one perfect position for pushing out your baby. Any position is fine except lithotomy (lying on your back). There are three reasons for this: (a) you must push against the force of gravity; (b) it tenses the pelvic floor, creating the need for an episiotomy while increas-

Positions for Pushing

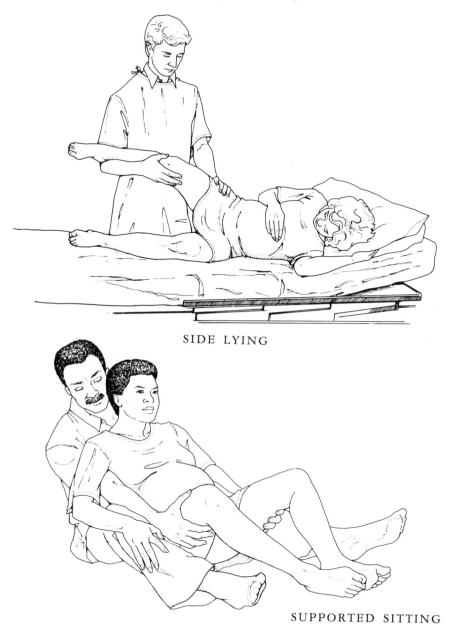

SIDE LYING

SUPPORTED SITTING

ing the chance of tearing; and (c) the baby receives less oxygen because the weight of the uterus presses on the vena cava and aorta, two of the body's major blood vessels.

All hospitals today are equipped to place women in a semireclining position by using pillows or raising the labor bed or delivery table to about a sixty-degree angle. If the baby is posterior, you will want to assume any position—squatting, side-lying, standing—that takes the weight of the baby's head off your spine. If you seem to be pushing to no avail, try another position. If you can't figure one out, you merely have to say, "I'm not comfortable, please help me find a better position." Difficulty with pushing doesn't necessarily mean your pelvis is too small or that you're not pushing hard enough; you just may be more effective in a different position.

Women commonly begin pushing in a semisitting position. This is one of the most adaptable postures because it's comfortable and you can move your legs easily. You can sit with your legs bent and your feet flat on the bed, or with your knees open and the soles of your feet together. Another variation is to allow your legs and feet to be held by your partner and the labor nurse. Or you can press your feet against your partner's shoulders, which will improve your leverage. The only leg position you should avoid is one in which you hold your knees against your chest with your feet off the bed. This tenses your perineum and is terribly uncomfortable. Unfortunately, this is a favorite among labor nurses and doctors. Simply insist that your legs be allowed to remain on the bed.

Most women throughout the world deliver their babies in a squatting position, and many childbirth experts consider it the best one because it opens the pelvis up most fully. To assume this position, you'll have to be supported on either side, most likely by your husband and the labor nurse. You could also squat unassisted for a while by leaning up against a wall or the back of your bed. In his book *Birth Reborn,* Dr. Michel Odent describes the reasons why women at his clinic in France deliver in this position: "Most women at Pithiviers give birth in the supported squatting positions. By far the most efficient from a mechanical point of view, since they maximize downward weight and minimize muscular effort and oxygen consumption and facilitate relaxation of the perineal muscles."

Two other good positions are all-fours and side-lying. The all-fours is recommended for back labor because it gets the weight off your spine. The side-lying requires someone to support your top leg, but its benefits include minimizing stretch on the perineum and facilitating blood flow to the placenta, especially if you lie on your left side. Both positions also make it easy for your partner to massage your back if the baby is posterior. Whatever position you assume, you should relax your legs between contractions. This will help prevent leg cramps.

How to Increase Your Effectiveness

To increase the ease and effectiveness of your pushing:

+ Assume an upright position
+ Relax your perineum
+ Breathe according to need
+ Contract your upper abdominal muscles
+ Round your pelvis
+ Don't get hung up on "technique"

When you push, try to take advantage of the force of the contraction and push as fully and continuously as possible. Short staccato pushes don't seem to work nearly as well as ones that maintain continuous pressure. If you are having trouble moving the baby, try to sustain each push for a slightly longer period of time. The breathing for pushing is described on page 97.

Vocalizing goes along with any great exertion, and pushing out a baby is no exception. We're not talking about bloodcurdling screams here, just ordinary grunts, groans, and yelps. Tennis players, weight lifters, and karate enthusiasts all make noises as they compete. Although your doctor or labor nurse may tell you this effort wastes valuable energy, it actually releases energy and is extremely helpful. Vocalization relaxes the pelvic floor and is a perfectly natural response during the second stage of labor.

It seems that most American obstetricians and labor nurses do a great deal of cheerleading during the expulsive phase. Sometimes husbands or anybody else in the room join in, resulting in a rather frenetic atmosphere not unlike that of an athletic event. Some women respond well to this urging; others don't. It's a matter of choice. If having three people scream, "Push, Push," helps you, that's fine. But if you find it rather confusing and overstimulating, have your partner ask them to stop so you can restore your concentration.

Dr. Odent doesn't believe in yelling at women while they are trying to deliver a baby. In *Birth Reborn* he writes, "Words are usually irrelevant at times like this and certain words—like 'push' or 'harder'—can actually have negative effects. Often the woman in childbirth knows exactly what she is feeling, and certain instructions may only conflict with her experience. I tend not to say anything. Or if I do speak, it will be something like, 'Good . . . good . . . let the baby come.' If the woman seems gripped by the fear of failure, I might suggest, 'Don't hold back; cry, shout if you want to.' "

Effective pushing usually entails a bit of trial and error. You should try different positions and different breathing patterns. Don't be dismayed if you don't get the hang of it right away. Some women take twenty or thirty minutes before they can get comfortable and begin to push effectively. Ideally, you should have spoken to your doctor before delivery about pushing positions and gotten his approval to experiment a bit. As long as everything is progressing normally, your doctor or midwife should permit you to discover the best position and technique for you.

In her book, *The Experience of Childbirth,* Sheila Kitzinger beautifully describes the importance of sensitivity to contractions during the second stage. "The important thing to remember is that one should listen to contractions in order to remain sensitive and aware of their exact nature, and be alert to any change in their character. The urge to push varies from contraction to contraction. One pushes exactly when and as long and as strongly as each indicates. It is a little like the orchestra responding to the conductor's baton. The contracting uterus is the conductor."

If There Are Problems

If pushing should continue past two hours, your doctor or midwife may begin to get concerned about the baby's well-being and the reason for such a long second stage. If this is your first baby, you will probably be given a maximum of about two and a half hours to deliver him naturally. After that point, your doctor will want to get the baby out. Three things will be monitored to make sure it is safe to continue pushing:

- *The strength of the baby's heartbeat.* Even if you've only been pushing for fifteen minutes, the baby's heartbeat will be checked. If there's any sign of a serious drop, there may be a problem with the placenta or the umbilical cord. If this happens, your doctor or midwife will decide whether a forceps or cesarean delivery is indicated. This choice will depend on the station of the baby.
- *The condition of the mother.* Maternal exhaustion can be a big problem at this point and is perhaps the number one cause of forceps deliveries. Your blood pressure and pulse will be taken to determine how well you are holding up.
- *The amount of progress being made.* This means ascertaining the station

and position of the baby. If the baby is descending, you will probably be allowed to continue. If after two hours, however, the baby still isn't engaged, this could mean your pelvis is too small (cephalo-pelvic disproportion, or CPD). It could also mean the umbilical cord is exceptionally short or that the baby's chin is not properly flexed, thereby obstructing his passage. In these cases, a cesarean would probably be performed.

On the other hand, some women, particularly those who have had children before, can push out a baby in ten seconds flat. For these women, the trick becomes *not* to push, especially until the doctor or midwife arrives on the scene. Here the thing to do is to pant or blow out hard for as long as you can. (See the correct breathing pattern for offsetting the urge to push on page 96.) This is difficult because the uterus is working against this distraction, intent on expelling the baby. If the baby is coming quickly and you are home, call your doctor or midwife or 911 and stay put. Don't ever allow anyone to instruct you to hold your legs together. This is a dangerous technique and can cause brain damage.

CROWNING

This is the moment when the baby no longer recedes into the vagina at the end of each contraction, but remains visible, revealing a silver-dollar-size swatch of hair. If you will be using a delivery room, this is when you will probably be transferred.

Crowning can be extremely painful if no episiotomy is performed. The baby's head is stretching the perineum to its maximum degree, and there is a burning sensation. You will be instructed to stop pushing; the doctor or midwife will support the perineum; and the force of the uterine contraction will ease the baby's head out. Once the baby's head has emerged, there will be a tremendous feeling of release and relief and the baby's shoulders and body will immediately follow.

If an episiotomy is performed, it is done at the moment of crowning. If it is done before this time, there will be excessive bleeding. Though the pressure of the baby's head against the perineum creates a numbing sensation, a local anesthetic is always given before the episiotomy is done. The injections are administered in a few locations in order to numb the entire area and are felt as a slight burning sensation. In this way the perineum will already be anesthetized for the stitching.

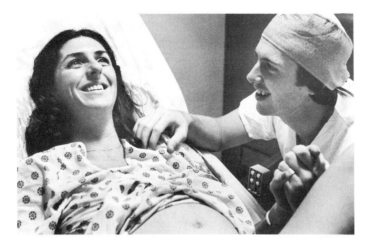

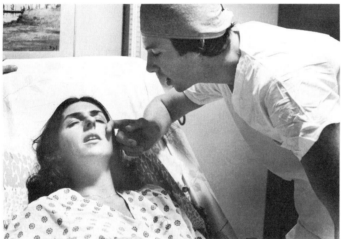

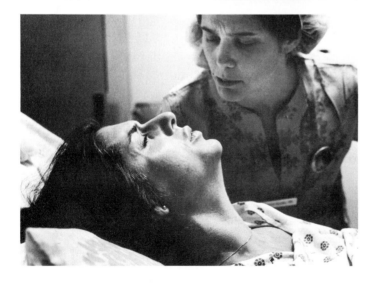

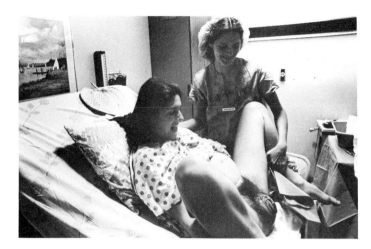

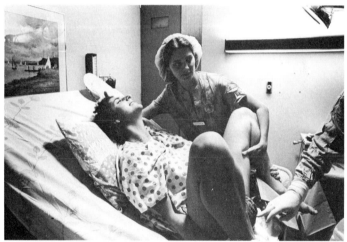

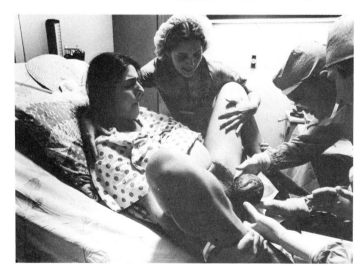

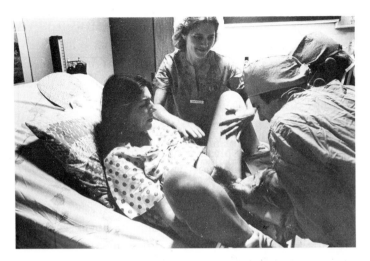

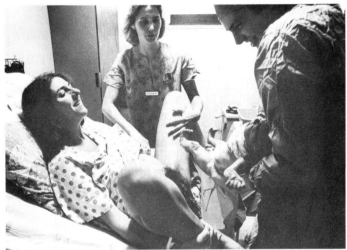

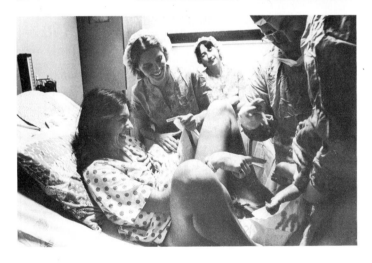

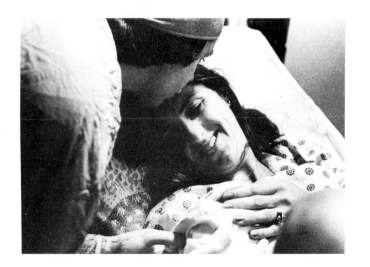

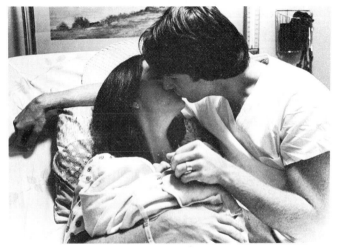

EPISIOTOMY

The episiotomy is the second most common surgical procedure in the United States today, following the cutting of the umbilical cord. Episiotomy became an accepted part of childbirth during the 1920s and '30s, the era when women changed their place of birth from home to hospital. Obstetricians are trained to do episiotomies routinely, and it is performed in 62 percent of all deliveries, with about 90 to 95 percent of all first-time mothers receiving them.

Whether or not you have an episiotomy will depend more on your choice of doctor or midwife than on any particular circumstance. Some doctors do them 100 percent of the time for first deliveries, some 50 percent, and some only 10 percent.

The depth of an incision or tear is measured in degrees, from the shallowest to the deepest. The first degree is the most superficial and involves only the outer skin and the vaginal mucous membrane. A first-degree tear requires one or two stitches or none at all. The second degree will include the submucosal tissue and the perineal muscle. An episiotomy is a second-degree incision, requiring many stitches as each layer is sewn. Third-degree tears (which can occur with or without an episiotomy) continue into the rectal sphincter muscle; a fourth-degree tear extends into the anterior rectal wall as well.

There is no such thing as a small episiotomy. Most are about one and a half to two inches long because the incision has to be big enough so that you don't tear past its end. The cut can be one of two types:

- *The mediolateral* is made on a diagonal. It is usually performed because the perineum is particularly short or because this type is the doctor's personal preference. The mediolateral is considered to be less apt to tear into the rectum, but it is also more painful, more prone to infection, and harder to repair. It also heals more slowly because the muscle fibers must rejoin on the bias instead of in the central body of the perineum.
- *The midline,* or median, is the type most commonly done in the United States. It is a straight cut, directly toward the rectum.

You should try to dissuade your doctor from performing a routine episiotomy, because it's an unpleasant part of childbirth that can spin the web of intervention and complication. It's the reason for doing a pubic shave. It necessitates the use of sterile drapes during delivery, which can

EPISIOTOMY

◆

"I had a nine-pound baby the first time, so an episiotomy was necessary. The healing was so painful I was glad there wasn't time for one this time! I did tear a little bit, but the healing was nowhere near as painful as that huge cut the first time."

◆

"It healed right away, but the doctor was wrong—I felt both the cut and the stitches."

◆

"I tore anyway, even with an episiotomy. Very uncomfortable healing process."

◆

"I didn't have one, and after delivery needed only one stitch."

◆

"This was my biggest fear, but I never felt a thing."

◆

"To me, the stitches were more painful than the labor."

◆

"My doctor was washing me down for an episiotomy when my daughter went flying into her arms. All I ended up needing was one stitch."

◆

"The doctor insisted on doing a small one, just to give himself something to do, I think."

◆

"The doctor did one that went off to the side and it was painful for three weeks."

continued

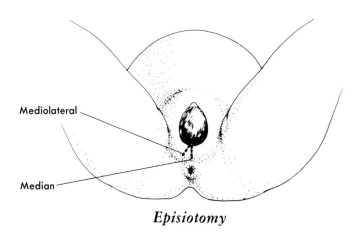

Mediolateral

Median

Episiotomy

obstruct your view and prevent you from touching the baby as he emerges. The incision can become a site for infection, which may require you to take the precaution of cleansing yourself with a Betadine solution after urination. The perineum will swell, itch, and hurt, requiring the use of ice packs, sitz baths, anesthetic sprays, and perhaps even analgesics. It often compounds the pain of hemorrhoids, making it very difficult to feel relaxed and comfortable in any position after birth. It affects your ability to regain your strength, to take care of your baby, and to make love with your husband.

In 1981, U.S. government doctors David Banta and Stephen Thacker conducted a review of the medical literature concerning episiotomy and concluded that "the data on benefits of episiotomy are very poor and offer no convincing argument to support the routine use of that procedure. . . . Moreover, there are significant risks associated with episiotomy that have not been adequately studied."

We object strenuously to the routine use of episiotomies. However, there are some clear-cut instances in which episiotomies should be done. They include the following:

+ When a woman is pushing uncontrollably and it's impossible to guide the baby's head out slowly. The potential for tearing in this instance is great, so an episiotomy is preferable. To avoid being cut, you must have enough control to stop pushing and to simply let the force of the contraction ease the baby out.
+ Some few women have tough perineums, with little pliability or elasticity. This may be the natural condition of the perineum or the result of poor nutrition or lack of exercise. Tension in the pelvic floor muscles can also cause a tight perineum. This may be the result of poor body position (especially if you are lying on your back) or an inability to let go emotionally as well as physically.
+ Forceps deliveries always require episiotomies because the normal vaginal opening isn't large enough to accommodate the instrument.
+ If the baby is in distress and needs to be delivered quickly, an episiotomy will be performed.
+ If the mother's condition (toxemia or heart disease) necessitates a short second stage with a minimum of pushing, an episiotomy will be necessary to enable speedy delivery of the baby.

Your doctor may try to convince you that episiotomies are necessary, using the following arguments:

+ *It's better than tearing.* Women who responded to our questionnaire expressed great dissatisfaction with their episiotomies, but time and time again they said, "Well, it was better than tearing." In fact there is a good chance that you may not tear at all and that if you do, it's likely to be a small tear that does not require repair (unlike a deep incision).

All episiotomies cut through muscles, but tears often don't. In June 1984, the *British Medical Journal* published a study on routine mediolateral episiotomy. In this research, a control group of first-time mothers were delivered without episiotomy unless it was deemed medically essential: 21 percent did not tear, 25 percent had a first-degree tear (which does not require stitching because it heals spontaneously), and 47 percent experienced a second-degree tear. There were no third-degree tears. In this study, almost half (46 percent) of the women sustained less damage than they would have with a standard episiotomy, and almost half of that group did not tear at all. The remaining 47 percent with second-degree lacerations were no worse off than they would have been with an episiotomy. One interesting result was the finding that only 8 percent underwent episiotomy for medical reasons, as compared with 89 percent in the six months prior to the study.

The tear you do not want is a third- or fourth-degree one, which extends into the rectum. There is no guarantee that an episiotomy will prevent third-degree laceration, and in fact episiotomies themselves often tear and extend into the rectum.

• *It's easier to repair a clean cut than a jagged tear.* Yes, it is easier to repair a clean surgical incision rather than an irregular third- or fourth-degree tear, but this does not hold true for a small tear. Also, there's a good chance that if you don't receive an episiotomy, you won't require any repair at all.

• *It's good to sew you up nice and tight because this will enhance future sexual pleasure.* No study has shown that a tightly sewn perineum guarantees sexual satisfaction to either party, and in fact, it can decrease sexual pleasure because it can make intercourse very painful. The Kegel exercises (see page 124) are more effective than episiotomy in regaining vaginal tone.

• *An episiotomy can save your baby from being brain damaged.* An episiotomy is not a rationale for avoiding brain damage. The reasoning behind this notion is that an episiotomy can shorten the second stage of labor, thus saving the baby's head from pressure against the perineum. The study in the *British Medical Journal* stated that it "produced no evidence of . . . trauma to the baby's head, or greater damage to the pelvic floor, when episiotomy was not performed." If your doctor cites brain damage as a reason for episiotomy during a normal delivery, he probably distrusts natural childbirth altogether.

♦ *An episiotomy can prevent uterine prolapse later in life.* There has been no proof that episiotomy prevents future uterine prolapse (a condition in which the uterus falls into the vagina). Prolapse most frequently occurs in women who have had many children or in women whose pelvic muscles have been weakened by mid- or high-forceps deliveries. In fact, most of these women have received episiotomies.

♦ *An episiotomy is necessary if you have a big baby.* No one has to stretch your belly to accommodate a large baby, so why should anything be done to your perineum? The difficulty in delivering a large baby has more to do with the size of your bony pelvis than the soft tissues of your vagina. Skilled doctors and midwives can and do deliver large babies over intact perineums.

If you do have an episiotomy, you will be given a local anesthetic, such as lidocaine. There is often a tingling, burning pressure that is felt as the baby is about to be born. This sensation can act like a natural anesthetic, but you should definitely have a shot of the real thing, because you will need it for the repair. Even with the injection many women can feel the stitching, and it will take about twenty or thirty minutes to be sewn. You should do your Lamaze breathing and distract yourself by holding the baby.

How to Avoid an Episiotomy

Avoiding an episiotomy isn't simply a matter of asking your doctor or midwife not to do one. First and foremost, you need to be in a proper position. A medical student recently told us, "I used to believe episiotomies weren't always necessary, but yesterday I saw a woman tear very badly." When we asked about the mother's position, the student said, "Lithotomy, of course." You cannot be on your back with your legs spread wide apart and expect not to tear. Instead, you must be sitting, squatting, or lying on your side. Your doctor or midwife should be skillful, and of course, there can't be any medical necessity. Lastly, delivering over an intact perineum is a team effort, requiring patience and cooperation between you and your doctor or midwife. You must be able to push or stop pushing on command, allowing the baby to be born slowly and gently. You will also need reassurance that the burning sensation you will feel is normal, and temporary. You must be convinced that a little extra effort now will save a lot of pain and difficulty later.

Most midwives advocate massage as a means of relaxing the perineum. Olive oil can be worked into the skin to increase elasticity, and the gentle rubbing and stretching techniques are performed throughout the entire second stage of labor.

Another method to avoid episiotomy is the Ritgen maneuver: A towel is held over the mother's rectum as upward pressure is exerted on the baby's chin through the perineum. This action permits a careful and deliberate delivery of the baby's head.

Still another technique is "ironing the perineum," which means the muscles are slowly stretched by applying finger pressure against the inside wall of the vagina during the final stages of labor. None of these methods have been scientifically tested, however, for efficacy. Many practitioners manage to avoid episiotomy by doing nothing more than supporting the baby's head as it is born.

SEEING YOUR BABY

This is absolutely the best part. It's the moment when labor and delivery are finally over and you can see your baby at last and know if it's a boy or a girl. Normally, the sequence of events goes something like this: The baby's head is born and the doctor or midwife immediately suctions out mucus with a bulb syringe. With one more push the shoulders are delivered, and then the body. Somebody yells, "It's a boy!" or "It's a girl!" and either you or your husband or both begin to weep. The baby is checked over and suctioned again, then he is placed on your chest with the cord still intact. If his color is normal, you should be permitted to hold the baby for a while. At some point during the first few minutes, he'll be footprinted and tagged for identification so that there's no possibility of mistaken identity later on in the nursery.

Cutting the Umbilical Cord

One possible variation in this scene is the timing of the cutting of the cord. Approximately one-fourth of all babies are born with the cord wrapped around their neck. Usually, the doctor or midwife can simply unloop it over the baby's head, but if the cord is too tight or wrapped twice, it will have to be cut right away. To do this, the cord will be clamped in two places and cut in the middle. It's a painless procedure for both parties because the cord contains no nerve fibers.

If there is no complication with the cord, it's likely that your baby will be allowed to rest on your chest for a few minutes before cutting. This delayed clamping permits the baby to continue to receive oxygen and helps the uterus contract, which aids the natural expulsion of the placenta. Sometimes the father is asked if he would like to cut the cord, and we applaud any doctor or midwife who would make this lovely gesture.

Another school of thought on cord cutting is to wait about three minutes to allow the cord to stop pulsating completely in order to permit a complete transfer of the remaining placental blood to the baby. Receiving this additional blood has been shown to prevent anemia in later infancy, but in order to be successfully implemented, the baby must be held below the level of the uterus for the entire three-minute period. This prohibits the immediate skin-to-skin contact that is desired by most parents. Late-clamped babies have been shown to be more red, more irritable, and more wakeful during their first few days of life. And these babies also have a higher incidence of newborn jaundice from the extra blood cells they have received. Late clamping is a controversial procedure that some people strongly support. You should discuss it with your pediatrician and obstetrician before delivery.

Feelings Immediately After Birth

No matter how many preparations you have made in advance, it is still a shock actually to be holding your baby. The room might be all set up at home and all the baby clothes bought, but somehow it's still a surprise when the fantasy becomes reality. You may have watched the entire birth, but it's still hard to associate the newborn in your arms with the active being that was just inside you. For most first-time parents, the pregnancy is one experience, being a parent is another.

How you feel after birth depends to a great extent on the course of events during your labor and delivery. But if everything has gone well and you've counted ten fingers and ten toes, you will probably experience the most incredible "high" of your life. Ten minutes earlier you may have been ready for a tubal ligation, but now you're already thinking about the next time. You will finally understand why women say that the pain of labor is worth the reward of birth.

There can be mixed emotions, too. You may be exhausted, but also wide awake; ecstatic that labor is over, but sorry you're not pregnant

♦

"I felt like the only woman who had ever given birth. I wasn't sure how other women got their babies, but I was sure they hadn't done what I had."

♦

"I was thrilled and felt that I could stand up against a den of lions to protect my child."

♦

"I felt pride in accomplishment, and relief—and loneliness. My body was 'alone' again."

♦

"Ecstasy! All the pain was immediately forgotten. I wanted to laugh and cry and hug everyone in sight. My doctor came over and gave me a hug and a kiss, too."

♦

"I felt distance toward the baby, not close to him right away."

♦

"Exhilarated! I felt as if I'd run a marathon and come in first. My baby is the equivalent of a gold medal!"

♦

"Absolute elation, and a love that filled my entire body. I wanted that moment to last forever. The pictures show me being very tired, but I had lots of energy. Very self-satisfied and in awe of my little miracle."

♦

"Relieved. I didn't feel that interested in the baby, I just wanted to sleep."

♦

continued

♦

"I was exhausted physically and emotionally. In the recovery room, I felt very lonely and isolated. I didn't feel like I had a baby because I didn't get to see her. I wish I could go back and make them let me hold her as soon as she was born. I missed out on it because no one thought of me at that moment."

♦

"Hungry, happy, and satisfied. At the same time, though, I felt as if I'd been run over by a cement truck (or given birth to one!)."

♦

"I felt like Mother Earth. I was overwhelmed by maternal love and felt I had accomplished the greatest thing a person can ever do in life."

♦

"I was amazed she was a girl. I wanted a girl very much and couldn't believe God was so kind. And then I was flooded with relief that she was healthy and looked so strong and aware."

♦

"I was so full of adrenalin I could have climbed a mountain. I was giggly and excited and madly in love with my daughter."

♦

"For as long as I live, I'll never forget how it felt when she came slithering out of my body. It's a feeling that words can't express, and I thank God I didn't grow up in my mother's era, when they put you out and you missed all that."

♦

"I never felt as close to my husband in our four years of marriage as I did then."

♦

continued

"The midwife handed Bert the scissors to cut the baby's umbilical cord. This act summed up for me the last nine months of growing this child. He was no longer of me, but rather a person unto himself."

◆

"My husband turned to me with tears in his eyes and said, 'Thank you. Thank you so much!'"

◆

"The moment my daughter was born, she was placed on top of me. She just looked at her father and me and moved her arms and legs, taking in the new world. We were still connected by the umbilical cord. The most exhilarating feeling came over me."

◆

"The doctor placed Christopher on my tummy, where he took one look at me and *howled!* Then I knew everything was okay."

◆

"The highlight of my birth experience was when I tentatively reached out and touched my son for the first time."

◆

"I first felt sorry for our baby when I heard him cry at birth. It must be a real trauma being born! Then there was excitement, a feeling of everything being unreal, probably a little fear, and a sense of wonder. When I saw him, I *knew* him; he looked familiar."

◆

"I couldn't believe she was actually there and not inside me any more. The lump had become reality."

continued

♦

"I was amazed at how large and alert the baby was, how good I felt, and how strange it was to finally look at the person I had known for nine months."

♦

"When I first saw her, she looked exactly like my mother-in-law, and I thought, 'Oh, my God, after everything I went through, this is what I get?' But that night, in my room, she was the most beautiful thing I had ever seen."

♦

"Aaron was born with a cleft lip and palate. I bawled my eyes out for a minute. Then my husband brought him to me, and we all fell in love with each other as a family. It was the most emotional moment of my life."

♦

"The baby was a girl, which my husband openly wanted and I secretly wanted, so I was thrilled because of that. She had ten fingers, ten toes, all normal, which is always a concern. She was just so beautiful, beyond words!"

anymore; you may want to hold the baby, but also want some time by yourself to adjust to the fact that the work of pushing is done.

It's no wonder that your body may exhibit a typical shock reaction. It's common for women to feel suddenly cold, with chattering teeth and uncontrollable trembling. This is normal and will subside after a time. Ask for blankets and have your partner put the socks from your Lamaze bag on your feet.

Your Newborn's Appearance

You may be a little alarmed at first by your baby's appearance. Many infants emerge in a rather limp state and are bluish gray in color. This is normal. Within seconds, however, the lungs will fill with air, and the baby's skin will become oxygenated and pink. Some babies come out screaming and kicking, whereas others are quiet and watchful, so don't be concerned if yours isn't making any noise.

There are a number of other possible characteristics of the newborn that may startle you, including:

- A creamy white skin covering called *vernix* which looks like cold-creme, but protects the baby's skin during his nine months in water.
- A coat of fine downy hair, called *lanugo,* that falls off within a few days.
- The baby's genitals will be swollen, and often the breasts will excrete tiny drops of milk, called *witches' milk.* Girl babies can also produce a small amount of menstrual-like bleeding. These symptoms are all caused by the mother's hormones and are short-lived.
- Most babies are born with blue-gray eyes, which may later change color.
- Many babies have slightly misshapen or pointed heads due to the molding of their skull bones during the passage through the mother's pelvis. You can see perfectly-shaped cesarean babies in the nursery, but it may be several weeks before your baby's head becomes completely round.

The Apgar Evaluation

During the first few minutes after birth, your baby will be watched carefully by the nurses in the delivery or birthing room to make sure he is adjusting normally to the new environment. One minute after birth, and then four minutes later, your baby's health will be evaluated by five vital signs: color, heart rate, reflex irritability, muscle tone, and respiration. This test is known as an *Apgar exam,* named after Dr. Virginia Apgar, an anesthesiologist (see chart). Each category can receive a maximum of two points, making ten points the highest score. There is usually an improvement between the first and second score. A typical one- and five-minute Apgar would be 7/9. Although Apgar scoring is pervasive, it is not a completely reliable assessment because it is subjectively determined. The obstetrician or midwife who delivers the baby also gives the Apgar rating, and therefore is essentially grading his own performance.

If a pediatrician is present, however, he will determine the Apgar

APGAR SCORING CHART

SIGN	0	1	2
HEART RATE	Absent	Slow (below 100)	Over 100
RESPIRATORY EFFORT	Absent	Weak cry, hypoventilation	Good strong cry
MUSCLE TONE	Limp	Some flexion of extremities	Well flexed
REFLEX RESPONSE 1. Response to catheter in nostril (tested after oropharynx is clear)	No Response	Grimace	Cough or sneeze
2. Tangential foot slap	No Response	Grimace	Cry and withdrawal of foot
COLOR	Blue, pale	Body pink Extremities blue	Completely pink

scores. This would happen under special circumstances, such as after a cesarean or a difficult forceps delivery. Don't put too much store in these numbers. It's only a gross assessment of the baby's condition, and a more detailed examination will be performed later in the newborn nursery.

Eye Drops

The first hour after birth is a time of amazing alertness for your child. He can hear perfectly and will turn his head toward you as you speak. A baby's eyes can focus on an object eight to twelve inches away; this means your baby can see your face as you hold him in your arms. For this reason, many parents ask to delay the administration of silver-nitrate eye drops. The drops prevent blindness caused by the transmission of maternal gonorrhea and are mandated by law in most states. They also irritate the eyes, causing a type of conjunctivitis, which can last for a few days. The baby's eyes become puffy and red, and he can't see as well as he did at birth. For this reason, couples commonly request that the drops be given in the nursery after the newborn exam, after they've had adequate time in the delivery or recovery room to get acquainted. Many hospitals now give a topical application of erythromycin or tetracycline ointment instead of the silver nitrate drops because they are considered less irritating.

Bonding

From reading our questionnaires, we were distressed to learn that parents and babies are still being separated after birth. The hospital's rationale is that the baby's body temperature can be maintained only in a warmer. This isn't true. A baby can be kept warm enough if he is held close to his mother or is well swaddled and not losing body heat through an uncovered head. Some hospitals provide tiny caps to keep babies warm.

We encourage you to savor this special postpartum time and to make it last as long as possible. If the baby is healthy, this is the time to enjoy the reward of all your hard work. It's also the beginning of your relationship with your baby, and these first moments might make a difference.

Drs. M. H. Klaus and J. H. Kennel of Case Western Reserve University created a body of work on the emotional connection between a mother and her newborn immediately after birth. They called this process *bonding,* and although some of their claims for long-term results have been called into question, their appealing idea has caught on. It is mutually satisfying for both parents and baby to have this special time to become acquainted. Routine separations have been eliminated, and bonding has been incorporated in most hospitals.

Bonding is great, but it's not a prerequisite to a good future relationship. It's the optimal thing to do, but if you have a cesarean under general anesthesia or if the baby must be taken to the nursery, this separation won't impair your ability to love your child. Some people will not feel instantly comfortable or in love with their baby, and that's normal. Some people are so swept away by labor and delivery that it's difficult to switch the focus to the baby, and that's normal too. However you feel after birth, be assured that just about every person is capable of forming a strong attachment to his or her children.

Nursing After Delivery

Nursing immediately after delivery has become part of the bonding process. The nipple stimulation and the skin-to-skin contact will help the uterus contract and expel the placenta, and you can get a tremendous high watching your child performing this first instinctual act. You shouldn't feel pressured to nurse immediately, however, if you're too tired or the baby just prefers to look around. You can try later in the recovery room or back in your own room in a few hours. The more important thing is just to hold your baby and bask in the knowledge that everything has turned out well.

THE INFLUENCE OF LEBOYER

In the past decade, procedures in the delivery room have been influenced by the work of the French obstetrician Frederick Leboyer. Gone (we hope) is the practice of welcoming the baby into the world by dangling him by the feet and slapping him on the buttocks. Instead delivery practices have been shaped by Dr. Leboyer, in accordance with his techniques of "gentle birth": low lights, delayed cord clamping, soft voices, no routine suctioning, skin-to-skin contact, and a warm bath. *Birth Without Violence* was published in France in 1974, and since that time Leboyer's approach has been adapted by doctors and midwives throughout this country.

His philosophy is to make birth as atraumatic as possible and to ease the baby's transition from the mother to the outside world. This means re-creating an environment that closely simulates the intrauterine world: a subdued atmosphere and the continuation of physical contact with the mother. Delayed cord clamping permits the baby to begin breathing at his own pace. The purpose of the bath is to return the baby to the familiar sensation of being suspended in water.

The bath is usually the hardest part to arrange in a hospital because of concern about possible heat loss. For this reason it is most commonly done in birthing rooms and in alternative-birth centers. We know of several hospitals that permit the Leboyer bath in the delivery room, but in general this can be difficult to get because delivery rooms are kept quite cold.

Your doctor or midwife is the person who can arrange for a Leboyer delivery. You should discuss any desire for a gentle birth with this person well before labor.

THE PLACENTA

The delivery of the placenta is considered the third stage of labor, and it is usually painless. After the baby is born, the uterus will continue to contract, and this shrinking will cause the placenta to detach from the uterine wall. This process has been likened to a postage stamp peeling off a deflated balloon. With one final push it will be expelled. The uterus will continue to contract, sealing off the placental site and shrinking until it is about the size of a grapefruit.

Normally, the placenta appears anywhere between five and thirty minutes after birth. Some doctors want to speed up this delivery because they are eager to begin the episiotomy repair. In order to accomplish this, the doctor or nurse may try to push very hard on the top of your stomach to initiate a strong contraction, or may tug on the umbilical cord. These two techniques are dangerous and should never be performed. They increase the chance that a bit of the placenta may break off, remain attached, and thus cause hemorrhaging.

It's rare when the placenta does not emerge. If this happens, your doctor or midwife may have to reach into the uterus and extract the placenta manually. You will probably be offered a whiff of nitrous oxide if manual extraction is necessary because it will hurt.

Giving a shot of Pitocin right after delivery of the placenta is quite routine; however, many women are unaware this is done. Pitocin really isn't necessary unless your contractions are too weak to close off the placental site, which can occur after a very long labor or if your uterus has been weakened by having many children. Two good ways to encourage natural expulsion of the placenta are putting the baby to the breast (or any form of nipple stimulation) or gently massaging the abdomen. Many doctors feel legally protected if they administer Pitocin, and they reason that there's no harm in giving it prophylactically. On the other hand, Pitocin contractions can be more painful, and it's another instance when an intervention is given ''just in case.''

Once the placenta has been expelled, labor and delivery are finally complete, and the postpartum period has officially started. Any perineal tears or episiotomy will be stitched, and your legs and belly will be washed. You will then be moved to the recovery room or allowed to remain in the birthing room. In either location, your husband and baby will usually be permitted to remain with you for an hour or so. Pregnancy is over, and parenthood has begun.

CHAPTER 11

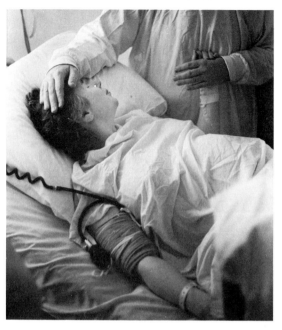

Medication

The ideal birth is an unmedicated one. Natural childbirth produces healthier babies and allows new mothers peace of mind unattainable with a medicated birth. Unfortunately, only about 10 percent of all women in the United States today experience labor and delivery without drugs or anesthesia. We think this is deplorable because of the risks associated with medication and because the quality of the birth experience can be compromised by unnecessary or poorly administered drugs.

Many women today abstain from smoking, drinking, or taking drugs during pregnancy and claim to be concerned about the effects of medication on the baby. They should be, because no drug has been proved to be both free of risk and effective. As stated in the medical textbook

Obstetrics and Gynecology, by Wilson, Carrington, and Ledger, "Many drugs have been given to make labor and delivery less painful, but unfortunately, all have disadvantages that limit their usefulness. The 'perfect' agent must provide relief from pain while it neither interferes with the progress of labor nor adds to the maternal or fetal risk. Such an agent has not yet been discovered."

We're not against the use of drugs or anesthesia during labor when needed. Obviously if there are complications, medication will be indicated. We are, however, adamantly opposed to its routine use and its prescription as a substitute for emotional support. There are several interdependent reasons why thousands of women expect to have natural childbirth but end up with something quite different. They include the following:

+ *Having a baby can be very painful,* and many women are not prepared for any sensation beyond a mild menstrual cramp. They feel angry and betrayed when labor gets tough, and this reaction undermines their ability to cope. The normal reaction to something new and overwhelming is to become frightened; this fear makes the pain worse, which makes the fear increase, triggering the vicious cycle of fear-tension-pain.
+ *Doctors are trained to relieve suffering,* and that means giving pain relief. They are not taught to sustain their patients emotionally, although in childbirth, that's what's really needed. Many doctors can't accept pain as a normal part of birth and they feel obliged to offer women drugs. If, every time an obstetrician was asked for medication, he spent just ten minutes talking to a woman and her partner, breathing with them, or offering reinforcement for their efforts, the use of medication during childbirth would decline precipitously.
+ *A woman in labor needs constant support,* especially during transition. She needs a sensitive doctor or midwife, good nurses, and an excellent partner. If any of these components is missing, her chances of having natural childbirth are diminished. Encouragement during transition is critical because that's the time when a woman asks for medication—and she gets it. This is a shame, because this phase of labor is relatively short and anything taken now will impair her ability to deliver naturally.
+ *Our society accepts and even promotes drug use.* Americans are not accustomed to experiencing pain, and therefore it seems strange not to take medication when something hurts. There's no point in with-

holding pain relief from terminally ill or postoperative patients, but childbirth is different. It is not an illness, and it is finite.

There are four primary types of pain relief available in hospitals: *analgesics,* which inhibit the reception of pain stimuli and therefore raise the pain threshold; *local* and *regional anesthetics,* which interrupt the transmission of pain signals along nerve fibers; and *general anesthetics,* which produce unconciousness. All drugs pass through the placenta and affect the baby to some extent, although the specific effects depend on the particular drug, how it is given, the dosage, and when it is administered.

Medication is a subject that should be discussed with your doctor ahead of time, preferably at the beginning of your pregnancy, so that you know whether he truly supports natural childbirth. In any event, you should discuss medication again, sometime near your due date, so that you can find out what you might appropriately receive if there are complications. Most doctors have favorite drugs, and the choice will also depend to a great extent on the practices of the hospital. Still, you should be informed about possible choices in the event that medication is required.

ANALGESICS, TRANQUILIZERS, BARBITUATES, AMNESTICS AND INHALANTS

Drugs used during labor or delivery include analgesics, tranquilizers, barbituates, amnestics, and inhalants. They are administered either singly or in combination, to alleviate pain. By far, the most commonly given medications are the analgesics.

Analgesics

These drugs, also known as narcotics, are taken during the first stage of labor. They can be administered through an intravenous or by an intramuscular injection. The effects of intravenous administration can be felt within minutes, but it will wear off more quickly than a narcotic given by intramuscular injection. It takes 10 to 15 minutes for an analgesic to take effect if it is given intramuscularly (drugs are rarely given orally during labor because the digestive system has slowed down, which impairs the drug's absorption).

MEDICATION

♦

"Before labor, I was absolutely opposed to medication, thinking that women who received it were 'chicken.' Now I feel that you do what you have to do. I feel fortunate to have made it through labor and delivery without medication. I feel proud, not heroic."

♦

"I was all for medication. I thought painkillers were the answer. Never again! I felt manipulated and out of control."

♦

"I didn't want any medication and didn't receive any. I feel this is best for mother and baby. However, I no longer feel that a drug-free delivery makes you a better mother or a stronger woman."

♦

"My husband and I talked about going drug-free a lot and really 'psyched' ourselves up for it. I think that helped. If I had gone into labor feeling, 'Oh well, if it hurts, I'll take something,' I probably would have."

♦

"Once I started having labor pains, I realized there was no way I could have natural childbirth."

♦

"I wanted medication, but I was seven centimeters dilated when I got to the hospital, so I couldn't have any. It really wasn't all that bad, and I'm glad I didn't take any."

♦

continued

♦

"Never felt that I wanted to have medication before or during labor and delivery. I knew that I wanted to be done with the job, but that medication wasn't a solution."

♦

"I wanted a 'proper' entrance into the world for my daughter. To me, doped up is not the way to be born. Secondly, I was totally selfish. I didn't want to miss anything because I was 'out of it.' "

♦

"The second she was here, I could enjoy her, enjoy the moment. Felt great, got to my room, and sent my husband for pizza. It was such a truly wonderful experience. Even two hours after she was born I said labor was awful, but I was really glad I hadn't opted for medication."

By far the most popular narcotic of all is Demerol, but Nisentil and Dolophine are also sometimes prescribed during labor. Nisentil is fairly widely used because it is as effective, but shorter-acting than Demerol. It is given in doses of 40 to 60 milligrams (mg).

We have devoted most of our discussion of narcotics to Demerol because it so widely available and so popular as a method of pain relief during labor. The use of Demerol is so widespread that many people do not fully consider its proper use, its risks, or its side effects. Demerol (meperidine is its generic name) is a depressant of the central nervous system; it can be administered by an intramuscular injection or through an intravenous line. It is normally given in doses ranging from 25 to 75 milligrams, which last anywhere from two to four hours. A shot of 25 milligrams takes about 15 minutes to take effect, whereas the same dose put into an IV line is felt immediately.

The good thing about Demerol is that it will relax you enough to let

ANALGESICS

♦

"My labor was long and hard. When my doctor decided to stick with a vaginal delivery, they offered me some kind of drug, which I took. I was able to sleep between contractions and keep control."

♦

"When I finally asked for relief from the pain and got a shot, my attitude got better."

♦

"The Demerol relaxed me and allowed my cervix to dilate and my delivery to go quickly. My goal was to deliver as easily and as safely as possible for both myself and the baby. I had Demerol both times, and both my children were alert and active."

♦

"I wish I had not finally accepted the Demerol. It didn't do anything except make me sleep a little and not push with every contraction."

♦

"All Demerol did was make me vomit!"

♦

"The medication took away what control I had and left the pain."

♦

"The pains were just as strong after I took some medication, but in between them I could just collapse. The pain was easier to bear, and time didn't make much sense."

♦

continued

◆

"Demerol was not properly presented to me. My doctor told me it would help the pain, but instead I was practically unconscious between contractions, which seemed to intensify and worsen."

◆

"If I'd known I was going to deliver so soon, I wouldn't have taken it."

◆

"My doctor said it slowed my contractions."

◆

"The medication made me see double and slur my speech. It frightened me, but I was already into transition and I could not articulate this to anyone."

◆

"I had Demerol. I'd rather have done without it, but I now understand its usefulness."

◆

"Next time I will not use drugs unless it is absolutely necessary. My son did not begin breathing normally, and I attribute this to Nisentil."

you doze between contractions. It will not take away the pain, it will just put you in a state in which you don't care about it so much. Women have reported feeling slightly drunk under the influence of Demerol and losing their ability to speak and react at a normal speed. The bad thing about Demerol is that it can prolong labor because it relaxes smooth muscles, thus reducing the effectiveness of uterine contractions. It can also make you nauseated; approximately two women out of ten will vomit from the drug.

Demerol will affect the baby's central nervous system as well. After birth, breathing may be depressed, the heartbeat slowed down (bradycardia), body temperature lowered (hypothermia), and relaxation of the smooth muscle may produce poor muscle tone and a delayed sucking reflex. These reactions can occur because any drug taken by the mother passes quickly to the baby's brain and blood through the placenta. Because the baby is so small, he metabolizes and transfers back drugs to his mother's bloodstream at a far slower rate than he receives them. This is an indisputable fact, and while you may be correctly told that Demerol won't harm your baby, you should know it will affect him.

We're not advocating a ban on Demerol. We're merely saying it should be used intelligently and not prescribed as casually as it is today by so many doctors. There are two clear-cut instances in which an analgesic can be a real boon to a troublesome labor. They are when:

- You've been up for two days with false labor. Finally, you are in true labor, admitted to the hospital and only three centimeters dilated. The problem is now exhaustion and how you'll handle the demanding parts of labor to come. Demerol may give you the ability to doze between contractions and catch some needed sleep. It can allow you to recover the energy necessary for an unmedicated delivery.
- You arrive at the hospital and you're three centimeters dilated. Three hours later you've reached five centimeters. Three hours later you're still five centimeters. The pain is becoming unbearable because you know your contractions aren't doing anything. This situation is called a plateau, and it's not uncommon. It can have a physical as well as a psychological basis. Before taking a drug you should try walking, putting pressure on spleen #6, a shower, or a good cry. If none of that helps, Demerol may help you to relax and allow labor to progress.

The key to Demerol is in the timing. It is not considered good medical practice to give analgesics during early labor because of the likelihood that contractions will be diminished in strength and frequency by the drug. On the other hand, medication should not be given near the time of delivery because at that point an infant is at the greatest risk of respiratory distress. To be used most safely, Demerol should be taken during active labor. The tricky part is determining when active labor is taking place and how long it's going to last. Many women spend several hours in active labor, but others dilate from four to nine centimeters in forty minutes. If a woman takes Demerol and then dilates rapidly, it can mean that she may be too sleepy and unfocused to push out her baby without the help of forceps, or that the baby will have trouble breathing at birth.

We expect that your doctor will attempt to coordinate the administration of any drug with your anticipated time of delivery. But as one expert, Dr. Howard Shapiro, states in *The Pregnancy Book for Today's Woman,* "Unfortunately, predicting the time of birth is often difficult if not impossible and occasionally a baby may be born with more than the desired amount of medication in its bloodstream." If this situation occurs, it can be remedied, according to Shapiro, by injecting a so-called narcotic antagonist, Narcan (naloxone hydrochloride), into the blood vessels of the umbilical cord.

Obviously, it's best to avoid an analgesic if you can. But this is difficult, because many obstetricians prescribe them at the first expression of pain or discomfort, and women believe their doctor knows best. Many women feel proud that they made it through labor and delivery on only a little Demerol. We feel that pride is justified and we're not trying to make you feel guilty for taking an analgesic. We just want you to recognize the risks of Demerol and to know you have a real choice concerning its use.

Tranquilizers

Tranquilizers include: Valium, Vistaril, and Phenergan. They are used either singly, or in combination with narcotics, i.e. Demerol and Phenergan, to decrease nausea and increase the effectiveness of the narcotic. Tranquilizers may be given to a woman who is particularly tense, to help her to relax her muscles and experience less pain. One drawback is that tranquilizers can make you feel so relaxed you are unable to breathe through contractions or actively participate in labor.

Barbiturates

Barbiturates are rarely used during labor because they have a depressant effect on the baby (which may last for several days). Some common barbiturates are: Seconal or Nembutol. They do not provide direct pain relief, but have a sedative effect which can produce sleep.

Amnestics

The most well known amnestic is scopolamine, a cerebral depressant. Used in combination with a narcotic, scopolamine was the most popular drug for childbirth during the 1950s. It was sometimes referred to as twilight sleep because it induces a confused, excited state which is remembered as a state of dreamless sleep. Side effects of scopolamine include euphoria, amnesia, fatigue, restlessness, excitement, hallucinations, and delirium.

Scopolamine does not eliminate pain, it just removes the memory of it. A labor passed under its influence often seems nightmarish in retrospect. Women given scopolamine often lose their ability to speak coherently and they must be closely watched or restrained so that they don't harm themselves.

Today scopolamine is rarely used in obstetric practice, although it is not obsolete. This is one drug you should never take under any circumstances.

Inhalants

This type of analgesia is often available in the delivery room to increase comfort during a painful delivery. It might be used during an episiotomy repair if the local is not fully effective or if the placenta has to be manually extracted. Inhalation anesthesia is most typically a combination of oxygen (50 percent) and another gas (50 percent), such as nitrous oxide. The mixture must contain at least 30 percent oxygen or the baby could experience oxygen deprivation. The gas is inhaled through a mask and is administered in small doses. It has no pronounced effects on either mother or baby, since it is used for such a short period of time.

LOCAL ANESTHETICS
The Pudendal Block

This procedure blocks sensation to the external organs—vagina, vulva, and perineum—making it useful for pain relief during delivery but not for labor. There is controversy about whether it provides adequate pain relief for a forceps delivery. It is administered by injection next to the pudendal nerves, located near the ischial spines, on either side of the vagina. It is easily administered by an obstetrician, and a dose of three to five milliliters of lidocaine or mepivacaine lasts about an hour.

The main disadvantage to the pudendal block is that it can interfere with the urge to push. The most serious complication is the rare, accidental injection into a blood vessel. Symptoms would include slurred speech, numbness in your tongue, or a metallic taste.

The timing of the pudendal is very important because it should be done after full dilation but before active pushing. If there is a delay in giving it, there will be too much pain and trouble to make it worthwhile.

The Perineal Block

The perineal block provides pain relief for the cutting and repair of the episiotomy. It consists of a series of injections of local anesthetic into the perineum. Anesthesia can be complete, but often there are areas (especially in the deepest layers) that retain sensation.

REGIONAL ANESTHETICS

Today there are four types of regional anesthetics available: epidurals, spinals, saddle blocks, and paracervicals, with epidurals being the most popular. All numb sensation in specific areas, but they are administered differently and have varying effects. The paracervical is the only one given by an obstetrician; all the others are performed either by an anesthesiologist or a nurse anesthetist (a nurse trained in the use of anesthesia).

Most hospitals maintain a staff of anesthesiologists, and the one on call will usually be the one to attend you. However, you may request a particular person if you know his reputation. A staff anesthesiologist may be a stranger to you, but your obstetrician will probably know this person from previous deliveries.

Should a regional anesthetic be necessary, your obstetrician and anesthesiologist will discuss your choices with you and make a recommendation. This will be based on the medical condition of you and your baby, the skill and preference of the anesthesiologist, and your expected time of delivery. You will obviously be at an advantage in this situation if you have discussed these considerations in advance with your doctor.

All of the medications used for regional anesthesia cross the placenta. Their effect on the baby is determined by the specific drug used, the amount given, and the route of administration, the metabolism of the mother, the timing of administration, and the general health of the baby. In addition, the baby would be indirectly but substantively affected by the medication if it impairs the mother's blood pressure or circulation.

The use of regional anesthesia is usually contraindicated for women with previous back surgery, bony deformations of the spine, skin infections near the site of the intended injection, a history of bleeding problems, or low blood pressure. It is impractical if a speedy delivery is necessary.

The Epidural

The epidural has been nicknamed the "Cadillac of anesthetics" because it is considered to be the safest and most effective. The epidural can be used during active labor and transition, pushing, and delivery by forceps or cesarean section. It numbs but does not paralyze the lower half of a woman's body, leaving her clear-headed but pain-free. Epidurals are not available at all hospitals, however, particularly smaller ones, where there are no round-the-clock anesthesiologists. To many people epidurals represent childbirth at its best—awake and aware, but numb from the waist down.

Epidurals can vary considerably in their effects, and this depends largely on the amount of medication used. It also depends on the individual metabolism of the person receiving the anesthetic. The same dose epidural can be given to five different women, and they will experience five different degrees of pain relief.

Low dose, or *segmental,* epidurals can "take the edge off" contractions, but leave some sensation in the lower abdomen and perineum. A *standard,* or *lumbar,* epidural will completely anesthetize the region from the top of the belly to the tips of the toes. Obviously, the deeper the level of anesthesia, the greater the potential for side effects. These include:

- Weakened and slowed-down contractions. For this reason Pitocin is frequently given in combination with the epidural. Epidurals are usually not be given until active labor is well established, with dilation to at least four or five centimeters. If contractions do weaken, there is a good chance they will establish their former intensity after about thirty minutes, but few doctors will wait for this to happen. Often Pitocin is routinely added to the intravenous line once the epidural is in place.

REGIONAL ANESTHETICS

♦

"I had an epidural an hour before my daughter was born. It turned a night that was fast becoming hysterical into an event that I could participate in."

♦

"The numbing effect of the spinal went up to my lungs. I felt I was suffocating. This was the worst feeling I've ever had."

♦

"I thought I was only about six centimeters dilated and didn't think I could stand transition, so I had an epidural. It turns out I was fully dilated! So here I was completely numb for the pushing. I was a good pusher, so the doctor didn't need to use forceps, but I couldn't feel anything, which was kind of strange. I should have had the epidural an hour before. It was a waste at that point."

♦

"My husband and I are both pro-medication. He didn't want to see me suffer, and I wanted to enjoy the birth. I would have the next one exactly the same way if I could. The epidural is the greatest thing since peanut butter. I would never fear labor again."

♦

"After my son was born, I wanted to kiss the guy who invented regional anesthesia. I thought it was the greatest thing in the world. It allowed me to enjoy the birth, without pain."

♦

"My spine hurt for weeks."

♦

"I went through nine hours of excruciating pain, determined to go 'natural' all the way. I was totally unprepared for the waves of back pain that followed each

continued

contraction. After nine hours I was on the edge of hysteria, and my husband was frantic with concern. We decided to go with an epidural—one of the smartest moves I've ever made."

♦

"I received an epidural after nine hours of induced labor. I seemed to be stuck at seven centimeters. About thirty minutes after the epidural, I started dilating again."

♦

"The pain I endured with back labor totally overwhelmed my breathing techniques, leaving me scared and on the verge of losing control. Intellectually, I know I made the right choice in going with the epidural, but I felt guilty afterward because I didn't tough it out."

♦

"When the epidural wore off, it was like I couldn't even think straight, all I could see was pain. Next time, I'll tie the anesthesiologist to my bed."

♦

"Obviously, not everyone can go with no medication. However, those women who have 'saddle blocks' for a normal delivery are missing an exciting moment. By that time, the worst is over."

♦

"I had figured I would probably ask for the epidural. It was great not to hurt, but I hated that it slowed things down."

♦

"I had been up for over twenty-four hours, the baby was faceup, and I already had the urge to push. I was relieved when I finally got to five centimeters and

continued

♦

could have the epidural. I was exhausted and fell asleep when it started working."

♦

"I was not able to feel a sensation to push, the fetal monitor told me when a
contraction was beginning, and the nurse told me when it was time to push. The
baby was delivered with forceps."

♦

"Medication helped me enjoy the birth. It's no fun being in pain. The last ten
hours were spent laughing and enjoying the process. The epidural allowed me
to be more aware and understanding of my surroundings."

♦ The increased incidence of neonatal jaundice. It's unclear whether
  this is the result of the epidural, the Pitocin, or a combination of
  effects.

♦ The increased use of forceps. For labors without epidural anesthesia,
  the rate of the use of forceps is from 4 to 21 percent; for labors with
  the standard lumbar epidurals, the rate of use is 65 to 75 percent.
  Epidurals produce numbness, and therefore there is little or no urge
  to push. The epidural decreases the effectiveness of the muscles of
  the pelvic floor, preventing the baby from rotating naturally. When
  this occurs, the baby must be turned with forceps. A study published
  in the *British Medical Journal* in 1977 described the effects of lumbar
  epidurals given to 486 women; instrumental delivery (forceps and
  vacuum extraction) was five times more common, and malposition
  of the fetal head was three times more common when compared
  with a control group of women who did not receive epidurals.

♦ The increased risk of hypotension (lowered blood pressure). Epidurals cause your blood vessels to dilate, which can result in lowered

blood pressure. This decreases the amount of oxygen distributed throughout your body and to the baby. As a precaution, many doctors will give you extra fluids through the intravenous to increase your blood volume.

If you do need an epidural, you should request that you be given a segmental one, or one with the lowest possible dosage. This may permit you to retain some sensation in the lower perineum so that you can feel the urge to push and so that the baby may rotate naturally.

THE PROCEDURE

An epidural takes twenty minutes to administer and another ten to twenty minutes to completely take effect. If you request an epidural during labor, your doctor will have to write orders for one, and you will have to wait for the anesthesiologist to arrive. Your partner may be asked to leave the room while the epidural is being given, but he has the right to stay if you want him to. The procedure is basically bloodless and painless, so there's no reason why he can't stay to lend you moral support. If you don't already have an IV line in place, one will be inserted.

For the procedure, you will be asked to round your back by either lying in a curled position or sitting bent over. Your back will be washed with an antiseptic solution, and then you will be given a shot or two of a local anesthetic to numb the area in your back where the epidural will be given. This spot is known as the epidural or extradural space. (It is outside the last of the three membranes that cover the spinal cord and just inside the bone and ligament of the vertebral column.) The local will sting slightly, and then you will feel numb. Pressure is all that you will feel as the epidural needle, bearing the catheter (tube) is injected. The needle is withdrawn, but the long catheter is left in place and taped to the outside of your back and shoulder. By leaving the catheter in place, more anesthetic can be administered later if needed.

You will first receive a test dose of medication to determine if you are allergic to the particular drug being used. Then a full dose will be given. Depending on the dose and the drug used, the pain relief should last from forty-five minutes to two hours. The selection of the drug will depend on anesthesiologist's preference, the latest studies, the reason for the epidural, and the projected length of labor.

You will be immobilized with an epidural because although you can move your legs, they will seem heavy and weak and you won't be able to walk. You'll have to use a bedpan or have a catheter inserted into your

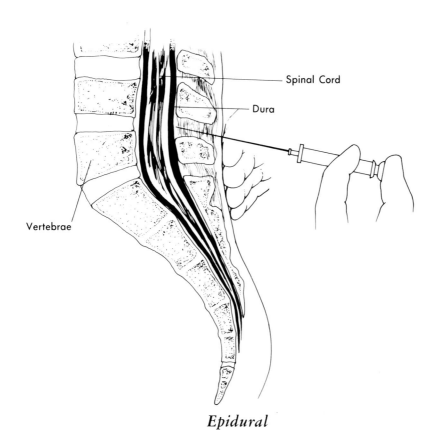

Epidural

bladder to empty it, because a full bladder can interfere with the descent of the baby's head. If forceps are used when the bladder is full, damage can occur, and the bladder can become infected.

Just like any other substance you receive or ingest, an epidural anesthetic crosses the placenta. Previously it was believed that epidural anesthetics did not reach the baby, but more recent testing of the neonatal blood after birth has found the anesthetic to be present. It is unclear what effect, if any, epidurals have on babies. A 1985 review of the literature on epidurals stated that the studies were far from consistent, although they did suggest a mild transient effect on newborn behavior.

Many women today take prepared-childbirth classes with the idea that they'll have natural childbirth if it doesn't hurt too much. If labor gets unbearably painful, they can always count on an epidural to bail them out. To some extent, this outlook becomes a self-fulfilling prophecy. Epidurals are enormously popular for this reason and also because they are encouraged by many obstetricians who consider them safe and effective. Granted, an epidural can salvage a labor that is doomed because of fear, unbearable back labor, or irregular and gruesome contractions. It can also turn a cesarean into a good birth experience because a woman is awake to meet her baby, and her husband is at her side.

Epidurals, however, are much more than just a tiny injection; they spin a web of intervention that turns normal labor into a high-tech affair. Your baby's heartbeat will be continuously monitored, you will be hooked up to an intravenous, and your blood pressure will be checked frequently. And, as we said earlier, the chances of receiving Pitocin and having a forceps delivery are much greater than if you didn't have the epidural.

Many women request epidurals during transition, but this is the worst time to receive one. You will have to hold still for the procedure during your worst contractions, and by the time it takes effect, you will be fully dilated and too numb to push effectively. You might take a nap while waiting for the anesthetic to wear off, but it's a rare doctor who will not rush from one stage of labor to the next. You will be forced to push whether you feel like it or not.

To avoid this happening to you, you should ask for a cervical check before receiving an epidural. Contractions can seem unbearable because labor is progressing rapidly. You may gain some perspective, however, if you learn you've just dilated four centimeters in thirty minutes and are finally at nine.

The Spinal

A spinal takes about three to six minutes to administer and lasts approximately an hour and a half. It numbs and paralyzes the lower half of the body, from the chest to the toes. The legs cannot be moved to change position, and the abdominal muscles will be immobilized for pushing. Spinals have been replaced by epidurals for the pain of labor, but they are still used today for forceps or cesarean deliveries.

Preparation for the spinal is the same as it is for the epidural. You will be asked to round your back and it will be washed and a local injection will be administered. A test dose will be given for allergic reaction and to assure that the needle is in the proper position. This will be followed by a full dose. With a spinal, the injection is made directly into the spinal canal and cerebrospinal fluid.

It is important not to cough or move during the procedure in order that the anesthetic will not be moved higher within the spinal canal. If that were to happen your blood pressure could drop precipitously and your breathing would be impaired. The spinal anesthetic bathes the nerves, blocking the passage of pain sensation to the brain. As it takes effect, a warm tingling sensation will spread from the toes to the abdomen.

Spinals have some advantages in comparison to epidurals, particularly when time is a consideration. They require less skill to administer, less anesthetic is needed, they take effect more quickly, and they are faster to administer. Spinals also have a slightly higher success or "take" rate: 95 percent versus 93 percent for the epidural. Their primary drawback is that maternal side effects are greater than with the epidural.

Hypotension is the most common complication. There is a widening and loss of tone in the maternal veins due to the interruption of the sympathetic nerve impulses that control blood pressure. This is exacerbated if the woman lies on her back; she must lie on her left side. Spinals can also cause difficulty with respiration because sensation to the intercostal (rib) muscles is affected by the anesthesia. Breathing may seem labored or shallow, and you may feel you can't breathe. You should be sure to inform your doctor right away if you experience this reaction. In the most extreme case, you would be put on a respirator until the anesthetic wears off. In most instances, however, you should be reassured that if you can still talk, you can still breathe.

The most infamous complication of the spinal is the spinal headache, caused by a loss of cerebrospinal fluid due to the injection. In this situation, the spinal fluid leaks out the hole made by the injection, causing a change in spinal pressure and hence the headache. This used to be a more common problem, but today a finer-gauge needle is used, creating a smaller hole. A study of 9,277 spinals administered showed an 18 percent incidence of headache when a large 16-gauge needle was used; when a smaller 24-gauge needle was substituted, the headache rate dropped to 6 percent.

After receiving a spinal, women are advised to remain supine for eight hours following delivery to avoid developing a headache. There is some controversy about whether this actually helps prevent the occurrence, but there's no question that it's the only position to assume once you've got the headache. Pain medication is also helpful, along with the knowledge that the headache is finite, usually lasting one or two days.

If a headache from a spinal or epidural is severe, a procedure called a blood patch can help. This is administered by an anesthesiologist and consists of an injection of 10 to 15 milliliters of your own blood into the site of the puncture. The blood will then create a seal over the leak. A saline solution may also be substituted. The procedure is not without risks, so its use depends on individual circumstances.

Which Anesthetic for Cesarean Section?

There are advantages and disadvantages to both epidurals and spinals for cesarean delivery. As we've said before, if you find yourself in a position to choose, you'll probably be guided by the preference of the anesthesiologist and the practice of the hospital. In addition to what we've already told you, some of the things to consider are

- Epidurals cause less of a drop in maternal blood pressure.
- Because a catheter can be left in place, epidurals can easily be topped off if anesthetic effect decreases.
- A thicker gauge needle must be used to administer an epidural, and if there is a puncture in the dura, the headache that ensues can be worse than a spinal headache. It is estimated, however, that this complication occurs in only 1 to 2 percent of all cases.
- The epidural can also result in spotty coverage, only affecting half the body or leaving "windows," or small areas that are not anesthetized.

The Saddle Block

If a woman is given a spinal and then remains sitting for ten minutes, the method of anesthesia becomes a saddle block. This is because the drug settles to a lower body level than if it were administered while she was lying down. A saddle block numbs the vagina, perineum, and upper thighs. With the exception of the vagina, this is the area that would rest on a saddle, hence the name.

This is an effective anesthetic for a forceps delivery or a painful second stage. An advantage to the saddle block over a full spinal is that some feeling in the abdomen remains so it does not completely impair the ability to push. It does not seem to be a very popular method of anesthesia. Since it can interfere with the normal descent of the fetal head, it should only be given if the baby is well engaged in the mother's pelvis.

The Paracervical

This is the only regional anesthetic that is administered by the obstetrician. It relieves the pain of contractions, but does not affect the pain of back labor or numb the vagina or perineum. The paracervical consists of two injections, into the nerves on either side of the cervix, so it is usually administered no later than active labor, when there is enough cervix to use as a guide. The anesthetic effects can last anywhere from forty minutes to two hours, depending on the particular medication used.

This type of regional anesthetic has largely been replaced by the epidural because of a 25 to 30 percent risk of fetal bradycardia.

GENERAL ANESTHESIA

General anesthesia is most commonly used today for emergency cesarean sections. If the baby is in distress or the mother is hemorrhaging, there won't be time for a spinal or epidural; with a general anesthesia, a baby can be delivered in less than ten minutes. A general anesthetic is also used for nonemergency cesareans if this is the anesthesiologist's preference or if there are contraindications for a regional anesthetic.

If you know in advance you will be having a general anesthetic, you will probably be admitted a day early to the hospital and be prohibited from eating or drinking anything for eight to twelve hours prior to delivery. If you need an emergency cesarean, you will be given some kind of antacid, such as sodium citrate, Maalox, or Tagemet, to neutralize stomach contents.

The reason for these precautions is that the greatest risks of general anesthesia are respiratory irritation or infection or death from the aspiration of acidic stomach secretions. The latter can occur whether you have fasted or not and is called Mendelson's syndrome. It is the leading cause of anesthetic obstetrical deaths.

The Procedure

Once you are in the delivery room, you will be given oxygen to breathe. The mask may smell unpleasant, and it may be uncomfortable to have your nose and mouth covered, but it will help if you try to relax and breathe normally. Then a barbiturate will be injected into your intravenous line, and this will put you to sleep in just fifteen to twenty seconds.

A muscle relaxant will then follow, which will cause temporary paralysis. Now a plastic (endotracheal) tube can be inserted down your throat and the anesthetic gases are administered through the tube, causing unconsciousness. The tube also reduces the risk of inhaling stomach contents. When you awaken, the tube will be gone, but your throat may be sore for a few days.

MEDICATION CHART

MEDICATION	ADMINISTRATION	PURPOSE
Analgesics Narcotics (Demerol, Nisentil)	IM or IV	Decrease perception of pain. Promote relaxation during labor.
Barbiturates (Seconal, Nembutol)	IM, IV or oral pill	Induce sleep (rarely used during labor).
Tranquilizers (Phenergan, Valium, Vistaril)	IM or IV	Reduce anxiety and/or nausea during labor. (Is often used in conjunction with Demerol.)
Inhalants (nitrous oxide)	Inhalation	Pain relief during delivery.
Amnestics (scopolomine)	IV or IM	Erase memory of experience.

You may be confused, groggy, or nauseated when you wake up and you may have a poor sense of time. The grogginess may last for a few hours or a few days, depending on the amount of anesthetic used and your own metabolism. Once the anesthesia wears off, there will be a sudden return of sensation, and you may need pain medication right away in the recovery room.

ADVANTAGES	DISADVANTAGES
Increases relaxation. Can take the "edge off" contractions. Effects can be counteracted with an antagonist (Narcan).	Can cause respiratory depression in newborn. Can slow contractions. Often causes nausea and vomiting. Safe dosages too low for effective pain relief. Sleepiness can reduce ability to cope with contractions or push effectively.
Can reduce fear and anxiety.	Has a depressant effect on baby. Cannot be counteracted by an antagonist.
Has no effect on contractions. Can increase relaxation.	Provides no direct pain relief. Can cause maternal hypotension.
Rapid onset of action; rapid recovery when gas is discontinued.	Does not provide total pain relief.
Does not affect uterine contractions. Eliminates memory of labor and delivery. No known adverse effect on newborn.	Response is unpredictable, ranging from euphoria to wild, irrational behavior (especially common reaction in the presense of pain). Does not relieve pain so must be used with other medications. Father cannot be present. Mother has no active participation or memory of experience.

MEDICATION	ADMINISTRATION	PURPOSE
Local Anesthesia		
Pudendal (Xylocaine, Nesacaine, Marcane)	Two vaginal injections into area of the pudendal nerves.	Numb vagina, vulva and perineum.
Perineal Block (same as above)	Injection into perineum.	Numb perineum for episiotomy incision and repair.
Regional Anesthesia (Marcane, Xylocaine, Carbocaine)		
Epidural	Single injection or through catheter placed in epidural space.	Pain relief during labor and/or delivery. Anesthesia for cesarean delivery.
Spinal	Injection into spinal canal.	Anesthesia for vaginal delivery. Anesthesia for cesarean delivery.
Saddle Block	Same	Numb vagina, perineum and upper thighs.
Paracervical	Injection into vagina, into tissue on either side of cervix.	Pain relief during labor.
General Anesthesia Combination of medications	Inhalation of anesthetic gases or IV medications.	Produce unconsciousness.

ADVANTAGES	DISADVANTAGES
Provides pain relief for normal delivery or episiotomy repair; Relaxes perineum.	Not adequate pain relief for forceps delivery.
Provides pain relief for episiotomy repair.	None.
Safest and most effective regional anesthesia. Eliminates pain without affecting awareness. Mother can still actively participate.	Often causes maternal hypotension. Often decreases strength and frequency of contractions. Eliminates urge to push. Increases likelihood of fetal malposition and need for forceps. Anesthesia can be "spotty" or only take on one side. Can become a spinal and cause headache.
Requires less skill and is easier to administer than epidural. Provides excellent pain relief	Greater maternal side effects compared to other regional anesthetics, especially hypotension. Possible spinal headache.
Provides effective pain relief for pushing. No effect on contractions.	Can interfere with normal descent of baby.
Can be administered by obstetrician.	Can cause fetal bradycardia. Cannot be given past 8 cm dilation.
Fastest anesthetic for emergency cesarean or difficult vaginal delivery. Provides complete pain relief.	Greater risk of complications for both mother and child than regional anesthetics (or natural delivery). Possible depression in newborn. Father cannot be present for delivery. Mother is not awake.

CHAPTER 12

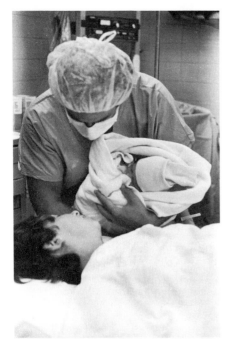

Variations on Normal Labor and Delivery

No one wants to read this chapter because no woman wants to think about her labor deviating from the norm. If your pregnancy has been enjoyable and free of problems, the possibility of complications seems hard to accept. Often women who have been healthy can't even contemplate something going awry. If things have gone smoothly so far, you think, why jinx my luck by worrying?

We're not asking you to worry. We're only hoping that you'll extend the process of childbirth preparation to include a consideration of forceps and cesarean deliveries. This sort of discussion should not be considered frightening, nor does it condone medical intervention. Knowledge reduces fear, and talking about complications does not produce them. There are many reasons why the cesarean rate has practically quadrupled since 1970, but discussion isn't one of them.

In 1983 the national cesarean rate was 20.3 percent and climbing. If you don't learn something about this method of delivery, you'll be sticking your head in the sand. If there are five couples in your Lamaze class, one of them is likely to have a cesarean, and it could be you. According to the responses to our questionnaire, most people decided to have their baby in a hospital, just to be safe. For that same reason, you should read this chapter—just to be safe, and to know the choices you will have to make if a cesarean or forceps delivery becomes necessary. Preparing for labor makes you better able to make decisions, and preparing for complications does the same thing. If you're informed, you are able to participate more actively in your child's birth and better understand the entire experience, no matter what the circumstances.

FORCEPS

The need for a forceps delivery is apparent only during the second stage of labor, after you have dilated completely and are trying to push the baby out.

Forceps are paired metallic instruments, frequently compared in design to salad tongs; they are used for rotation and/or extraction of the baby's head. The analogy to tongs isn't really precise, however, because the blades come apart. They are placed around the head individually and then, once in place, they are joined together.

There have been more than six hundred types of forceps designed, but all of them are used primarily for two purposes: exerting traction (pulling out the baby) and turning the baby's head to a better position. Forceps deliveries are classified according to the station and position of the baby's head when they are applied, and not according to the type of instrument used, as you might think.

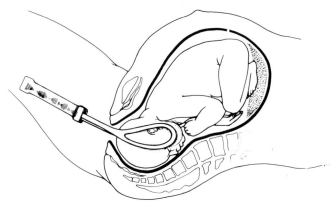

Forceps

Types of Forceps Deliveries

The three varieties of forceps deliveries are

- *Low-,* or *outlet, forceps.* This is the most common type of forceps delivery, occurring just before the baby's head crowns. The head, however, is visible without opening the labia. This is the safest method of forceps delivery, provided it is performed by a skilled obstetrician.
- *Midforceps.* In this situation, the baby's head is higher up in the pelvis, although it must be engaged for the procedure to qualify as a midforceps delivery. Any delivery requiring rotation of the baby's head becomes a midforceps delivery, regardless of how low the head is resting in the pelvis. It's sometimes difficult for an obstetrician to predict how difficult a midforceps delivery will be; some are quite easy, whereas others can be traumatic for mother or baby. The risk of the delivery is greatly increased if the doctor has incorrectly judged the position or station of the baby's head.
- *High-forceps.* This operation has become extinct in the past fifteen years because of the increased safety of cesarean sections. A high-forceps delivery is an outmoded and dangerous procedure. In this delivery, the baby's head is not engaged and may be floating high in the pelvis. A cesarean section is virtually always preferable to a high-forceps delivery.

"It took longer to sew me up than for her to pop out! The forceps badly bruised my daughter's face."

♦

"The doctor was very careful. My daughter never had any marks at all."

♦

"The procedure looked too violent to my husband, and he felt the baby must be experiencing pain from the use of the forceps. They caused a small red spot on the baby's face, but it is all gone now."

♦

"I hated it! It was the most painful part of the whole birth. I think my doctor was in a hurry and just wanted to speed things up."

♦

"The forceps were not painful, but there was a lot of pressure. At the time I didn't care what they did as long as I could have the baby."

♦

"I was initially upset when my doctor got out the forceps, but was happy because they sped up the delivery and my baby came out unharmed."

The Procedure

Most forceps deliveries require the use of an anesthetic. Pudendals, epidurals, and spinals are the ones most commonly given. If there isn't enough time to give anesthesia, the doctor may offer you a whiff of nitrous oxide (laughing gas). To enlarge the vaginal opening, an episiotomy is always done. Other requirements for delivery include an empty bladder (to create maximum room in the pelvic cavity), and ruptured membranes (so that the doctor will not lose traction by having to place the forceps over the amniotic sac).

If the doctor is doing a low-forceps delivery, you will be asked to push as he pulls during each contraction. His hands may shake and it will appear that he's exerting a lot of force. He is pulling hard, but the whole thing probably looks much scarier than it really is. In a couple of pushes, the baby's head will emerge, and you'll be almost there. Sometimes a sensitive doctor will bring the head down with forceps and then let you push out the baby yourself.

Indications for Forceps

Women who have little or no medication during labor usually don't need forceps. For them, pushing is hard work, but it also brings relief, and usually after about an hour the baby is born. There are, however, several reasons why forceps are necessary. They include

- *Fetal distress.* Forceps can be a godsend when fetal distress is detected and the baby needs to be born quickly. In that case, you would probably be given several whiffs of oxygen to boost the baby's supply and moved to the delivery room immediately.
- *Helping the mother's own expulsive efforts.* This use of forceps increases as epidurals become more available and more popular. A woman with no sensation in her pelvic floor has much less ability and desire to push. Approximately 65 to 75 percent of the women who receive epidurals for pain relief also require the use of forceps. This rate contrasts with the use of forceps in 4 to 21 percent of deliveries without anesthesia. Other reasons for an inability to push are exhaustion after pushing for a long time, poor uterine contractions, or an abnormal positioning of the baby's head.
- *The need for extra traction to offset a cord difficulty.* Sometimes a short cord or one that is wrapped around the baby's neck or shoulders can prevent the head from descending naturally. This phenomenon is indicated when the head crowns but repeatedly slips back into the vagina. There may also be some fetal heart deceleration. When this occurs, your doctor will need to use forceps. You may wonder if he's rushing things, but in this case you need this assistance. You could go on for another hour and the head would still be retreating after

each push. The baby is not in danger, because the cord is quite elastic, but a forceps delivery is necessary in order for the baby to be born without further stress.

- *Exceptional medical problems of the mother.* A woman with heart disease should avoid the physical strain of pushing. Also, a woman with a detached retina should not raise her intracranial pressure by strenuously bearing down.
- *A premature infant.* The head of a premature baby needs more protection than that of a full-term infant. To reduce stress to the head, forceps may be used to shorten the delivery.

The Risks Involved

Naturally, there are risks involved with the use of forceps, and as with any other medical intervention, you must weigh them against the benefits. Forceps can lacerate the mother's cervix, vagina, or bladder. And they can cause facial nerve damage in the infant as well as hemorrhage within the head. The risks of complications are greater with high- and mid-forceps deliveries than with low ones. Often, with outlet forceps the baby sustains only temporary bruises or indentations where the metal touched his head. To minimize these risks, it's very important that a woman be fully dilated and that the doctor be experienced. Unless there's a true emergency, don't allow your baby to be delivered by an intern or resident who is just learning how to do a forceps delivery. As we said earlier, you're under no obligation to be a good sport or to provide educational opportunities for young doctors.

Low-forceps deliveries are considered safer. However, in *The Pregnancy Book for Today's Woman,* Dr. Howard Shapiro states that many doctors now believe that if an easy outlet-forceps delivery cannot be performed, a cesarean section should be done instead, because there is less risk of maternal and infant trauma. Shapiro cites the research of Dr. Emanuel Friedman, who noted two infant deaths per one thousand spontaneous deliveries, compared with eleven deaths per one thousand deliveries with midforceps and twenty-nine deaths per one thousand deliveries if midforceps were used at the end of a long labor. Children who were delivered by midforceps also had a much greater incidence of hearing and speech disorders at age three—the impairments occurred at a rate of thirty-three per one thousand, compared with six per one thousand among children who were born by normal vaginal delivery.

Avoiding a Forceps Delivery

When all is said and done, sometimes it's a bit of true grit or super willpower that enables women to deliver without assistance. Often all it takes is the mention of the word *forceps* to give a woman that extra ounce of energy to push the baby out herself. A delivery-room nurse was recently quoted as saying, "You see this all the time with these birthing-room/natural-childbirth mothers—you just mention forceps and they get those babies born."

No woman can exercise total control over her labor. Although you may not have wanted a forceps delivery, there are times when it is necessary. To give yourself the best shot at natural childbirth, don't have epidural anesthesia. Take it easy during early labor so that you can decrease the chance of exhaustion much later on. Assume a comfortable position for pushing (not on your back) and try using a mirror or some visualization to give you that extra edge. Another technique is to have the doctor or midwife place two fingers just inside the vagina. This pressure will help you find exactly where to push. Sometimes the transfer to the delivery room can make a difference because it's a change of scenery and it means you really are getting closer to the end.

VACUUM EXTRACTION

Vacuum extractors are suction pumps used in lieu of forceps. They have been popular in Europe for many years, but have never achieved the same status here because of the risks associated with the metal cup that was attached to the baby's head. The machines with the metal cup have now been replaced by a more sophisticated device, which utilizes a cup made of soft silicone rubber.

The indications for using extractors are virtually the same as those for forceps:

- Proper position of the baby. Not recommended for brow or face presentations.
- No demonstrated CPD (cephalo-pelvic disproportion).
- Adequate dilation and effacement of the cervix.
- Ruptured membranes.
- Engagement of the baby's head.

Unlike forceps, however, the extractor should not be used for breech deliveries or when unusual amounts of traction are required.

The machine works on the principle of a vacuum, which is created by pistons in the motor. The rubber cup fits on top of the baby's head, and suction is applied only during a contraction. The extractor cannot be used if fetal-scalp sampling has been done because of a risk of excess bleeding. One of the biggest advantages of the extractor is that unlike a forceps delivery, it's not always necessary to perform an episiotomy.

Vacuum extractors have a bad name with many doctors because of the high risk of scalp lacerations and hematomas (blood clots under the skin) associated with the old metal cup. The original machines also had a long

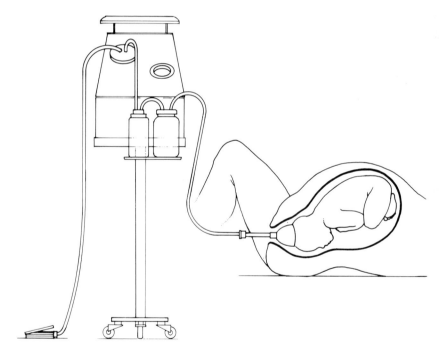

Vacuum Extractor

start-up time—anywhere from four to thirty minutes—and therefore were not suitable in cases of fetal distress. The machines in use today can achieve a vacuum in thirty seconds.

The up-to-date extractors are not widely available, however. We spoke to representatives of the two major manufacturers, who said they had placed many machines in hospitals lately, but only on a trial basis. Advocates of the vacuum extractor claim certain advantages in comparison with forceps: (a) A local anesthetic can often be used instead of a regional, thereby allowing the mother to push more effectively; (b) the cervix doesn't have to be fully dilated for the cup to be applied; and (c) the severity of injuries to mother and baby is less. One study stated that extraction with the silicone cap was a safe substitute for midforceps deliveries because there was no risk of vaginal and cervical tears from the metal blades of the forceps. It also cited reduced risk of hematoma to the baby.

We spoke to Dr. James Ottolini of St. Louis, an obstetrician who has performed more than one thousand deliveries with the extractor and is considered an expert in its use. "The extractor is like any other machine," he said. "Extractors are only as good as the people who use them, and that's a shame because there are many things they can do." Dr. Ottolini likes to use the extractor for the vaginal delivery of twins. The second twin, who is generally smaller and less robust than the first, can be delivered by suction in a matter of minutes. Dr. Ottolini said he consistently gets Apgar scores in the eight to ten range for the second twin, an outcome that is considered quite good.

Another of his unusual uses of the extractor is during a repeat cesarean section. "Often the baby is quite high and not engaged, and getting him out can be like bobbing for apples," Ottolini explained. The doctor uses the extractor to locate the head and then pull it into a more accessible position. "The effectiveness of the extractor enables me to make smaller incisions in the abdominal wall and in the uterus," he said.

The extractor has all but replaced forceps in Ottolini's practice. He believes its use during a delayed second stage can reduce the likelihood of a cesarean. "Often when a regional anesthetic is used, there can be a long second stage, with the mother experiencing difficulty with pushing. If I can bring the baby into place with the extractor, I'll know for sure there's no CPD, so it's just a matter of letting the epidural wear off and letting her push the baby out herself.

"One of the extractor's best uses is as a substitute for low-forceps, a delivery that normally requires an episiotomy. The pull on the head can be controlled beautifully. I use it gently, almost like a shoehorn. With the mother's cooperation it's a gentle, controlled delivery."

Obviously, not every obstetrician can match Dr. Ottolini's expertise and experience with the vacuum extractor. As with forceps, an extractor is best used by someone with considerable skill.

CESAREAN SECTION

The Statistics

In the United States today, more than one out of every five babies will be born by cesarean section. The national cesarean rate for 1983 was 20.3 percent of all deliveries, which represents almost a fourfold increase from 1970, when the rate was just 5.5 percent. This incredible jump has been described as a cesarean epidemic and is denounced by radical feminists and conservative obstetricians alike.

This surge of cesarean deliveries has a lot to do with the operation becoming safer and with the hazards of midforceps and difficult breech deliveries becoming better known. But there are also many unnecessary cesareans being performed. It's sometimes difficult to determine when a cesarean is truly needed because the issue of the baby's safety often overlaps with the doctor's fear of malpractice or his desire for convenience.

The cesarean rate differs from state to state and from hospital to hospital. One would think that large hospitals and teaching hospitals perform the most cesareans. In the past, studies have shown that the bigger the hospital, the higher the rate. Cesarean deliveries are so prevalent today, however, that there is no longer any direct correlation between hospital size and rate of cesarean section. The Massachusetts Department of Public Health did a study in 1984 disproving the notion that smaller hospitals have a lower cesarean rate. The study found state cesarean rates in 1982 to range from 31.22 to 7.63 percent and revealed that small community hospitals in the greater Boston area had the highest rates. In fact, of the ten Massachusetts hospitals where the most cesareans were performed, only two of them were referral centers specializing in high-risk cases. The principal author of the study, Letitia Davis, said that the most striking thing about her findings was that the tremendous variability among hospitals cannot be explained by known risk factors.

Putting the statistics aside, your chance of having a cesarean depends

Cesarean Delivery

♦

"Feeling the doctor take the baby from my womb was an experience I couldn't begin to describe! It was so moving to see my child. I felt so many emotions—tears, laughter, the whole nine yards!"

♦

"What I didn't understand, and still don't, is why they let me labor for twenty-two hours."

♦

"When the cesarean became necessary, I was caught off guard and was totally unprepared to make any decisions about what was happening. I didn't even realize that there were decisions to be made. I just went along with the doctor, nurses, and policies."

♦

"Once I accepted the fact that I had to have one, the entire experience was fulfilling and not at all disappointing. My husband was allowed to be with me the whole time, and then he was with our baby, which was wonderful. I felt very supported by my husband and the staff."

♦

"The hospital staff treated me like a piece of meat. I accepted the cesarean section, but not their attitude."

♦

"I had to ask for everything—bikini incision instead of vertical, spinal anesthesia instead of general."

♦

"Obviously I did not get what I wanted when I had a cesarean section after nineteen hours of labor, but at least I have a tape recording of her first cry and

continued

some pictures from right after she was born. There are no words to tell how disappointed I was, and for the first few months I was very depressed. I felt deprived of my bonding experience and wondered what my poor, new, trembling little baby must have thought. I wonder how different things might have been with a vaginal delivery, without the aftermath of the pain and disappointment from the cesarean."

◆

"I was relieved. I was afraid of labor."

◆

"I felt cheated. I kept apologizing to my husband, as if I were to blame."

◆

"Made the most of it and had a really good time! My husband was with me, the staff were super-supportive. There was a very warm and joyous atmosphere."

◆

"I was absolutely devastated. I think my doctor lied to me to cover up for his associate, who attended the birth. There were many other women on the floor who had cesarean sections, but I was the only one with a vertical cut. My family and friends could not understand my feelings, since everyone was alive and well at the end, but it's a tremendous sense of loss."

◆

"During the operation I was tied down and paralyzed. It was the most terrifying and humiliating experience of my life."

◆

"I got to experience early labor without medication, which I wanted to do. But I will never know what it actually feels like to push a baby out."

continued

♦

"I chose general anesthesia. After twenty-four hours of labor, I just wanted to be asleep and have them deliver my child."

♦

"I think it was unnecessary. It was my doctor's idea, and I was too tired to fight anymore."

♦

"I don't feel guilty about any part of my delivery. Fear of surgery is natural, but the guilt is totally unnecessary."

to a great extent on the individual cesarean rate of your doctor or midwife. This is one of the most important questions to ask a doctor during a preliminary consultation, and just about every obstetrician, whether his rate is high or low, will be proud to tell you. If 8 percent of his deliveries are cesarean, the doctor will say that he doesn't believe in intervention and that a patient, natural approach is best. If his rate is 25 percent, the doctor will talk a lot about better babies and the benefits of technology. Midwives can't perform cesareans, but any midwife should be able to give you the percentage of her patients who require surgical delivery. (Midwives, unlike obstetricians, screen their patients in advance to turn away women who are high risk, with increased chances of having a cesarean.)

Reasons for Cesarean Delivery

In 1979, the Department of Health, Education, and Welfare contracted Dr. Helen Marieskind to evaluate the rising cesarean rate. Her report, released in 1980, stated that there is no evidence that supports a correlation between lowered infant mortality and morbidity rates with the rise in the rate of cesarean sections. In her research, Dr. Marieskind interviewed more than one hundred doctors, and from their comments she compiled a list of the twelve factors contributing to the tremendous increase in cesareans. The primary reasons, in order of significance, were the following:

1. Threat of malpractice
2. The policy of performing repeat cesareans
3. The nature of current obstetrical training, which encourages cesarean delivery (that is, for breech babies)
4. The belief that cesareans produce better babies
5. Changing and expanded indications for cesareans, that is, twins and breech

In the same year, 1980, another federal agency, the National Institute of Health (NIH), also studied the growing phenomenon of cesarean birth. The NIH convened a special task force of nineteen members, which issued a 536-page report. One of their most important findings was that four diagnostic categories account for about 80 percent of all cesareans, and about 80 to 90 percent of the increase in the past fifteen years. The categories are

- Dystocia
- Repeat cesareans
- Fetal distress
- Breech presentation

Some women will know in advance that they may need a cesarean, but most receive the news during labor. You simply cannot know beforehand what kind of birth experience you are going to have. Even if you think you are an unlikely candidate for surgery, you should review the following conditions so that if one of them arises, you will better understand what is happening

DYSTOCIA
Dystocia is a catchall category that includes failure to progress, *cephalopelvic disproportion* (CPD), and relative CPD. *Failure to progress* means that contractions either stop or fail to produce dilation. This can occur because the uterus is stretched out and unresponsive, because of an odd

presentation, or because a woman is tense, fearful, or exhausted. *CPD* means that the woman's pelvis is too narrow to permit the baby to pass through. This condition can slow down dilation, but it is most apparent during expulsion, because pushing fails to move the baby. Except in rare cases, CPD can't be accurately diagnosed until labor begins. True CPD is believed to occur in only about 2 percent of all births, but it is frequently mislabeled and blamed for failure to progress.

The task force recommended that before performing a cesarean for failure to progress, several other alternatives be tried. They include rest, hydration, relaxation by sedation, walking around, and stimulation of contractions with Pitocin. We certainly endorse any of these measures in an attempt to avoid a cesarean. In addition to the task force's recommendations, we would suggest nipple stimulation, massage, visualization, relaxation techniques, and changing body positions. Labor is greatly influenced by a woman's state of mind and her energy level. Fasting, exhaustion, tension, and laboring in the supine position can all make dilation falter or stop.

REPEAT CESAREANS

Perhaps the most controversial recommendation of the NIH Task Force was that repeat cesareans not be performed routinely. It suggested that women who had previously had a cesarean by means of a low transverse cervical incision (see page 295) be permitted to attempt a vaginal delivery for subsequent pregnancies, if the condition that necessitated the first cesarean is not present. This recommendation has great potential for reducing the escalating cesarean rate, because repeat operations account for nearly one-third of cesareans performed. As more primary ones are done, the likelihood for more secondary ones increases. Vaginal birth after cesarean has recently attracted considerable publicity, but in practice approximately 98 percent of the women in the United States with a previous cesarean now give birth by repeat cesarean.

FETAL DISTRESS AND FETAL MONITORING

Many people believe there is a meaningful correspondence between the growing reliance on electronic fetal monitoring and the rising cesarean rate. The task force did not make a direct correlation between these two developments, but did state that probably no more than 1 percent of the total cesarean rate is attributable to fetal monitoring. The study did not deal with the indirect effect of this technology, particularly on dystocia. Several studies have demonstrated that normal fetuses undergoing stress and those who are compromised and truly distressed may show the same abnormal pattern on the fetal monitor. To differentiate between these two very different situations and thus avoid unnecessary cesareans, fetal-scalp sampling is necessary. Unfortunately, this test is unavailable in more than half of all American hospitals, and it is often underutilized even when it is available.

BREECH DELIVERIES

Breech deliveries, the last major contributing factor to the high cesarean rate, are a controversial subject. Many doctors strongly believe that breech babies should be delivered by cesarean because numerous studies have shown the outcomes of cesarean deliveries to be superior to vaginal deliveries. However, a vaginal delivery of a breech baby is sometimes possible (see chapter 7). This is not a black-and-white issue, so it's difficult to generalize. The decision really hinges on your doctor and what type of delivery he is comfortable performing. The choice of vaginal or cesarean delivery is complicated, and this is something that should be discussed at length with your doctor or midwife.

HERPES

An active case of genital herpes makes a woman a prime candidate for a quick cesarean section. If vaginal delivery occurs, the infant has a 50 percent chance of contracting the virus during the passage through the infected birth canal. If the baby gets herpes, he has a 60 to 90 percent chance of either dying or sustaining damage to the central nervous system. If you have herpes, your doctor will determine whether it is active by checking carefully for lesions and by taking viral cultures for several consecutive weeks prior to delivery.

PLACENTA PREVIA

A rare condition, occurring in roughly one out of every two hundred pregnancies, placenta previa means a placenta partially or completely covering the cervix. It is diagnosed by bright red bleeding that is painless, usually occurring during the last trimester or during labor. Vaginal delivery is sometimes possible if the placenta is not completely blocking the cervical opening, but in most cases a cesarean must be performed. With placenta previa, the primary risk is maternal hemorrhage. There is also the possibility that the placenta can become compressed by the baby's presenting part, thus cutting off the oxygen supply, or that the placenta will prevent the baby's descent into the birth canal.

PLACENTA ABRUPTIO

This is a type of uterine hemorrhage caused by the complete or partial separation of the placenta from the uterine wall. It is more rare and more serious than placenta previa because it can pose an immediate threat to the baby's oxygen supply. Its severity depends on the degree of placental separation, because oxygen and carbon dioxide can be adequately transferred across a semidetached placenta. Often this condition begins before the onset of labor, but it is not apparent until labor begins. Be aware of any sudden onset of continuous and localized pain.

POSTMATURITY

This occurs in 4 percent of all pregnancies. The condition is also known as placental deficiency syndrome because of the placenta's inability to function efficiently. Postmature babies actually lose weight and they suffer from a diminished supply of oxygen. If you go past your due date, your doctor or midwife will probably perform a nonstress and perhaps a stress test to assess the condition of the fetal-placental unit. (See chapter 7 for more on these procedures.) If it seems that the placenta is aging and therefore not providing proper food and oxygen, labor will be induced. If induction does not stimulate effective labor, a cesarean will be done.

CORD PROLAPSE

Women carrying babies in the footling or incomplete breech position have the greatest risk of cord prolapse. It can also occur when the membranes have ruptured and the baby is not well engaged in the pelvis; the cord slips down in the uterus and becomes prolapsed or wedged between the baby and the cervical opening. With each contraction, the cord is squeezed and the baby's oxygen supply is interrupted to some extent. Sometimes the cord will actually slip out of the cervix into the vagina. Cord prolapse is an extremely dangerous condition, requiring an emergency cesarean.

MULTIPLE BIRTHS

In 40 to 50 percent of all twin births, one of the babies presents in the breech position. Babies born in multiples are likely to assume odd positions. If the first twin is breech and this is your first pregnancy, a cesarean may be necessary. But if the first baby is vertex (head down), vaginal delivery is possible if your doctor or midwife is willing.

MALPRESENTATION

Malpresentation means anything other than the normal vertex position. The most common variation is breech (see chapter 7 for a full description of the varieties of breech and the standards for normal delivery). Another odd position is *transverse lie,* in which the baby is stretched across the uterus at a forty-five- to ninety-degree angle to the mother's spinal column. In this instance, cesarean section is advised, because the shoulder usually enters the cervix, blocking the passage for the rest of the body. Babies can also demonstrate a *brow presentation,* in which the head is not tucked into the chest, or a *face presentation,* in which the head is extended and the face is forced to enter the birth canal first. Some of these presentations necessitate a cesarean, but frequently they are accompanied by complications, such as failure to progress or fetal distress.

PREMATURE RUPTURE OF THE MEMBRANES (PROM)

This is a common complication of pregnancy and it does not necessarily require a cesarean. After the membranes rupture, there is increased chance of infection. To minimize risk, many doctors prefer delivery to occur within twenty-four hours. If your water breaks and labor does not start on its own, your doctor may insist on performing an induction, and if that fails, a cesarean. We consider this to be an aggressive approach and would prefer to allow labor to start naturally with scrupulous care paid to hygiene in order to prevent infection. (For a complete discussion of PROM, see chapter 8.)

TOXEMIA OR PREECLAMPSIA

Toxemia, also known as preeclampsia, is a dangerous and somewhat mysterious condition that can occur at any time during pregnancy, but most commonly appears in the third trimester. It is heralded by a trio of symptoms: high blood pressure, protein in the urine, and edema (swelling from water retention). The cause is unknown, but many people believe it is linked to diet. Mild toxemia can often be controlled by medication and bed rest. Its cure, however, is delivery. If left untreated, toxemia can progress into a condition known as eclampsia, which can cause maternal convulsions, coma, or even death. If the disease does not respond to more conservative measures, labor will be induced or a cesarean will be performed.

DIABETES

Preexisting diabetes must be carefully monitored during pregnancy to make sure it doesn't worsen. Also, diabetic women are apt to develop toxemia. Babies born to diabetic mothers have an increased chance of respiratory distress syndrome due to the delayed maturation of their lungs, and stillbirth if the baby goes to term. (This doesn't apply to those women who develop gestational diabetes during pregnancy.) For this reason, many doctors will deliver early by induction if possible, or by cesarean. The NIH Report on Cesarean Birth noted improved treatment for diabetic women and their babies, resulting in diabetic pregnancies being extended closer to term and more mothers delivering vaginally. Still, cesarean birth occurs in approximately 75 percent of all diabetic pregnancies.

HYPERTENSION

Hypertension alone does not necessitate a cesarean. Excessive pressure on the blood flowing to and through the uterus can impair the supply of nutrients and oxygen to the baby because of the associated narrowing of the blood vessels. If your blood pressure remains high throughout pregnancy, the baby may not be properly nourished and your doctor may want to induce labor. Some women develop gestational hypertension during pregnancy, but this condition responds well to good nutrition, medication, and rest.

The Risks Involved

Even though cesareans have become much safer to perform in the past fifty years, they are still major surgery, with risks for both mother and baby. Cesarean births have a maternal mortality rate two to four times greater than that for vaginal birth. If a woman has had an internal fetal monitor prior to a cesarean, her chance of intrauterine infection is 35 to 65 percent. (Without the monitor, the rate of infection is 20 to 40 percent.) There is also the possibility of hemorrhage, infection of the incision, and injury to the bladder and ureter. For the baby, jaundice is the most common complication after cesarean delivery, followed by respiratory distress syndrome (RDS). Cesarean babies do not have fluids squeezed from their lungs during normal delivery and therefore experience greater difficulty breathing. Also, some babies have RDS because they are delivered too early, before their lungs have had time to mature fully. Cesarean babies can also appear sluggish after delivery because of the drugs or anesthesia given to the mother during labor and delivery.

The Operation

In many cases, the decision to do a cesarean is made during labor and it is made with your involvement. Although there may be some urgency to deliver the baby, there is usually enough time to discuss choice of anesthetic and incision and to understand what's happening to you. You will be asked to sign a consent form for surgery and you will be given a routine surgical prep—urinary catheter, intravenous, shave of the abdomen and upper pubic area, and cleansing of the abdomen with an antiseptic. Most of this will be done in the labor room. When you're ready, you'll be wheeled to the operating room, which is usually located on the same floor.

FATHERS IN THE OR

Recently, hospitals have begun to permit fathers to be present in the operating room during cesareans when regional anesthetic is used. This is a privilege that most parents want but many hospitals are reluctant to grant. It has become a battle analogous to the one fought in the late sixties, which won fathers admission to the delivery room. We're confident, though, that the forces of reason and economics will triumph again, and soon all hospitals will allow couples to be together for the birth of their children.

If your hospital allows fathers to be present during cesareans, we encourage your husband to be with you. You will be draped, so he won't have to actually see the operation if he doesn't want to. If you have regional anesthetic, he can talk to you, and you can share the joy of delivery together. He will also be able to hold the baby right after birth. If you need a cesarean and the hospital will not permit your husband to be present, at least ask your doctor. There's always a slight possibility the expression of your desire may fuel the momentum for future change.

ANESTHESIA

If time permits, you will be offered a choice between general and regional anesthesia. The most popular regional anesthetic today is an epidural (see chapter 11 for a complete description), and we would encourage you to have it instead of being put to sleep. There are several advantages of an epidural compared with general anesthesia:

+ You are awake and able to see the baby seconds after birth.
+ You're not groggy for several hours and you won't be nauseated as you might following general anesthesia.
+ You won't have a sore throat because it isn't necessary to insert a tube to maintain an open airway.
+ It's a safer procedure for both you and the baby.
+ You will be able to hold and nurse your baby in the recovery room.

The only objection women sometimes have to receiving epidurals for cesareans is that a slight tugging of the uterus can be felt as the baby is lifted out. However, this is not painful, just disconcerting. If you've had a long labor and need a cesarean, you may feel ready to end your misery and just be put to sleep. This is an understandable reaction, but your partner or doctor should gently persuade you to have the safer regional anesthesia. Some women, however, are repulsed by the idea of remaining awake for surgery and won't consider an epidural. This is a personal choice and yet another matter that should be discussed in advance with your doctor or midwife. Even though it may seem a bit negative to bring up the subject of anesthesia during an office visit, it's a good idea. As one of our friends said about her cesarean experience, "When it came to picking the anesthetic, I felt like I'd been handed a menu, but I was in no position to make a choice."

The great advantage to general anesthesia is the speed with which it can be administered. If there is a true emergency, such as cord prolapse or sudden fetal distress, there won't be time for explanation or discussion. Although these situations are terribly frightening, you are given an opportunity to see your hospital in its finest hour as it responds to a medical crisis. If necessary, you can be hooked up to an intravenous and be given general anesthesia in five to ten minutes. Undoubtedly, you will feel scared and your husband powerless as he waits outside the operating room. At this moment, the only thing to do is to place yourself in your doctor's hands with complete faith in his ability and concern for you. Within a few minutes, your baby will be born, and about an hour later you will wake up in the recovery room to find that everything has turned out all right.

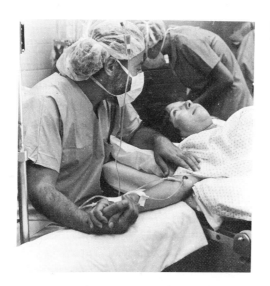

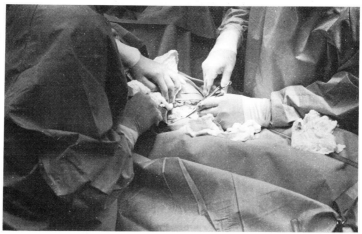

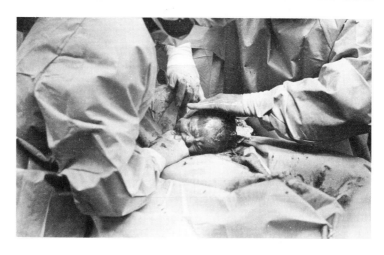

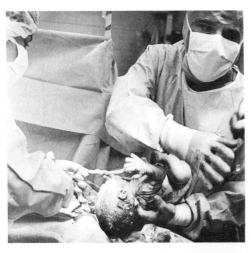

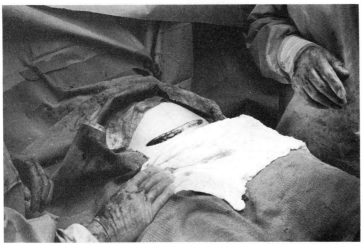

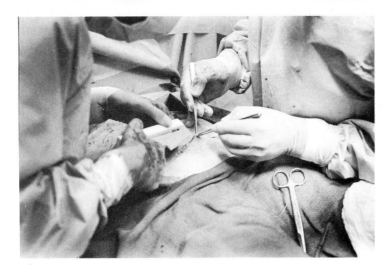

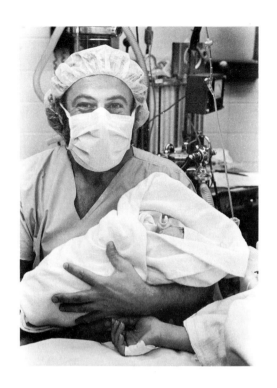

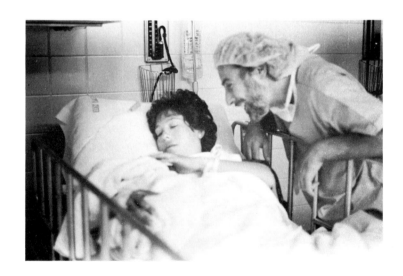

THE OPERATING ROOM

If you pictured yourself delivering your baby by natural childbirth in a cozy environment, the transfer to the operating room can be a jolt. Once a cesarean becomes necessary, there is no more talk of dimming the lights or getting the champagne ready. Suddenly the medical team goes into action, fast.

Usually there is quite a cast of characters in the operating room during a cesarean: your obstetrician, who will be performing the surgery; an assisting surgeon; the anesthesiologist; an attending pediatrician; and various nurses. The operating table is narrow and uncomfortable, the room is cold, the lights are extremely bright, and the whole situation is unfamiliar. The setting may be a little alarming, but you can comfort yourself with the thought that you are in the right place and that your baby will be delivered soon. A cesarean does not provide a natural delivery for your newborn, but if complications occur, this is no longer a priority.

THE INCISION

During the surgery, the anesthesiologist will stand by your head. Right before the anesthesia is administered, you will be given some oxygen to give the baby a little boost. As soon as the anesthesia has taken effect, your doctor will make the incision. Unless there is an emergency, he will do a low transverse incision, known as the bikini cut (its scar is low enough to be hidden by a bikini).

This type of incision has all but replaced the classical vertical one (see drawing) because it is more aesthetically pleasing and has much less chance of rupturing in subsequent pregnancies. The classical incision is still performed in about 5 percent of all deliveries, and in those instances it's done because of extreme emergency, unusual position of the baby, or because placenta previa prevents the use of a bikini incision. An occasional doctor will do a low vertical incision, known as a semiclassical, but this type is also more prone to rupture than the low transverse incision. It's not likely that you'll be dictating the type of incision your doctor should perform, but there may be some room for discussion about this choice, either during an office visit or just prior to surgery.

Your Baby Is Born

Within five minutes, the baby will be out. He will be thoroughly suctioned and quickly evaluated for Apgar scoring. If your husband is there,

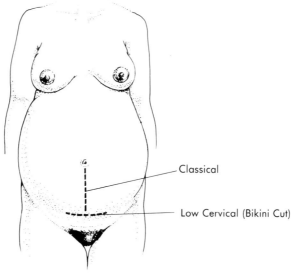

Classical

Low Cervical (Bikini Cut)

Cesarean Incision

he should be able to hold the baby at this point. Then the placenta is manually extracted, and the layers of muscle and skin are stitched. The sewing-up process takes time, approximately forty-five minutes to an hour. The inner layers are sewn with absorbable thread, whereas the outer ones will be done either with absorbable thread or with stitches or staples that will later be removed.

Recovery at the Hospital

THE RECOVERY ROOM

Soon after the operation, you will be taken to the recovery room. If you had a general anesthesia, you'll be in and out of consciousness and won't really be aware of what's going on. If, however, you've had an epidural or other regional anesthesia, it can be a good time to become acquainted with your baby. This first meeting may have to be arranged by advance special permission, however, because many hospitals routinely whisk cesarean babies out of the delivery room to the nursery, where they are kept for observation. Cesarean babies do have greater breathing difficulties than vaginally delivered ones, but if your baby is doing well, the pediatrician should be able to arrange for you to have him in the recovery room. If you're sleepy and unresponsive, your husband can spend some time with the baby, either in the nursery or in your room. There's no reason why your cesarean should prevent your husband from seeing and holding his child.

The recovery room can be a good place to try nursing. You should put a pillow over your stomach to protect it from little kicking feet. Or, you might use the football hold (see illustration) to avoid resting the baby on your abdomen.

While you're in the recovery room, you will probably be offered some Demerol for relaxation. Some women feel a bit shaky and disoriented after a cesarean, but that doesn't mean they need a narcotic. Demerol at this time is not medically indicated, so this depends entirely on how you feel. You should feel free to say no thanks.

The amount of time you spend in recovery will depend on the type of anesthesia you received and on your condition. You may be nauseated or vomiting if you had general anesthesia. If you're in good shape, however, you could be in your own room within a few hours.

YOUR PHYSICAL RECOVERY

The first forty-eight hours after the surgery are not going to be any fun. If at all possible, get a private room. You will be very tired, especially if you had a long labor, and your incision will feel excruciatingly tender. Getting out of bed will be painful, and just five minutes on the phone will exhaust you. For all these reasons, we suggest either having your husband stay with you continually for the first twenty-four to thirty-six hours or hiring a private-duty nurse. This is worth the money because you'll greatly appreciate a professional sponge bath and experienced hands helping to turn you in bed. The staff may forget to tell you about turning, but it is important that you not lie frozen in one position. Since movement will be painful, you'll appreciate help.

You'll also need help when you're required to stand and walk a few steps about twelve hours after surgery. Moving about helps prevent thrombosis (blood clots in the arteries), and it will hasten your general recovery and give you a great feeling of accomplishment. You may not be happy about walking, but you have no choice. Try using the Lamaze breathing again, and remember, your stitches are quite strong; you are not going to come apart.

Sometime after surgery you will have the catheter removed, and the intravenous should come out a day or two later. If you received nonsoluble stitches, they will be removed around the fifth or sixth day. If you

Nursing After Cesarean

Pillows used to cover incision

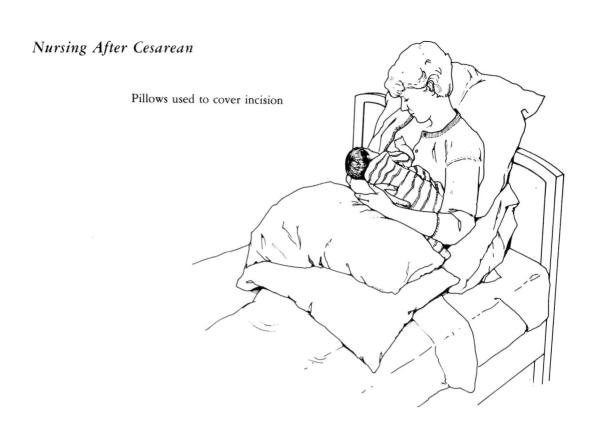

Pillows used to support baby (football hold)

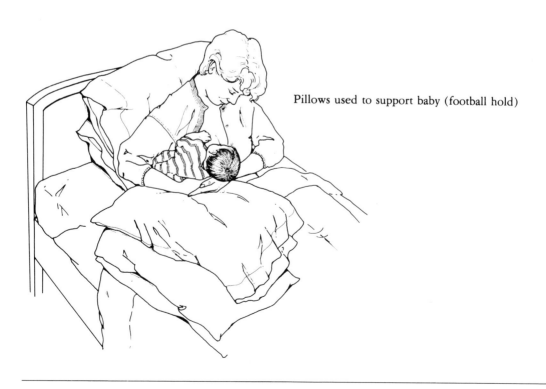

have staples, they may come out sooner because they promote better healing. Soluble stitches are simply absorbed.

Gas pain is a common problem following any abdominal surgery and occurs because the digestive system has been inactive. The best remedy for gas is walking about and getting some exercise. Pain medication may further slow down intestinal functioning, so it's better to avoid it if you're having trouble with gas. A suppository or little enema may also relieve gas pains.

You will be put on a liquid diet for two or three days until the doctor is convinced that your intestines can handle food. Drink *lots* of liquids, beyond thirst, for this will help your recovery.

It is important that you do some deep breathing or coughing on a regular basis to avoid fluid building up in your lungs, which could lead to pneumonia. Deep breathing is especially important if you had general anesthesia. Start this exercise right away for maximum benefit. As an added bonus, it should help with gas pains.

If you did not come to the hospital prepared for a possible cesarean, you may need to send your partner out for stick-on sanitary napkins so you won't have to wear a belt. Forget the bikini underwear, which will cut right across your incision, and switch to something bigger for the next few weeks.

The pain from your surgery will manifest itself in unexpected ways. Your incision is tender for a while, but you also have several layers of stitches inside that hurt in different places. The nerves in your skin have been cut, so you will feel numb until the nerve connections grow back. (This takes time but will happen.) Your pubic hair will be uncomfortable when it starts to grow back. These aches and pains all take time to subside. Do not expect to feel the way your friends who have just had vaginal births feel, and do not expect to be "all better" in six weeks.

The average hospital stay following a cesarean is twice as long as one after a normal delivery: 6.2 days versus 3.1 days. Toward the end of this time you will start feeling much better, and there's no reason you shouldn't have your baby with you as much as possible. Nursing is more difficult after a cesarean, but there are many women who manage it. If your stomach is just too tender to have anything resting on it, you should try the football hold, as we just suggested, or nursing while lying down, propped on one arm. Also, you may need painkillers during the first few days, so ask for them. There's no reason to be uncomfortable after delivery. To minimize the drugs' effect on the baby, take them right after you nurse. We urge you to accept pain relief because at this point your milk isn't in and only trace amounts will appear in the colostrum. It makes sense that nursing will proceed most smoothly if you're not in pain.

An estimated 30 percent of cesarean mothers will run fevers of at least 100.4 degrees. This is not a serious medical problem, but nevertheless women with even slight fevers are often separated from their babies because of a slim possibility that the babies could become infected with a disease that could contaminate the nursery. We think this policy is unduly conservative and a serious overreaction to a common situation. There are many experts who agree with us, among them Dr. Audrey Naylor, a pediatrician and lactation specialist at Mercy Hospital in San Diego, California. She believes that only in "very rare circumstances" should a baby be taken from a nursing mother and that those circumstances would include an active case of tuberculosis or hepatitis.

"In developing nations, where infectious diseases pose a serious problem, studies have shown that when a nursing mother and baby are separated, there has been a significant increase in newborn infections," Dr. Naylor said. "When the mother and baby are allowed to remain together, there has been a decline in newborn infections, and this has been demonstrated even in very crowded clinics where mothers are sometimes forced to share a bed." She feels, however, that more caution should be taken with mothers who are bottlefeeding, because those babies do not benefit from the antibodies contained in breast milk.

This is one hospital regulation we encourage you to fight. Losing your baby, even though temporarily, can undermine your recovery by making you angry and upset. Try to enlist the support of your pediatrician and your doctor or midwife. If you're given the argument about infection contaminating the nursery, see if you can keep the baby with you and have your baby be given his daily bath and exam in isolation. Your child stands a greater chance of getting anything you might have if he is not allowed to nurse and receive the antibodies your body is manufacturing.

Recovery at Home

Having a cesarean means having help when you get home from the hospital. There's no way around this. There are many things you shouldn't be doing at first, such as lifting or going up and down stairs, and if you do, you'll delay your recovery by weeks. If your husband can't take off from work, someone should be with you for at least the first full week. You will be totally preoccupied taking care of your baby and regaining your strength. Dishes, cooking, and cleaning can be performed by a surrogate, paid or otherwise, until you're back on your feet. You will be extremely tired, and routine chores will be exhausting. Walking around the block or entertaining for an hour will send you to bed for a nap.

THE EXERCISE ROUTINE

You have a longer road to recovery than the new mothers who have had vaginal deliveries. Your big challenge during your hospital stay is simply getting to the point where you can stand up straight. As you begin to feel better, however, you should try to help your body recover from both pregnancy and surgery by doing the following exercises. In a few weeks you will once again be able to lie on your stomach and get out of bed like a normal person.

Take things one step at a time, following the progression below. Each day add one new exercise to the ones you are already doing, keeping in mind that as a postoperative patient you need to conserve your energy. Numerous short periods of exercise during the day (four five-minute sessions) are better than one long, tiring one (twenty minutes all at one stretch).

For the first week, do these exercises lying in bed. After that, move to a firm surface, such as the floor, and add the pregnancy exercises, which are gentle. Once you have had your postpartum checkup, you can begin the postnatal exercises in chapter 14 (see page 351).

Foot Circles
Circle one foot to the right twenty times and then to the left twenty times. Repeat with other foot.

Foot Pumping
Flex and point your foot twenty-five times as if you were pumping the brakes of a car. Repeat with the other foot.

Pelvic Tilt
Lie on your back with your knees bent and your feet on the bed. Exhale, contract your abdominal muscles, and flatten your lower back into the bed. Repeat ten times.

Knee Bends

Lie flat on the bed, legs straight. Slide one heel along the bed toward your hips. Straighten your leg by sliding your heel away from you. Alternate knees, ten times each leg.

YOUR EMOTIONAL RECOVERY

For cesarean mothers, disappointment is a natural component of the postpartum experience. Women who have had cesareans frequently express feelings of failure because they feel they have flunked the ultimate femininity test—giving birth. They can also become embittered because they've been deprived of their fantasy Lamaze birth, a dream they worked so hard to achieve. On top of that, they worry about letting down their husbands and families. The icing on the whole sorry cake can be strong feelings of self-hate, fueled by a sense of betrayal by a body that didn't perform properly.

The worst part of all this is that every time you get worked up and begin to feel really bad, you then feel guilty because you have a healthy baby. The depression and sorrow never get fully expressed because they are always held in check by the guilt/gratitude response. You can end up in a terrible depression, which is really a case of normal postpartum depression compounded by a case of cesarean depression and simple fatigue.

Negative feelings following a cesarean should be expressed and accepted. This expression is crucial or they're likely to surface again during a subsequent pregnancy. They can even become transformed into resentment toward the baby, who put you through all this. We strongly recommend joining a cesarean support group, which will provide a format and a sympathetic atmosphere for you to express your feelings. You can find one by writing to C-SEC at 22 Forest Road, Framingham, Massachusetts 01701. This group's acronym stands for Cesareans/Support Education and Concern, and it can refer you to a cesarean support group or help you establish one. You might also check women's centers, YWCAs, or churches for a referral.

In time you will be able to handle more things by yourself, but in the very beginning you must remember that you are recovering from surgery. Do not expect to keep up with the new mother down the street who had an easy delivery, and do not expect anyone who has never been in your position to know what it is really like. It is up to you to set the boundaries and to forgive yourself for any perceived shortcomings.

CHAPTER 13

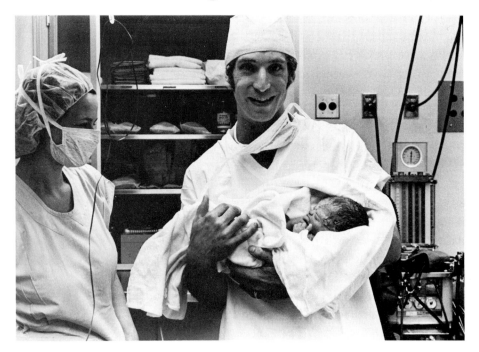

Being a Partner

This chapter is for you, the partner. For whatever reason, you may not do a lot of research about pregnancy and childbirth, and you may not look at the rest of this book, but we hope you will read this section. It will give you an overview of the whole process of childbirth, help define what you as a partner can do—both in advance and once that process begins—and, if you have doubts, give you an idea of how lucky you are to have this opportunity.

WHY SHOULD I ATTEND THE BIRTH?

It wasn't until the mid-1970s that men were permitted by hospitals to be with their wives during childbirth. Before that time, husbands were banished to a smoke-filled waiting room or ordered to wait it out at home. Although some of you may not want anything to do with natural childbirth, you're lucky to have a choice about participating. Fifteen years ago, men were treated like imbeciles who were only capable of chauffering the precious cargo to the hospital and then passing out the cigars. Today it is universally accepted that husbands and wives belong together during labor and that men have an important and unique contribution to make.

In this chapter, we direct the majority of our comments to fathers and refer most frequently to the partner as husband. That is because the great majority of Lamaze students are married couples. It seems unfairly restrictive, however, to consider husbands the only proper companions for labor. Women can be assisted by a husband, a boyfriend, a mother or sister, a friend, or a professional labor companion. The Lamaze method is so sound that the partner's role can be successfully assumed by anyone.

The term *coach* is often used to identify the primary Lamaze labor companion. To us, *coach* suggests gung-ho athleticism, with an implication that women should play a secondary role. We therefore prefer the word *partner,* because it more accurately reflects the shared experience of childbirth and the joint effort of working together toward a common goal.

The best reason to be with your wife during childbirth is that it can be the most exciting and profound experience of your life. As you can see from the responses we received to our questionnaire, partners felt joy, amazement, and awe. They felt closer to their wives as a result of sharing the birth experience and had a chance to see and touch their baby immediately.

The second best reason to be at the birth is that your wife wants you there. If the roles were reversed and you were giving birth, you'd feel just as apprehensive and you'd want her at your side. Psychologist Deborah Tanzer has studied the components of a good birth experience and found that a husband's presence and participation are necessary to pro-

♦

"Ten seconds after our son was born, the doctor handed him to me, umbilical cord still attached. I looked at my baby, and his eyes looked up at mine. I will never forget that first eye contact."

♦

"The best and most wonderful moment was the actual delivery. It's the most joyous thing I've ever experienced."

♦

"I gave my new son a Leboyer bath. My great reward was his sweet smile as I immersed him in the warm water."

♦

"Those first precious minutes. . . . She was beautiful and she stuck her tongue out at me. It was one of the happiest moments of my life."

♦

"I realized my father and my wife's father had never seen their children being born, and all I could think of was how unfortunate these two grown men were. I really feel it makes the man feel part of the birth to share this experience."

♦

"I had a whole new respect for my wife watching her go through labor and delivery. I wouldn't have missed it for the world."

♦

"You read things about pregnancy in books and magazines, but nothing, absolutely nothing, compares with witnessing the birth. I plan to be there for our next child, and every one after that!"

♦

continued

♦

"After my daughter was born, I just melted. It's bringing tears to my eyes just remembering what it was like, seeing her being born. It's beyond me how my parents' generation did not allow the father to participate in this, an experience I wouldn't have missed."

duce a peak experience for the mother. Her ability to feel joy and ecstasy is directly related to her husband's involvement.

Your job is to support your wife emotionally and physically. You will try to free her from distractions and to increase her comfort by massaging her back or offering her sips of water. You'll be doing whatever you can to make labor enjoyable and endurable. Being there means that you're willing to share everything with her, her pain as well as her joy. Labor can get pretty intense. You won't get any breaks for coffee, and it may be hard to find the time to go to the bathroom. If things go well, however, it should be one of the greatest moments of your life.

FEARS ABOUT CHILDBIRTH

In the final months of pregnancy, it is normal for you to feel fearful or anxious about many aspects of labor and delivery: the hospital environment, the pain of labor, the health of the baby, and the role you will play. Fears about fainting in the delivery room may haunt you, as well as worries about your being completely superfluous. You can feel quite shaky as idiotic people recount childbirth horror stories and Lamaze classes make you aware of some of the things that can go awry. Try not to worry. Complications are rare, and after it's all over, you may be more enthusiatic about Lamaze than your wife—many women have trouble forgetting the pain and exhaustion of birth, but their husbands savor the experience as a romantic and thrilling memory.

Fears about Childbirth

♦

"I was afraid that it was going to be bloody and disgusting, but actually it was beautiful."

♦

"I was worried that all wouldn't go according to plan for a natural childbirth."

♦

"I feared an unknown complication over which we would have no control."

♦

". . . not getting my wife to the hospital in time."

♦

"My major concerns were about the baby being stillborn or my wife dying in childbirth."

♦

"I was afraid I would faint or throw up when my wife needed me the most."

♦

"I was afraid I would forget how to do something and make my wife even more nervous."

♦

"I feared feeling helpless in the face of anxiety and suffering."

♦

"The biggest fear I had was of being intimidated by the doctor/nurse/hospital routine. . . . The midwife encouraged me to help and was not fearful of my usurping her authority."

Participating in childbirth is a scary idea to most first-time fathers. Many men enter as reluctant participants, but emerge as enthralled advocates of shared childbirth. You don't have to be a particularly demonstrative or emotional man to support your wife during labor—all kinds of men do it, and all kinds of men are thrilled by the experience. Some even feel sorry for those who have missed the births of their children. Others become proselytizers for the Lamaze method. Whatever your feelings, being with your wife during the birth of your child will increase your mutual respect and love. She cannot help but appreciate your presence, and you certainly will appreciate her willingness to work so hard for you both.

Visiting the Doctor or Midwife

Your chances of enjoying your child's birth are increased if you have been emotionally involved in your wife's pregnancy. On a tangible level, this means accompanying her on some visits to the obstetrician or midwife. Ideally, you should have participated in the selection of this person. If you did not attend the initial interview, you should meet the doctor or midwife as soon as possible at a routine office visit. A bonus will be the opportunity to hear a unique sound: your baby's heartbeat. Also, you will feel more at ease during labor if you are familiar with the person responsible for your wife's care.

ATTENDING LAMAZE CLASSES

It seems to be a rare expectant father who reads books on pregnancy and birth. We commend you for reading this chapter and urge you not to wait until Lamaze class to gain further information. Reading clears up misconceptions, decreases anxiety, and provides a point of reference to your wife's pregnancy. There's no reason you shouldn't finish the rest of this book or tackle any others your wife can recommend.

We assume that you will be attending a Lamaze course with your wife or your partner. At the outset, many men have to be persuaded to go to classes, but most of them actually end up enjoying the course. Classes are great for several reasons:

- You feel less anxious, because you learn how to help and participate in your child's birth

- You participate in discussion, which helps clarify your expectations about birth
- You meet other men in the same situation
- You develop a sense of camaraderie with the other couples at a time when you sorely need it
- You can talk about your feelings and worries if you want

Practicing the Breathing Patterns

As the due date approaches, you should be diligently practicing the breathing patterns with your wife; this is of critical importance. Since tension is the normal reaction to pain, it takes a lot of conditioning to change that reflex to one of relaxation. Even though we'd prefer to resist sports metaphors, natural childbirth is analogous to a strenuous athletic event: It requires stamina, proper attitude, and the confidence that comes with training.

It seems that men are often more lax about practicing, although women can be too, albeit for different and more complicated reasons. We have analyzed men's feelings about not practicing and have come up with four classic excuses for avoidance. They are

- It's better if you breathe by yourself, and then, after you get the hang of it, I'll do some with you.
- You're doing just great, you don't need my help. I'd probably just mess you up.
- Your pain threshold is incredibly high. I don't think you're going to need to do any breathing at all.
- We don't have enough time now. I brought work home with me, and then later, if it's not too late, I want to repaint that rocking chair for the baby's room.

All of these excuses are bogus, of course, because you can find the time and energy for something you care about doing. If you really want to help your wife during childbirth, you're going to have to practice now. You've got to learn the breathing techniques because she may forget them. In addition, you must become acquainted with her particular rhythm in order to guide her through the vicissitudes of labor. By practicing now, you'll know which words and suggestions are most effective. For example, if she needs to slow down, you'll know that

A T T E N D I N G   L A M A Z E   C L A S S

◆

"It's amazing how much I didn't know. I learned a lot."

◆

"Lamaze helped us both feel more confident, and it made me feel like, 'It's my baby, too!' "

◆

"I didn't like going to the classes, but the information was helpful."

◆

"The classes forced us to take the time out of our schedules to talk about things we had been thinking about all along."

◆

"Lamaze taught us to rely upon ourselves to control the situation, rather than letting the doctor control it."

◆

"I felt foolish lying on the floor practicing breathing patterns. It was like getting ready to go over Niagara Falls by sitting in the bathtub."

◆

"The sight of blood had bothered me in the films, but didn't during delivery."

◆

"I liked the friendship and support of all the other men in the class. I could say exactly how I felt about everything, and I wasn't the only one to feel that way."

◆

"Lamaze classes opened my eyes to techniques that were not easily understood from books."

continued

"The classes helped prepare me for a situation that for many years was considered women's work."

◆

"There was nothing to dislike. The camaraderie of the couples was great. The patience and insight of the instructor were wonderful."

◆

"I had distanced myself emotionally from the birth because I was scared about what might or might not happen. The classes helped me keep in touch."

simply saying "slow down" doesn't work, but telling her to take deeper breaths does the trick.

THE FINAL STRETCH

The last month of pregnancy is not a particularly enjoyable time for either parent-to-be. Both of you are getting anxious and impatient, your wife probably feels like a lethargic blimp, and your sex life is a thing of the past. You can gain a lot of points at this time by extending a little sympathy. A foot massage, a cup of tea in bed, an unexpected hug, or drawing a hot bath will assure her of your empathy and love. There's no way you can really know what it feels like to be pregnant, but imagine carrying around six five-pound bags of sugar twenty-four hours a day, and you'll have some idea of the effort involved. We know all of you are filled with goodwill, but it doesn't hurt to make a daily demonstration of that spirit.

There are lots of practical things you can do right now to prepare for the baby and make things easier for your wife. If you've never been domestically inclined, this is a good time to learn to make an omelet or run the washing machine. These skills will be appreciated now, but will be invaluable in a few weeks when things get hectic. You should also try to have a little fun at this point because in a month or so you won't be going out too much. This is a good time to go to the movies, visit friends, or do whatever you enjoy.

Labor Begins

You may have a vivid fantasy about the way labor will begin, such as the water breaking while the two of you are waiting on a movie line or fierce contractions developing in the middle of the night and the baby emerging a few minutes later. Try to abandon this type of thinking and just relax. Many couples spend the final weeks as if they were waiting for a bomb to explode. Often it is only in retrospect that you know when labor began, and though early labor can be very exciting, the onset is not always announced with a flourish.

If labor begins during the night, you should make your wife a stiff drink or some cocoa or draw a warm bath (unless her water has broken), and you should both go back to bed. You may be tempted to start timing contractions or packing the Lamaze bag, but you should both conserve energy for the hard part. If she's having mild contractions and doesn't need to use her breathing, there's no reason for you to be up. (Your wife may have other ideas, but we don't see any point in two people being tired.) You should return to bed and sleep until you're truly needed, or just too excited to sleep.

As we say many times in this book, most couples go to the hospital much too soon. Ideally, you should spend early labor at home, and active labor should be well established before you leave—contractions approximately four to five minutes apart, lasting forty-five to sixty seconds. Remain calm and tell yourself, repeatedly, that first-time mothers spend an average of eight to nine hours in early labor. The chances of your baby being born at home are slight, and there's a strong possibility you will encourage unnecessary intervention by arriving at the hospital too soon.

Early labor is a time for watching television, taking walks, fixing light meals, and relaxing. Unless it's the middle of the night, call your doctor or midwife to say labor has begun and describe how things are going. Escort your wife to the office if she needs to be seen. We don't advise calling anyone else because you will then be obliged to issue updates, a task you won't have time for later on. Try to enjoy this exciting time

"I'll never forget the excitement, anticipation, and togetherness I felt with my wife during our drive to the hospital at sunrise."

together, making sure both of you maintain energy by eating and drinking. Though you may not feel you are doing anything important for your wife, your presence and your support are more help than you know.

You will both be working harder as labor progresses and its intensity increases. You may be breathing with her and you should certainly begin timing contractions as the pace picks up. (Time the intervals by clocking from the beginning of one contraction to the beginning of the next. For example, contractions are said to be five minutes apart when there is a one-minute contraction, followed by a four-minute rest.)

The decision about when to go to the hospital can sometimes be a hard one, but in general, allow your wife to decide. It's easy to get fidgety and nervous waiting around, and you're likely to jump the gun. Only she can determine how much stronger her contractions have become and whether she thinks things are progressing. Although that doesn't sound very scientific, it's the best standard available, and you've just got to trust her. If, on the other hand, your wife is agitating to leave as soon as contractions begin, try to slow her down, but don't force her to stay. Some women are just not comfortable laboring at home, and it's better to give in than to fight. If you're really in dispute, call your Lamaze teacher or obstetrician.

AT THE HOSPITAL

At the hospital, you will assume yet another job, that of your wife's advocate. For those of you who are married to women who have no trouble speaking for themselves, this role may seem slightly redundant.

It's not. The hospital can be a threatening environment where individual needs can take a backseat to efficiency. Women in labor shouldn't be expected to fend for themselves as they normally do. Therefore, it is up to you to maintain physical and emotional continuity, to provide comfort, and to make sure no one disturbs your wife. In order to accomplish this, you've got to stay by her side, especially at such critical points as admission, internal exams, and transition.

We're not suggesting that anyone in a hospital will purposely undermine your wife's efforts. We're merely saying that innocuous remarks, such as, "First labors take a long, long time" or "You're going to get tired out if you keep up that breathing," can shake her confidence. Hospitals, even the smallest ones, are noisy, busy places, and teaching hospitals are the worst in terms of impersonality and chaos. If your wife's breathing is repeatedly interrupted by a resident's questions or if her concentration is shattered by a parade of people through the room, you must intercede. It's your job to answer questions for her during a contraction. It's your job to make the room quiet by closing the door, and if necessary, it's your job to limit personnel to only the truly essential people—the doctor and labor nurse.

It's extremely common for labor to falter or even stall once a woman gets to the hospital. This is because it's hard to make a smooth transition to a new place, even in the best of circumstances. You must provide the link from the reassuring home environment, as well as run interference with all the obstacles a hospital can present. It's your job to remove the distractions and to encourage your wife to relax and focus on her labor. It makes sense that a woman who is well trained and calm will dilate much more quickly than one who is not.

If you need to leave the room to get some coffee or clear your head, you can ask the labor nurse to take your place. In general, labor nurses are terrific, and usually they are well versed in Lamaze. This means that if you forget a particular breathing pattern or want some new suggestions for back labor, they will guide you. If you're feeling overwhelmed or helpless, don't hesitate to ask for help. Just remember that even the nicest, most competent nurse cannot replace your presence.

Active Labor

During active labor you will just be trying to maintain an even keel. Many couples quickly develop the hang of breathing in conjunction with the fetal monitor, and this can work well. You see a contraction beginning and you alert your partner before she even feels it. Later, you can announce when the contraction has peaked, and this knowledge can help her cope with the rest of the contractions. If labor is progressing nicely and the two of you are working well together, the fetal monitor can seem like the greatest invention since the wheel. It is, however, a quirky piece of technology with definite limitations.

The monitor shouldn't control your labor. If your wife wants to walk around, that's what she should do, and the monitor can be used intermittently—on for ten minutes, then off for twenty. If she wants to change positions in bed, this should also be encouraged, and the monitor can be readjusted. She should be disconnected approximately every hour to go to the bathroom. Don't panic if your baby's heartbeat suddenly disappears; most likely the belt has slipped off or the baby has moved out of range.

The Plateau Phenomenon

Most of the time, the pace of dilation accelerates as contractions increase in intensity and frequency. Sometimes, however, cervical progress can come to a halt, even though good, strong contractions continue unabated. We call this the plateau phenomenon, and though it usually happens around five to six centimeters dilation, it can also occur as late as eight or nine centimeters.

Contractions, even if they hurt, are usually bearable as long as they are accomplishing something. But the same contractions become unbearable if they cause only pain and no dilation. If your wife reaches five centimeters dilation and remains at the same point for the next three hours, you must intervene in some way. No one knows for sure why these plateaus occur, but tension often plays a large part. To help her relax you can

+ Restore calm and order to her environment. Turn down the lights, get her into a more comfortable position, and ask anyone else in the room to speak quietly or not at all.
+ Help her into a shower. Water can be very soothing.
+ Change her surroundings. Sometimes a walk and a change of scenery works wonders. Go visit the newborn nursery if it's nearby.
+ Acknowledge her pain and reassure her that you are there to help. Try to make her feel less alone. Tell her, show her, that you love her.

BEING A LABOR PARTNER

♦

"I provided her with moral support and tried to comfort her as much as possible. She was super. I must confess, I'd rather be the coach than the player."

♦

"My daughter said she wouldn't have made it without me. The nurses said I was one of the best coaches they'd seen. I think my presence kept my daughter from being nervous, which helped with labor."

♦

"All she wanted me to do was rub her back and not leave her side. I did whatever she asked, and later she said I was great. I'm glad she didn't know what I was really thinking."

♦

"I'm not sure I helped at all. I was just there—but my wife says that's what counts!"

♦

"She did not feel alone."

♦

"I was the strong part of her that she wouldn't have known she had if I hadn't been there."

♦

"Initially I was pretty calm, but for the last hours, if they could measure anxiety, I would have been off the scale. I wanted to tell my wife to get up and let me lie down for a little while."

♦

"Anyone could have done the breathing and even the cheerleading, but my wife couldn't have yelled at anyone but me—which is what she needed to do."

HAVING A LABOR PARTNER

♦

"I needed my partner as a buffer between the hospital staff and me and as an advocate should any problem have arisen that required a sane decision."

♦

"My husband pulled me through. He was awake when I was tired, he was encouraging when I wanted to give up, he breathed with me when I couldn't think straight, and he was kind when I was irritable."

♦

"He was beside me the whole time. He kept telling me to *open my eyes,* forcing me not to crawl inside and lock up with all the pain."

♦

"My husband protected my right to rest between contractions by working out a system with the nurses. When the nurse came to check me, she'd look at my husband from the doorway and he'd gesture whether or not I was asleep."

♦

"His love and support were manifested in his touch, tone of voice, and caring for me physically. He is very goosey about vomiting, yet held a basin for me in a most calm and loving manner."

♦

"My husband was very supportive, helpful, and sympathetic. In all honesty, I was quite surprised. He is not usually an emotional man, and I saw a totally different side of him. I don't think I ever loved him more than at that time."

♦

"My husband was essential. I fell in love all over again. I can't imagine it without him. I leaned on him with each pain and felt his energy and support and love. The smell of his shirt was comforting. Labor was a very intimate experience."

- Remind her that she must ride the waves of the contractions, not try to control them. Tell her to allow herself to let go, to *give* birth.
- Encourage her to take 25 milligrams of Demerol. Often just this small amount can relax her when other techniques fail.

Transition

Active labor can seem unending, but you should be alert for the signs of transition, which is the last and hardest part of dilation. Transition means terrible crabbiness, a new and often irregular pattern to contractions, an urge to defecate, chills, nausea, and a desire to call it quits. Most women have a dread of this stage, and your wife may click on her denial mechanism as it happens to her. It is important to recognize transition because its intensity can make a woman feel like she's dying and doubt her ability to make it through one more contraction. It's your job to assure her that (a) this intense pain is normal; (b) labor will not get any worse; (c) this will probably last only a few more minutes; and (d) she is doing beautifully. This stage requires your most intense participation, and this is the time when most men must establish eye-to-eye contact and breathe right along with their partner.

Medication

Most men don't think too much about medication while they are taking Lamaze classes, except to register in their minds that their wives plan or don't plan on having it. The problem is that either point of view may have to be revised depending on the circumstances of the particular labor.

For example, your wife may expect to get an epidural once she has reached five centimeters dilation, but if labor progresses quickly, the doctor might advise against it. If you find yourself in this situation, it's critical that you know the Lamaze techniques. You will both have to work harder than anticipated, but you may discover that labor is easier and more thrilling than you ever imagined.

On the other hand, your wife may have planned on avoiding all drugs, but be taken by surprise at the intensity of the pain or worn down by a long labor and ask for relief. Even if she has a terrific power of imagination, she is not going to know in advance what transition contractions or back labor really feel like. You're going to be in a bind if she

TRANSITION

◆

"My husband didn't tell me what to do, he showed me. Because I was a bit irascible, he had to breathe with me. I could not have remembered the techniques had he not coached me. He rubbed my feet, hands, and the small of my back. And most of all, he knew I still loved him when I screamed, "Don't touch me! Don't ever do this to me again!""

◆

"When transition neared, my coach noticed a definite pattern with the contractions. He would tell me when to speed up or slow down my breathing. Most importantly, he kept telling me, 'You're doing great . . . just a few more . . . I know you can.'"

◆

"My husband was an angel. I couldn't have done it without him. He coached and praised and breathed and massaged and was handy with a cold washcloth. He suggested, 'five more minutes,' over and over again."

begs for medication during labor but you know she truly wants natural childbirth. She may even have enlisted your support during pregnancy, making you promise you will not allow her to have anything. Although this seems like a hopeless situation, there are several things you can do during labor to help her to attain her goal:

◆ *Try to determine if fear is making the pain seem worse.* Fear is a natural component of childbirth, but it is commonly overlooked by childbirth educators, doctors, and couples themselves. Talk to your wife, attempting to determine her feelings about what she is experiencing. If she is scared, acknowledge this and try to assuage her anxiety. If she says, "I can't take it if it gets any worse," bring her attention back to the present, reminding her how well she is doing.

MEDICATION

◆

"He was supportive, reassuring, cool. He kept his head when I lost mine. I wanted to give in to an epidural or something, but he said, 'No, you're doing too well.' The baby was born within an hour."

- *Work on lessening the pain.* Change position, getting her to sit up or walk around the room just once. If you've been using cold packs, switch to hot or vice versa. If you haven't been paying much attention to the fetal monitor, use it to let your wife know when to begin breathing and when to relax. Work at establishing and maintaining eye contact—this helps many women. On the other hand, if you're sick of staring at each other, try some visualization. Pick out a beautiful and encouraging image and describe it so vividly, she can't help but relax. Try some back or foot massage. Ask the nurse for suggestions.

- *Take the next three contractions as a trial.* Give her a short-term goal and see if she can reestablish control with just a few contractions. When that's accomplished, ask her to try three more. Tell her you won't call for medication until she's tried to breathe through just a few more contractions. She may hate this idea, but she'll do it if you insist.

- *Get the doctor or midwife to perform an internal exam.* A particularly difficult phase of labor can produce great cervical progress. It may give your wife some inspiration to learn she's just dilated from three to eight centimeters in one hour, even though it was the worst hour of her life. Also, if the doctor or midwife will just emphasize how beautifully she is doing, this recognition can provide enough motivation to make it to the final stretch.

Medication is a tricky issue, because it is impossible to know in advance whether your wife will need it or how she will react to it if and when she gets it. While a drug-free birth is ideal, it is also true that a bit of relief at some point helps many women keep going and feel better about their whole birth experience. If your prelabor plans about medication begin to seem more and more inappropriate, then it's time to consider your options (see the medication chart on page 266). If your wife does need medication, you should be sure to inquire what she is being given and how much. You can also request that the drug be given in the smallest dose possible in order to minimize risk to the baby. There's a big difference between 25 and 75 milligrams of Demerol, and you should hold out for the lesser dose. It's always possible to give more medication if needed, but it's very difficult to undo the effects of too much.

Pushing

As transition moves along interminably, you should be alert for signals that dilation is completed. The end of this stage is sometimes accompanied by a strong urge to push. While this is very exciting progress, you should not permit your wife to begin bearing down until she has been examined by the doctor or midwife. If she pushes against an incompletely dilated cervix, swelling will occur, and dilation will actually decrease. To offset the urge to push, you must instruct your partner to blow out forcefully. At this moment, she'll probably be so dazed you may have to breathe along with her.

If you have your baby in a delivery room, you will be asked, somewhere near the end of transition, to change into a scrub suit and booties. The scrub suit replaces your clothing, but the booties go over your shoes with the strings tucked in. You'll also be given a kind of surgical shower cap to cover your hair and a mask. If your wife needs you at the moment you are requested to change, postpone leaving her until she regains her composure. You don't have to leave at that moment—you can wait until she is fully dilated or has begun pushing before you take the five necessary minutes to suit up.

The first thing you should do before your wife starts pushing is to check out the position of the labor or birthing bed. If you use a delivery room, your wife will do almost all her pushing in the labor bed, and then be transferred to the delivery room when the head crowns. The beauty of a birthing room is that pushing, delivery, and recovery take place in the same spot. Your wife should not be flat because that is the most disadvantageous position for effective expulsion. Ask that the back of the bed be raised, or find some pillows so that she can be elevated. You can also support her body by propping her up against you; she will be using you as a kind of backstop for pushing. An alternative position is holding one of her legs up while the labor nurse supports the other one.

Many women expect pushing to be the greatest and most fulfilling part of labor. While this is often the case, it's by no means a universal truth. Pushing can seem completely overwhelming, and for an occasional woman whose baby is wedged in an odd position, it can be painful. Many women are exhausted by the time they reach this stage, and consequently are shocked and dismayed by the intensity of effort required. It's been said many times that pushing out a baby is the hardest work a woman will ever do. We agree, and ask you to be mindful of that axiom when your wife acts bewildered, overwhelmed, or even resistant during this phase.

Confusion seems to go along with pushing because frequently women are instructed to bear down and breathe in a manner that contradicts the style learned in Lamaze class. If that happens, ask the doctor to allow you to use the method you've learned, leaving open the possibility of using his approach if yours doesn't work. If that suggestion isn't appreciated, at least make sure that your partner understands the new directions.

It seems customary for everyone in the delivery room to yell, "Push, Push," and this cheerleading creates a frenzied atmosphere. Some women appreciate the enthusiasm, but others don't perform well under this sort of exhortation. If your wife is hindered by the noise, ask for some quiet. Each woman has to feel free to give birth in her own way, to do it instinctively. You may not hear anything but her breathing, or she may grunt or yell. Either way, it is her lead that should be followed, not yours or even the doctor's.

You may be the most successful in encouraging your wife to push effectively. She has depended on your voice all throughout labor and she trusts it. Speak simply to her and issue one command at a time. If her face gets red and the veins in her neck stick out, remind her to let out some breath. First-time mothers usually push for about an hour before giving birth; second-time mothers take about half as long. If progress seems to be stalled, a squatting position may help. You can support one side of her body while the nurse helps with the other. Your wife may be less than enthusiastic about this suggestion, but it's worth a try. The doctor probably won't think of this position, but he should have no objection. Squatting is gradually gaining acceptance in the United States, although it is already successfully used by women in many other countries.

If an episiotomy is required, we suggest you don't watch. It's a simple incision, but it is bloody. It's not easy to watch anyone getting cut, and it's particularly difficult when it's your wife, and when it's in that spot. If, however, the doctor offers to let you cut the umbilical cord, you should. This is a painless procedure since there are no nerve endings, and it's a lovely symbolic act.

Your doctor may forget to ask your wife if she wants to watch her baby's birth, so you should remind him to position the mirror. In a standard delivery room, there will be a mirror attached to the overhead light; in a birthing room you will have to supply your own. Be sure your wife has her glasses if she needs them. Many first-time mothers refuse to look because they are so completely absorbed in pushing. Try to encourage your wife at least to glance at the mirror because she'll probably regret later on that she didn't actually witness the birth.

IF PROBLEMS ARISE

Obviously, not all labors go smoothly, and problems can pop up quite unexpectedly. Sometimes you can go to the hospital knowing there is a complication (for example, in the case of a breech presentation), but usually you are taken by surprise. While any complication can be scary, you will feel best if you understand what's going on and how it can be remedied. For this reason, we urge you to read one additional chapter, chapter 12, "Variations on Normal Labor and Delivery."

It's imperative that you trust your doctor or midwife, but the more you know about any situation, the more assured you will feel. If you're calm, your wife is also likely to be, and her composure can only help whatever is going wrong. The two most common impediments to a normal birth are the need for a forceps or a cesarean delivery. The following are some general suggestions about what you can do to help your partner if either of those interventions becomes necessary.

Forceps

Forceps deliveries are performed for three primary reasons: (a) an inability to push properly because of the numbing effect of regional anesthesia; (b) maternal exhaustion; and (c) the need to turn a baby in posterior presentation. If you are in a birthing room when the decision to perform a forceps delivery is made, you will be moved to a delivery room. An episiotomy is always done when forceps are used.

You may be frightened by the look of the forceps and by the doctor's hands shaking as he uses them. This is normal because he's exerting great force, and you shouldn't be alarmed. The best thing to do is to focus on your wife, trying to reassure her and encouraging her to work along with the doctor. She will have received an anesthetic, most likely a pudendal or several doses of a local, depending on the position of the baby. The doctor will pull with forceps only during contractions, and to maximize his efforts you should be helping your wife push as he tugs.

Once the baby is delivered, you may notice small red bruises or dents on the baby's face in the places where the forceps were applied. These are considered a normal complication of a forceps delivery and will disappear in a few days. It may take more than thirty minutes to stitch up the episiotomy, and that's because it has had to be made larger than usual to accommodate the forceps. During this time, you and your wife should be able to hold the baby, provided he is kept warm.

Cesarean Delivery

Unless you know in advance that your wife is going to have a cesarean, you're going to be shaken by this development, particularly if it's an emergency procedure. Obviously, your wife will also be upset, and it may be hard to remain steady for her sake. At this point, you're likely to feel yourself caring more for her than for the baby, who still remains rather abstract. You may also feel somewhat responsible, and thus guilty about this turn of events. If it's an emergency cesarean, things will be happening around you, and there will be very little you can actually do. If there's no emergency, your participation will be more important, and you will be included in any decisions.

The big question concerning your role during a cesarean section is whether you want to be with your wife and whether the hospital will allow you to be. If she can receive regional anesthesia and be awake, we believe there is great benefit in your presence. If she's going to be knocked out, there is less value, although it is wonderful to be able to see your baby immediately after birth.

A great many hospitals today permit fathers to witness the cesarean births of their children. If your particular hospital is not one of them, however, there may be little you can do on short notice to change that policy. There's no harm in asking, though, and it is possible you might get the permission of all those involved—doctor, anesthesiologist, pediatrician, nurse, or nursing supervisor—to be present.

Whether the operation is performed under regional or general anesthesia, you will not have to look at the actual procedure. Most likely, you will be standing or sitting at your wife's head and her abdomen will be draped, obscuring the view. If she's awake, you can talk to her, hold her hand, and just be a reassuring presence for the five or ten minutes it takes to make the incision and remove the baby. After the newborn has been assessed, you can hold the baby and show him to your wife. The stitching up can take as long as an hour, but after that, you can all go to the recovery room, where your wife will be able to hold the baby.

We know that many of you may feel squeamish about being in the same room where a cesarean is being performed, but your presence can be of invaluable support to your wife. Some of the women who filled out our questionnaires said the low point of their birth experiences was suddenly being separated from their husbands and having to go through the cesarean alone. Although you may feel hesitant now, imagine how anxious you'd feel waiting outside the delivery room for news of your child's birth and your wife's condition. We urge you to keep an open mind about being with your wife if a cesarean becomes necessary.

SEEING YOUR BABY

We don't have to say much about the birth itself because that is the wonderful exhilarating part, the moment when you know the baby is healthy and whether it's a boy or a girl. Many of the men responding to our questionnaire described witnessing the birth as the highlight of the whole experience.

After the baby has been suctioned and wiped off, he will be wrapped in a blanket and you or your wife can hold him. Now, while you are waiting for the placenta to be expelled, is the time for pictures. Don't hesitate to ask the nurse or the doctor to take a family portrait, because this is a rare moment you'll want to relive later on.

After Delivery

If you used a delivery room, you will probably remain there with the baby for about half an hour and then will be transferred to the recovery

S E E I N G   Y O U R   B A B Y

♦

"The moment he emerged, I could see he was a boy. His name had been chosen beforehand, so I was able to announce to my wife, who, not what, had come."

♦

"I bent down to kiss my wife, and our little girl looked right at me and smiled. I'll always remember that moment."

♦

"I finally realized that we had a tiny real live baby."

♦

"When he was completely out, the doctor, who had predicted a girl, said, 'It's a boy. Do you want me to put him back?' "

♦

"All I can say is I was glad they let me participate. I was allowed into the operating room for the C-section, was able to hold the baby right away, and went with her to the nursery for weigh-in, etc. Plus, they let me take all the pictures I wanted from the actual delivery to the time we left for home. I could visit my wife and child anytime from 7:00 A.M. to 10:00 P.M., and we could have the baby whenever we wanted. Our doctors and hospital staff were terrific, caring."

room. If you were in a birthing room, you should be able to stay with the baby for about an hour. Don't let the nurse rush your child away to the nursery. If the baby is healthy, there's no reason you can't have some time to get acquainted as a family. This good part is your well-deserved reward, and you should wallow in it.

Once your wife is in her room, you will want to open the champagne, eat the sandwiches you packed in your Lamaze bag, and make phone calls. This is also a thrilling time, so don't feel obliged to leave in order to let your wife sleep or so that you can go home to walk the dog. You may feel like eating Chinese food or pizza. Why not? This is a celebration, and we encourage you to experience it as fully as possible. If your wife has a private room, you may be able to have a cot brought in so that you can spend the night with her and the baby. Some men prefer to stay at the hospital, since returning to an empty house can be depressing after the excitement of birth.

◆ ◆ ◆ ◆ ◆ ◆ ◆ ◆ ◆ ◆ ◆ ◆ ◆ ◆ ◆

AFTER DELIVERY

◆

"I had the chance to get to know my son before he came home from the hospital. With the help of the hospital staff I became confident about handling and taking care of him. I felt he was mine, too."

◆ ◆ ◆ ◆ ◆ ◆ ◆ ◆ ◆ ◆ ◆ ◆ ◆ ◆ ◆

THE POSTPARTUM PERIOD

This is a time of indescribable highs and lows. There will be days when you believe your baby is the best thing that ever happened to you, and then a mere two hours later you will be convinced your life is ruined. We encourage you to seek solidarity with your wife and to use a team approach in solving problems. If you can view your condition as one of mutual bliss or mutual suffering, you will keep your spirits up and you may strengthen your marriage.

Most of the women who filled out our questionnaires reported that their husbands took a week or more off from work when the baby was born. Their reactions were uniformly positive, with many women making touching statements of appreciation. We encourage you to take as long off as possible because it can be tremendously helpful to your wife and because it provides a unique opportunity to get to know your baby. If your mother or mother-in-law wants to come to help out, that's fine.

But unless you all get along famously, things seem to work out better if the visit occurs after you've returned to work.

Most men seem to believe that women have an innate ability to care for babies, but this simply isn't so. Like anything else, baby care is an acquired skill. If you're both rank beginners, you can learn together and help each other with your nervousness. Some of you may not want to get too involved with the real dirty work, but we're convinced that the more you participate, the less excluded you will feel and the more you will enjoy. If your wife is nursing, she will obviously be doing the feedings, but that still leaves bathing, diapering, changing, playing, and soothing for you.

After a few weeks, when breast-feeding has been established, you may want to spell your wife for one night feeding and give the baby a bottle containing either formula or expressed breast milk. Some women may resist giving up a feeding, but it's really a sound idea. It allows you a special time with the baby, and some uninterrupted sleep can be an elixir for postpartum recovery. It also helps the baby become accustomed to a bottle, which is certainly desirable, since it will enable you to leave him with a baby-sitter.

Neither you nor your wife will be able to believe how much attention the baby receives and how little either of you get. We know you're both probably ready for a little recognition and nurturing, but unfortunately you're going to have to wait. If there's any extra emotional energy around, it should be diverted toward your wife. Right now she's feeling fat, bone tired, and overwhelmed by the demands of motherhood. A few weeks ago she was the center of attention, but at this moment she seems to be little more than a slave. If you do nothing else, try to boost her spirits by praising her performance as a mother and by expressing your appreciation for her efforts.

We know of one pediatrician in New York who instructs all new parents to engage a baby-sitter by the third week of their child's life. He feels it is absolutely essential that a couple reestablish itself by taking a breather. He says, "I know the baby will survive; I worry about the parents." We agree, but recognize it is difficult for some couples to put their anxieties aside and make that break. Your sojourn doesn't have to be lengthy, just take off two hours and go out for dinner. The baby can be watched by grandparents, a neighbor, or a good friend and will be fine. Leaving the baby is something everyone resists doing, but ultimately enjoys.

The postpartum period is a time to incorporate the baby into your midst and make the profound change from couple to family. This is more easily said than done. We think the best way to accommodate it is to concentrate on your marriage. If you are both loving, patient, and supportive, it will help cushion the jolt. Even the most wanted child disrupts the marital relationship, and you must compensate for this effect. If you can pull together, you will reap the benefits of greater communication and affection, and you will be giving the baby the best thing possible: a happy family.

THE PARTNER'S GUIDE TO LABOR

PHASE OF LABOR	SIGNS AND SYMPTOMS	PARTNER'S SUPPORT
Pre-labor	Baby engages, increase in vaginal discharge, fatigue, general discomfort, mucous plug is dislodged	Increase household participation; reassure her of your love; share your fears as well as your excitement; plan activities to fill time
Early Labor Average length: 8 to 10 hours	Backache, diarrhea, mild abdominal cramps, regular contractions 5 to 20 minutes apart lasting 30 to 45 seconds. Dilation to 3 centimeters	Encourage rest; check suitcase and Lamaze bag; fix light meals for her, heavier ones for you; help wife in bath or shower; phone doctor or midwife to report beginning of labor
Active Labor Average length: 3 to 4 hours	Stronger contractions closer together, some fear and surprise at intensity of contractions, need to concentrate on breathing and relaxation during contractions, contractions 3 to 4 minutes apart lasting about 60 seconds. Dilation to 7 centimeters	Help her to concentrate; encourage relaxation; give her liquids to drink; wash face and hands with washcloth; go to hospital and help with admitting procedures; arrange wife comfortably in bed or chair
Transition Average length: 1 hour	Strong contractions 2 to 3 minutes apart, lasting 60 to 90 seconds, irregular in intensity with double peaks	Set short-term goals, remind her it's okay—the pain is for a purpose; eye-to-eye contact for breathing; remind her

PHASE OF LABOR	SIGNS AND SYMPTOMS	PARTNER'S SUPPORT
	or plateaus at peak of contraction, bloody show, backache, irritability, nausea, feelings of despair, loss of perspective—thinks this will go on forever. Dilation to 10 centimeters	end is near; change clothes for delivery room
Pushing Average length: 1 hour	Urge to bear down, active pushing to crowning, relaxation to birth, second wind as realization comes that end is really near	Continue encouragement and instructions; assist wife to get in comfortable position; remind wife to watch the birth

CHAPTER 14

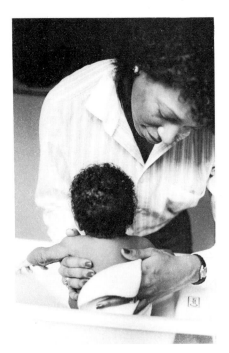

Postpartum

*H*aving a baby is a life crisis. Before having a child, you can't imagine the enormous physical, mental, and emotional adjustments you will be required to make. The postpartum period is a time when you and your husband will experience uncontrolled elation, unceasing fatigue, and endless ambivalence. It's a time when you'll feel more adult, more helpless, more burdened, and more thrilled than you ever thought possible. It's a needy time when everyone in the family will require mothering. It's also a time for living in the present, when immediate tasks sap your energy and long-term goals are put aside. But things do come together and caring for your newborn only gets easier. As you become more confident and organized, you'll understand why babies are called bundles of joy.

AT THE HOSPITAL

Your hospital stay can be one of the best parts of your postpartum period. Although most people don't like hospitals, they can be enjoyable for a new mother. There is service, attention, and general camaraderie on the maternity ward. It is here that you will experience the tremendous joy of calling all your relatives and friends to tell them about your baby's birth. It is here that you will feel an incredible sense of relief that labor and delivery have ended.

We encourage women to have their babies in their rooms at all times possible, a policy known as rooming-in. This concept works best if you have a private room and if the nursing staff supports it, which means they will take care of the baby in your room. It's wonderful to be able to gaze at your child anytime you want, and your constant availability gives breast-feeding a solid beginning. Rooming-in is not immediately feasible if you've had a cesarean (unless you have a private nurse), and not advisable if the hospital is so understaffed there's no one to help you with the baby.

Not every woman wants to spend all her spare time in the hospital ogling her baby. It can take a few days or a few weeks to develop strong parental feelings about your child. Some people fall in love at first glance, whereas others warm up slowly. Both reactions are normal. You may be slightly shell-shocked just after giving birth, and the sight of a red-faced, screaming creature can be strange.

YOUR PHYSICAL RECOVERY

After the baby is born, the hospital staff will be focusing a good deal of attention on you to ensure a complete physical recovery. Your uterus may have to be massaged to help *involution*—the return to its normal nonpregnant state. The nurses may do this, or you can do it yourself. If there's any discomfort, you can do some first-phase breathing. At this point, your uterus will feel like a hard grapefruit located just below your waistline, but within a week it will have contracted deep into your pelvis where you can no longer feel it.

In the forty-eight hours following delivery, you will be sweating and urinating a great deal as your body releases much of the fluid you have retained during pregnancy. You may feel exhausted, but not a bit sleepy because of the excitement of finally having your baby. This is a good time to unwind with relaxation exercises. Lie in bed; take slow, deep breaths; and allow your body to just melt into the mattress. Don't worry about not sleeping. You're experiencing one of the highest moments of your life, so let yourself enjoy it.

Your temperature will be checked regularly by a nurse. If you have a fever, this is a sign of infection and will be treated with antibiotics. Fever occurs most frequently following cesarean section. For the next few weeks you will be discharging *lochia,* a mixture of tissue, blood, and mucus. Immediately after delivery, the flow can be heavy, and for this reason you may want to wear a hospital gown so that your own clothing doesn't get soiled. If that strikes you as too institutional, you can always put your own robe over the gown. While the lochia is flowing red, you must always wear a pad, never a tampon, because of the possibility of infection.

The Episiotomy

By the time you're back in your room, you'll probably begin to feel the effects of the episiotomy, if you've had one. The pain varies greatly from woman to woman, but it is primarily determined by the size and direction of the incision. For the first twenty-four hours after delivery, you may want to apply an ice pack to reduce swelling. After that you can take warm sitz baths (a shallow warm bath in a tub or basin), which feel quite good. To decrease the possibility of infection and to ease cleaning, you will spray an antiseptic solution on your perineum after urinating. You can begin doing the Kegel exercises even though you may not feel any sensation in the perineum. By exercising the muscles of the pelvic floor, you will increase blood flow to the site and thereby speed healing of the incision.

Hemorrhoids

In addition to an episiotomy, you may also have to deal with hemorrhoids. You can treat these with sitz baths and witch-hazel compresses. The Kegel exercise will also help to relieve hemorrhoids. Doughnut pillows are not recommended because their uneven surface can create greater swelling. Though it sounds uncomfortable, sitting on a hard chair or other firm surface will help both the perineum and hemorrhoids to heal.

Breast-feeding

If you're breast-feeding, try to put the baby to your breast as often as possible. Your milk will probably not come in for two to three days, but that doesn't matter, because newborns need no more than water during that time. We advocate giving water because hospitals tend to be hot and therefore dehydrating and because water will flush out the liver, thus alleviating common newborn jaundice. The question of whether you give plain water or sugar water is highly controversial; you should discuss this with your pediatrician. From these first breast-feeding sessions, the baby will get *colostrum,* a yellowish liquid packed with antibodies that helps him adjust to life outside the womb. Moreover, it will stimulate the milk supply.

We don't believe in limiting initial breast-feeding to protect your nipples. They will either get sore or they won't. The determining factor seems to be complexion—fair-skinned women being more sensitive— rather than time spent at the breast. You may have been toughening up your breasts during the past few months by rubbing them with a washcloth in the shower, and that's fine. It's important, however, to position the baby correctly (his belly directly against yours) and to fix the baby's mouth entirely over the nipple and areola. To prevent soreness and cracking, the nipple should be placed as far back in the mouth as is comfortable. In addition, you should avoid washing with soap and water, which can dry out the nipples. If your breasts are tender, try vitamin E oil or lanolin. Both of these can be applied without having to be washed off before the next feeding.

When your milk comes in, your breasts will feel tingly and hard; this sensation can be unfamiliar and uncomfortable, but can be relieved by nursing.

If you're not going to breast-feed, you may be given a drug to dry up your milk. You'll be fairly uncomfortable as the milk comes in and your breasts become engorged, but cold compresses and an aspirin substitute can help. This is another instance in which some first-phase breathing will ease the discomforts of tightness and tenderness.

Coming to Terms with Your Birth Experience

One of the most important emotional adjustments you must make during the postpartum period is coming to terms with your labor and delivery. Every woman, even those who have had great childbirth experiences, knows something she would do differently next time if she could. This is because there are two things we can say unequivocally about childbirth: There is no average labor and no perfect birth.

Each birth has potential for unexpected snags: You may need medication; you may have to be induced; you may enter labor too tired to enjoy any part of it; or you may feel like a failure if you had a cesarean. When things go well, women tend to attribute it to luck, but when things don't, they usually fault themselves.

Birth is a confluence of factors. Of course, your preparation and motivation are important, but the size and position of the baby, the type and length of labor you have, the amount of support you receive, and the quality of your care all contribute to the experience. After all is said and done and you're home with the baby, you must accept what has happened. The most essential thing is to forgive yourself (and others) for whatever shortcomings you perceive and move on to other concerns.

In coming to terms with your birth experience you must accept all your feelings—the good with the bad. It is difficult to express negative emotions, because every time they emerge, you will take one look at your adorable baby and feel guilty for being anything but grateful.

Every woman should discuss her birth experience with her doctor or midwife while still in the hospital, so that she can clear up any doubts or misinformation about what actually happened. If someone has made a comment about your delivery that you didn't understand, ask about it right now, while the opportunity is there and the experience is fresh in your mind. Naturally, you will want to discuss the details of the birth with your family and friends. You may even want to write down your recollection of this important event. But after that, it is essential to accept what has happened and give up any lingering guilt or sorrow. Being hard on yourself is not going to change things, it will only diminish your enjoyment of the baby.

It's best to deal with your feelings now. This could mean seeking professional help or becoming involved with a childbirth-education group to change outdated hospital practices. You can plan to do things differently the next time, but know that perfection cannot exist in an imperfect world. You should resolve your conflicts or doubts about your first child's birth, so they won't interfere with your ability to enjoy a future birth experience.

YOUR PREMATURE BABY

A premature baby is one of those things you don't want to think about during pregnancy, but it does occur rather frequently—10 percent of all babies are born prematurely each year. A premature baby is one who weighs less than 5.5 pounds (2,500 grams) at birth. Some causes of prematurity are multiple birth, toxemia, placenta previa, placenta abrupto, and maternal illness. No cause is known, however, for approximately 60 percent of all premature births.

Until recently, all premature babies were thought to have been born too soon, but neonatologists now know that as many as 40 percent have suffered growth problems in utero. These babies are tiny but mature, and they are categorized as small for gestational age (SGA). It's important to distinguish between premature and SGA babies because they face different problems, requiring different treatment.

In the past twenty years, neonatology has become a sophisticated and effective science. Today its practitioners are skilled in treating babies as small as a pound and coping with their complex medical problems. If your baby is premature, he will undoubtedly be cared for in the neonatal unit of the closest large hospital. While you will be grateful for the expert medical attention, you're also likely to feel anxious, depressed, and not very much like a typical new mother. To ease the adjustment to your premature baby, we have compiled the following suggestions:

• Talk with other parents who've had the same experience. Sometimes informal support groups spring up among the parents of babies in the neonatal unit. Or at some hospitals, groups may be more formally organized by a social worker or volunteer.

• Look at pictures of babies who were premature but now are flourishing as toddlers and children. Some nurseries maintain scrapbooks of their alumni babies, containing encouraging "before" and "after" shots.

continued

◆ Make sure your husband is included as fully as possible in discussions and consultations with the neonatologists. His full participation and interest will help you emotionally, and you will feel more like a family, even though your baby is not at your side.

◆ When you are recovering from the delivery, move off the obstetric floor to a different section of the hospital. If that's not possible, at least get a private room, so that you are not continually confronted by normal newborns and glowing parents. Your needs are special at this time, and you probably won't want to socialize or watch other women interact with their babies. You're likely to feel a little shaky and sad, so you should make things as easy as possible on yourself.

◆ Involve yourself in your baby's care. In order to reduce your fear and general apprehension about the neonatal unit, you should learn the names and functions of the equipment used to support your child. Ask the nurses how to diaper and clean the baby in the incubator. Many hospitals encourage parents to hold their preemies during tube feedings, because it's been proven that babies relax and gain weight faster if they are held. If this is not your hospital's policy, make a special request.

◆ Try to breast-feed or prepare for breast-feeding by expressing your milk. Breast milk is the best food any baby can have, and by providing it, you will be doing something tangible for your child that no one else can do. Even if your baby is being fed intravenously, he will soon graduate to a feeding tube and then a bottle. If you can keep up your milk supply, you will be able to enjoy breast-feeding. An electric breast pump will make this job infinitely easier for you; you should be able to rent one.

◆ Don't delay in naming the baby. This is a small step that helps form an emotional bond to your child. As a measure of self-defense, many parents resist developing an attachment to the baby out of fear of losing him. Of course, this is a possibility, but naming your child may give you pleasure, and it's an act of affirmation in a very difficult circumstance.

The Blues

Whether you've had a vaginal or a cesarean birth, you might experience a kind of letdown around your second or third day after delivery. For some women, this is just a natural descent from an exhilarating time, but for others, it can be a real blue period, during which tears flow at the slightest provocation. Don't worry about feeling weepy and depressed; this sudden mood isn't going to last for the next three months. Right now your hormone levels are unstable, your episiotomy is aching, and your attempts at nursing may be more frustration than pleasure. Even though you're still in the hospital, you're zooming headfirst into a period of readjustment and you must have patience with your ability to take it all in.

We hope you haven't instructed your husband to bring an old pair of jeans to the hospital for the trip home. It doesn't matter if you've been in the hospital for one day or seven, you'll probably leave with the body you had in the fourth or fifth month of pregnancy. Trying to pull up a pair of size 10 pants over size 14 thighs is a good reason to cry, so don't set yourself up for this. The maternity dress you're the least tired of is the best thing to wear home. Checking out of the hospital can be unnerving with the challenge of dressing your baby for the first time and then the stress of decoding directions for the car seat—you don't need to start the day with a wardrobe crisis.

BEING HOME

There's no way you can really prepare for coming home from the hospital with the baby. Yes, you have a cute crib and a case of diapers, but that doesn't mean you're ready. What you really need is a wet nurse to breast-feed the baby, a fairy godmother to heal your episiotomy, and a caterer to take care of meals and snacks for all the company.

The first three months are difficult. You have to accept this, and try to get through them one day at a time. Sometime after the first month you'll experience a pure shining moment when you'll look at your child and realize why you had him. If you're reading this when the baby is colicky, and you haven't slept for more than two hours at a stretch and there are sixty baby presents to acknowledge, you must think we're crazy. Have courage; things do improve.

What you must remember about the postpartum period is that almost all first-time mothers find it difficult. Everyone has trouble getting a

HOME WITH BABY

♦

"It was a lovely, golden time. I remember the luxury of time—for me and for my baby. I stayed home from work for four months, and it was such a treat."

♦

"I felt tremendous loneliness and lack of support. My husband had just begun a difficult new job and was gone from dawn until dark, sometimes until 1:00 A.M."

♦

"It seems strange that the six weeks postpartum are supposed to be a time of recovery for the mother, since that is when the baby is most demanding and you get the least sleep!"

♦

"It was a lot harder than I thought it would be. My son cried a lot, slept little, and nursed every two hours around the clock. I was exhausted. He was a wild man. It was a true revelation to see how little control I had over the kind of person my baby was."

♦

"I seemed to live in a milky haze—a product of very little sleep, a cheerfully ravenous daughter, balmy spring weather, and the abrupt but not unwelcome transition from a high-pressure job to a role as house-mommy!"

♦

"I think I enjoyed the middle-of-the-night feedings the most. Getting up and holding and feeding that warm, soft little body while everyone else is asleep . . . it's a special time for mothers and babies."

♦

"My baby had colic. I'd never throw her out the window, but I wanted to jump myself."

continued

"It didn't seem like I was my son's mother. I was just a person who took care of him."

♦

"I loved the feeling of my son's breath against my neck when he was on my shoulder."

♦

"My husband, my son, and I slept in a double bed every night for our baby's first six months. I'm not sure which was more pleasurable, falling asleep together or waking up together."

♦

"Having to go back to work after two months almost made me afraid to get too close to my baby. I underwent more stress during that period than I have at any other time. It's the saddest thing a mother has to do. It would be nice to have longer maternity leaves."

♦

"The isolation was hard. I had no other friends or relatives with children, let alone infants. I found it difficult to go anywhere. The logistics of just getting out the front door are staggering!"

♦

"I went out to the garage and kicked the car tires until I wore off the frustration, then went back into the house. She was still crying, but I could handle it better."

♦

"I could have done without the constant unsolicited advice."

♦

continued

"I chose not to return to work and felt so misplaced. Getting used to the new routine wasn't an easy thing for me to deal with."

◆

"I usually looked forward to her naps . . . and then I would look forward to her waking up."

shower before 1:00 P.M., everyone has moments of resenting the baby, and everyone has times when things seem out of control. These experiences are normal, and you shouldn't feel you're the only new mother that's not organized and happy all the time. Just like pregnancy, the postpartum period is finite, and that fact makes it bearable. Once it's behind them, some women even become quite nostalgic about those grueling but exciting first days of motherhood when everything was new and confusing and wonderful.

The terrifying part is when you and your husband and the baby are at home with no nurses, pediatricians, midwives, or other new mothers to consult. The situation appears to be black and white: Either this baby will live or he won't, and it will all be your fault. Luckily, it only takes a few weeks before you and your husband realize that the baby will be fine, but that it's questionable whether *you* will make it. The first few weeks at home with a first-born baby are overwhelming. For this reason, most couples need support. Whether it's a baby-nurse, a mother or mother-in-law, a sister, a housekeeper, or even a teenage helper, you must have some assistance. Couples who are particularly insecure feel most comfortable with a baby-nurse, but this is expensive and can be superfluous if you are breast-feeding. Also, the nurse's expertise can make you feel even less competent. A family member is the best, but only if everyone gets along well. You don't need your husband bickering with his mother while you're learning to breast-feed.

The biggest problem you will face will be fatigue. We know that all of you have had times in your life when you've been exhausted, either from working nonstop or from pushing your body to the limit in some kind of athletic activity. Yes, you were tired, completely done in, but after a good night's sleep or a few days' rest, you felt better. Postpartum fatigue, however, is like nothing you have ever experienced. Having your sleep interrupted every few hours, night after night for several weeks or even months, produces a unique kind of debilitation. You go around in a dazed, clumsy condition that almost seems drugged, except you don't feel high. Studies have shown that a state similar to psychosis sets in after several nights of interrupted sleep—and these studies were done with subjects who weren't recovering from childbirth or caring for newborns.

The days are pretty bad, too. Taking on any new job is stressful, and in this one the responsibility is constant, and the training program nonexistent. Before giving birth, you at least had coffee breaks, and evenings and weekends. Now, you barely have three minutes to go to the bathroom. To avoid a nervous breakdown, you must be somewhat philosophical about your crying baby. There's just so much you can do after you've fed, burped, changed, and walked him and he's still howling. Infants cry a lot, and if you can accept that fact without feeling guilty, you will have made a major adjustment to the postpartum period.

If you don't have a baby who cries, you may have one who confuses days and nights, which means that he sleeps most of the day and is up almost all night looking for food and a good time. Of course, three-week-olds have no conception of night and day, and many people believe this is a problem that will correct itself. You can try waking your baby during the day in an attempt to teach him the difference, but don't get upset if the baby doesn't catch on.

Whatever your child's schedule, you'll probably have a difficult time trying to do everything you want—everything you had planned on doing during your maternity leave, plus all the other things that now take precedence. We don't want to be accused of sapping women's ambition, but there's just no way in the first few months that you can take care of a baby, yourself, your house, your social obligations, and maintain your career. Something has to give, and it will most likely be your health or your sanity.

During your first month at home, you should be mindful that you're still recovering from a strenuous physical experience, childbirth. If you begin to run a temperature, or experience back or abdominal pain, or the lochia becomes bright red or smells odd, you should call your doctor or midwife at once. These symptoms mean you may have an infection and need immediate treatment.

In order to protect your health, you must sleep while your baby does. Don't worry about returning phone calls or vacuuming; you've got to catch some rest while you can. Your enjoyment of motherhood during the first few months is directly proportional to the amount of sleep you get.

BREAST-FEEDING

Breast-feeding is one of those experiences you can't understand until you go through it. Sitting peacefully, your breasts are full, your baby hungry and pulling at your nipple, is one of the best feelings in the world. The flip side of that occurs when you're in the middle of lugging groceries in from the car, your older child is whining for a snack, the phone is ringing, the baby is crying for a feeding, and you're supposed to sit down, relax immediately, and feed him.

Breast-feeding has it all over bottle-feeding in terms of convenience and ease of preparation, but in a way it's an extension of the state of pregnancy because your body still is not your own. The preoccupation with good eating and rest remains paramount because you can't maintain the baby properly if you're skipping meals or feeling exhausted. While you're breast-feeding you'll be burning about 500 extra calories a day and some women find themselves drained by this effort. We encourage you to give breast-feeding a good try, if you're so inclined, because it's the most nutritious way to feed your baby and it has to be one of the loveliest parts of motherhood.

Contrary to much of the advice about breast-feeding, however, we do encourage you to give a relief bottle early on, say at ten days or two weeks. You won't subvert successful breast-feeding by offering the baby some formula and it will enable you to go out with your husband or leave the baby with a sitter. If you feel funny about the formula, you can express some milk, but by all means, try the bottle, so you are not tied down completely.

Today breast-feeding is undergoing a renaissance, and many women are made to feel tremendously guilty if they don't nurse their babies. Again, you've got to get past the well-intentioned advice and decide for yourself how best to feed your baby. Sheila Kitzinger recognizes the importance of a mother's attitude when she writes in *The Experience of*

BREAST-FEEDING

♦

"When the baby sucks strongly, with eyes half-closed and chubby arms flung across your breast, with no one to bother you, it makes it all worthwhile."

♦

"I loved breast-feeding. I nursed for eighteen months before my son quit. After my cesarean, it made me feel whole again."

♦

"I nursed for two weeks, and it just did not work out. I was absolutely exhausted, and the baby was so big he was not getting enough to eat, so he was fussy. After he was put on formula, he was fine, and so was I."

♦

"Since I was breast-feeding, the only things my daughter needed were me and air to breathe. It's such a warm, wonderful feeling."

Childbirth, "After all, it is not so much what she [the mother] feeds with as how she feeds him that matters. It is her loving touch that he needs, and unsuccessful breastfeeding can be a very frustrating and disturbing experience for both mother and baby. Whilst breastfeeding can be the best sort of feeding there is, unsuccessful breastfeeding comes a poor second to happy bottle feeding."

YOUR EMOTIONAL AND MARITAL ADJUSTMENT

Postpartum depression in the mild to moderate range is estimated to occur in 3 to 23 percent of all women. No one seems particularly concerned about these figures because they are thought to reflect hor-

"I had a severe depression, which lasted about two months. My husband was jealous of the baby, and I couldn't seem to get anything done."

♦

"I had trouble with depression. I couldn't communicate rationally. I had to go to the doctor, finally, and that helped—talking to someone who was objective."

monal changes, which correct themselves. We agree with this, but think researchers have always ignored or underestimated the effect of fatigue on a new mother's psyche. We don't mean to sound redundant, but fatigue is the number one problem during the postpartum period. It will make you grouchy, sensitive, foggy, prone to feelings of resentment, and it will probably affect your husband in much the same way.

There are, however, a lot of new feelings that go along with becoming a mother, and some of these emotions can be disturbing. For example, you may be vice-president of your company with your own secretary, but for now, you are the wet nurse and housekeeper. Of course, you want to take care of your baby, but there seems to be something slightly discriminatory about the fact that your husband can walk out of the house every morning while you're stuck there with a demanding infant and a pile of chores.

If you're just home on maternity leave, things are not too bad, because your predicament is temporary. Your worst problem may be finding someone else to take over the baby care. But if you've decided to take a year or an indefinite leave to raise your child, or even if you were not working at all before the baby was born, you must make a major adjustment to a new role. For women who are newly staying home, that means taking on a lot of the chores you used to share as a couple. This is because you're home and he isn't, and, because you both want him to spend his free time with the baby, not running to the cleaners. Being home also

How to Recognize
Serious Postpartum Depression

♦

Just about every woman experiences some postpartum blues after giving birth. An uncontrollable desire to weep, a feeling of helplessness, and a sense of being overwhelmed are common in the six weeks following delivery. Hormones and fatigue do contribute to mood swings, and these are normal during this period of difficult emotional adjustment. If, however, you continue to feel down for a few months, you may be suffering from serious postpartum depression, and you need help.

We asked Pat Shimm, who runs a support program for depressed mothers and their children at Barnard College in New York, to compile a list of symptoms of true depression. If you are still feeling depressed after six weeks, you should ask yourself if you

♦ Feel sad, blue, down in the dumps, withdrawn, lonely, helpless

♦

♦ Have trouble falling asleep at night, or wake up in the middle of the night and can't get back to sleep, or feel like sleeping all day
♦ Feel overly sensitive to comments of others about your ability as a mother
♦ Get angry and jumpy at every little thing
♦ Feel a loss of interest or pleasure in activities you previously enjoyed
♦ Find it hard to make decisions or concentrate as you did in the past
♦ Feel guilty and sometimes worthless
♦ Can't eat much food anymore, or can't stop eating all the time
♦ Worry about whether your depressed feelings are affecting your child's behavior
♦ Feel tired for little apparent reason, or feel like you're moving in slow motion

If you answer yes to three or more of these questions, there's a good chance you are suffering from real depression. If this is the case, Mrs. Shimm suggests you seek professional help immediately. Your doctor or minister may be able to

continued

recommend a therapist, or you can look in the Yellow Pages under mental health for some names. You might also ask your Lamaze teacher, because she may have helped previous students with this problem. Whatever happens, don't despair. Many women suffer from depression after childbirth, but they recover completely and resume full and active lives.

means you will pass a great deal of the day in your house with your baby, and that can be a big change from your bustling life Before Baby.

One of the things first-time mothers can't prepare themselves for is the work that motherhood entails. Just about every woman we know who has quit her job to take care of her child full-time says motherhood is more grueling. It's not that the work itself is so hard; this is another instance when the whole is greater than the sum of its parts. Everything —meals, cleaning, laundry, shopping, doctors' appointments, entertaining—falls on you, and you are responsible for every detail. If the baby is late for his polio vaccine, it's your problem. If the dog has fleas, it's your problem. If you've run out of soap, it's your problem.

Sometimes women have the stamina for all this work, but it's the responsibility involved in their new job that undermines emotional stability. You are the mother; this baby is your responsibility, and if you don't get moving and go to the store, there will be no diapers for your child. Even if you had a former job that was very high-powered and important, it didn't carry the total responsibility you have now. If you lapsed at work and made an error, your company may have lost an advantage or at worst, some money. Now the stakes are much higher. If your baby falls down the stairs, he could seriously hurt himself. The job of motherhood tolerates much less sloppiness, laziness, or irresponsibility than any other occupation.

Another negative part of full-time motherhood can be the pay. We realize that not all of your husbands are the warm, generous people they

HELP WITH THE BABY

♦

"My mother stayed with me for two weeks, and I could not have made it without her love and support. I hope I can do the same for my daughter someday."

♦

"My mother came, but I found it difficult to let her do the work. I still felt as if I should be the hostess."

♦

"I didn't have any help and I didn't need it. I had an easy birth and an easy baby, and I was home all day. My house was never cleaner and the meals never better."

♦

"My husband helped out, but his 'help' was sometimes more trouble than assistance. He is wonderful at fathering, but very questionable at householding."

♦

"I had a woman come in and clean. It saved my life."

♦

"I felt like I belonged in intensive care, but everyone expected me to carry on as if nothing had happened."

♦

"My husband was home for the two weeks following our daughter's birth, and he was a *tremendous* help. He gave me lots of attention and soothing words when I needed them, did all of the housework, and took care of our little girl. He also read my breast-feeding book to help me through the rough times."

♦

"I didn't want anyone to help me care for the baby. I wanted a cook and a laundress!"

continued

"It seemed to take two full months for my energy level to return to normal. I found it frustrating that I seemed to be able to do nothing except take care of the baby. I remember one day when my only goal was to dust the living-room furniture. At the end of the day, I had not been able to do even that."

♦

"My husband helped out a lot by putting the baby to sleep in the middle of the night. Also, it was nice having a second opinion on baby matters, since I knew about as much as he did."

should be, and you may feel odd about asking for money. Sometimes this is your problem, but often it is his. This is a shame, because if you or your husband could think rationally on the subject, you'd both realize that a housekeeper earning $50,000 a year wouldn't do as good a job as you. Try to maintain your dignity on this issue, but remember that your husband is under a fair amount of pressure. It's hard to be the sole breadwinner of a growing family, particularly a family that has become accustomed to being supported by two.

You don't have to be a family counselor to know that some marital relationships become a little shaky during the postpartum period. We know a good birth experience can be one of the greatest moments of a marriage, but unfortunately the feelings engendered by that event don't last for months. If you have a good marriage, you'll weather the postpartum period. Children by themselves cannot destroy a solid marriage. However, the stress of child rearing will most certainly exacerbate any existing weaknesses in the relationship and can bring on new ones. You simply cannot know in advance what kind of mother or father you will be, what kind of baby you'll have, or how you'll both respond to this life change.

No matter how sound your relationship, you'll probably lapse into some nagging and complaining. Even though you both appreciate the difficult changes you're going through, it's hard to be mature and accept all the turmoil with equanimity. It helps if you can figure out what specifically is bothering you. We've observed that couples seem to have certain basic resentments during the postpartum period:

Wife's Resentments:

He wasn't pregnant for nine months and doesn't have to wear maternity clothes even now.

He has a feeling of accomplishment at the end of each day.

He can leave for work each morning, where he talks to other adults and eats at least one uninterrupted meal.

He earns money for what he does.

He doesn't have to be reluctant to tell other people at parties about his job, because it's socially acceptable.

Husband's Resentments:

She doesn't know I'm alive now that the baby's here.

She's responsible for the household, and it's on the verge of collapse.

She's able to spend much more time with the baby than I can.

She's breast-feeding, and suddenly I'm the odd man out.

If you want your marriage to flourish along with your child, you should try not to be critical of each other's efforts with the baby. Unless you are a pediatric nurse or your husband is the oldest of seven children, neither one of you has probably had much experience with newborns. Every person has his or her own style of relating to children, and this should be respected. Short of strangling a baby in a receiving blanket or drowning him during a bath, there's very little serious harm that can be done. Couples commonly fall into a negative behavior pattern: You're both nervous, the baby is howling, and it's very easy to second-guess the person who is dealing with the child. To increase mutual enjoyment of the baby, avoid criticizing each other, and try to appreciate your individual styles of parenting.

There are a few basic things you can do to alleviate marital stress during the postpartum period. The first thing is to go out again as a couple, even if it's only for a walk. This seems obvious, but many new parents are unnecessarily afraid of finding a baby-sitter and leaving the baby for the first time. Nothing will happen except that you will relax a little and perhaps have an uninterrupted conversation. As we said earlier, breast-feeding will not be sabotaged by one relief bottle during the first few weeks, and the break will refresh you both. You should also consider sleeping through a feeding and allowing your husband or a sitter to give the baby a bottle. We're not suggesting this be done every day, but a few solid hours of sleep on occasion can improve your outlook.

In most cases, marital relationships improve as the postpartum period ends and as the baby matures. When your child reaches three or four months, your marriage begins to adjust as irritability and resentments subside. When he is six months old, you will be thrilled with your new family life, and when the baby reaches nine or ten months, it will be better than you ever thought possible.

Making Love Again

One thing that will boost your marriage a great deal is the resumption of your sex life. Most doctors give the go-ahead to have sex as soon as you have physically recovered. This can be at three, four, or six weeks postpartum depending on the scheduling of the checkup and the nature of the birth. Many couples, however, don't feel like making love for quite a while, and when they do, their sexual feelings don't always return simultaneously.

For women, lack of sexual desire in the postpartum period is usually hormonal; decreased estrogen levels affect libido and can contribute to vaginal dryness. This happens most commonly to nursing mothers; a lubricant such as K-Y jelly can solve this problem. For men, this same lack of desire is often related to seeing their wives give birth and then reconciling the pleasure of sex with the function of childbirth. You should be assured that both these stumbling blocks are temporary. Once you have your first menstrual period, your body's hormones will have returned to their normal level and your sexual desires should be rekindled. Rising estrogen levels will also increase vaginal secretions, and this will make sex more enjoyable for both of you.

You shouldn't feel there is something wrong if you don't feel like making love for quite a while after your baby's birth. The postpartum period is a time when you often feel affectionate but not sexual. Some women have desire at four weeks postpartum, whereas others don't until the baby is five or six months old. Sex therapists William Masters and Virginia Johnson studied 101 women in the third month after delivery and found 47 of them to have low or negligible levels of sexuality. The most commonly cited reason for this lack of desire was fear of permanent physical harm if sex was resumed too soon after giving birth. In the same study, the highest levels of sexual interest were reported by 24 nursing mothers. These women reported sexual stimulation while breast-feeding, but also indicated specific interest in resuming sexual relations with their husbands.

For some couples, the problems of when and where pose greater difficulties than any others. Your normal bedtime routine will probably be interrupted with a feeding, and once you're through with that you'll want to fall asleep immediately because you'll have to be up again in a few hours. Your daytime schedule will also be out of control, because it will be determined by your baby. If you used to go back to bed on Sundays after breakfast or nap on Saturdays before dinner, you don't anymore. The only feasible strategy seems to be catch as catch can.

As for where, the logical spot is the bedroom, but that's often where the baby is sleeping, and most couples are afraid of making the slightest noise. Obviously, there are two alternatives: the couch, and moving the bassinet out of the bedroom.

Sometimes fear of becoming pregnant again—especially if the baby was unplanned—is a new element in your sexual relationship. If you don't want to become pregnant again, you must use contraception as soon as you resume having intercourse. If you are not breast-feeding, you can take birth control pills. If you are breast-feeding, however, the hormones from the pills will be transmitted to the baby. Your other options include the diaphragm (you will have to be refitted at your checkup if you formerly used one), spermicidal foam, a cervical cap, a sponge, or condoms.

The main thing you need to enjoy lovemaking is a relaxed attitude. We know that spurting breast milk doesn't figure in most people's sexual fantasies, but if it happens, it's not a big deal. (You could try taking a shower first and expressing a little milk manually under the hot water, or feeding the baby just before making love.) The important thing to remember is that most sexual difficulties after childbirth are common and temporary. If you had a good sexual relationship before having a baby, you have an excellent chance of resuming it.

EXERCISE

When to Start

This may surprise you, but we don't think you have to start doing an exercise routine in the hospital the day after your baby is born. You should be doing your Kegels and walking around as much as possible, but your life will be complicated enough without worrying about doing leg lifts as soon as your baby takes a nap. There is a lot of recovery going on at this stage, both physical and emotional, and the feeling that you ought to be working out is just another burden for a new mother. Start as soon as you feel like it, but check first with your doctor or midwife.

Finding the Time

It is not going to be easy trying to fit an exercise break into your busy day, particularly if you have an unpredictable baby and no baby-sitter to spell you. The only advice we have is to make exercise a priority. If you allow the laundry to take precedence over your workout, you will never do another sit-up again. If you can prop your baby nearby in a carrier or put the baby on the floor with you, so much the better. If your baby doesn't tolerate this, wait until nap time, or get your mother-in-law to come over and babysit for half an hour.

Many new mothers have trouble setting aside time for their exercise routine because it seems like a selfish thing to do. If you are taking time to work out, then that's fifteen minutes you aren't spending on your baby, husband, house, dinner, or whatever. We urge you to think of yourself and your own well-being.

The Exercise Routine

The postnatal exercise routine consists of eight exercises, which should take a total of fifteen minutes to do. Four of these exercises are already familiar to you because they are holdovers from the prenatal exercise routine (see page 109); the other four are new. If you have the time, do the complete prenatal workout and add the four new exercises for a slightly longer session.

We've included exercises for the waist, hips, arms, back, and abdomen. These are good exercises for recovering tone no matter how out of shape you feel. The stronger you become, the easier they'll be to do.

(If you had a cesarean, skip these for the time being.)

SITTING SIDE STRETCH

To Start:
Sit tall, with your spine long and straight, your shoulders relaxed and open, and your head centered on the top of your spine.

Exhale:
Stretch your right arm over your head and bend to the left. Relax your head to the side and let your left elbow drop toward the floor. Feel the stretch along your entire right side.

Inhale:
Try to maintain the length along your right side as you unroll to the center position.

Total:
Six times to each side, alternating sides each time.

UPPER-BODY CIRCLES

This, too, is taken from the prenatal routine. Tension is even greater, now that there is a new baby to tend to, so do these circles slowly and gracefully. Breathe deeply and think only about how good it feels, not about chores or obligations.

To Start:
Sit tall, with your spine long and straight, your hands resting lightly on your knees.

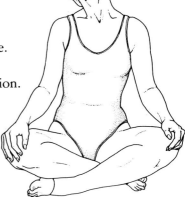

Shoulder Circles:
Circle your shoulders forward, up, all the way back, and down to center. Reverse. Eight times to each direction.

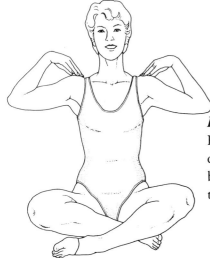

Elbow Circles:
Place your fingertips on your shoulders and circle your elbows forward, to the side, and behind you. Reverse direction. Eight times to each direction.

Head Circles:
Circle your head forward, to the side, around to the back, and to the other side. Drop your chin toward your chest and reverse direction. Four times each direction.

THE BICYCLE

The purpose of this exercise is to tone the abdominal muscles, so don't overwork your legs. Let your legs feel long and light, easily supported by the abdominal strength.

To Start:
Sit back on your elbows, keeping your chest high and your shoulders down. Maintain the pelvic tilt position throughout the exercise.

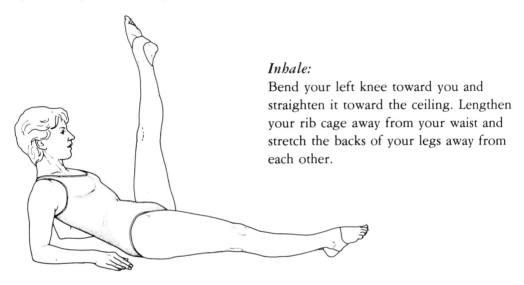

Inhale:
Bend your left knee toward you and straighten it toward the ceiling. Lengthen your rib cage away from your waist and stretch the backs of your legs away from each other.

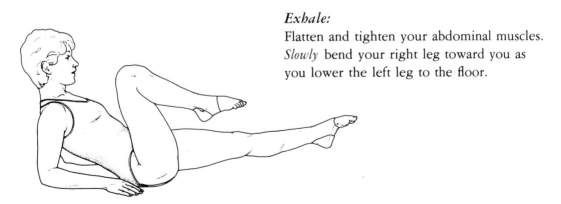

Exhale:
Flatten and tighten your abdominal muscles. *Slowly* bend your right leg toward you as you lower the left leg to the floor.

Total:
Sixteen times, smoothly alternating legs each time.

BACK MASSAGE

This exercise strengthens your abdominal muscles and relaxes the ones in your lower back.

To Start:

Lie on your back, with your knees bent and the soles of your feet on the floor, hip width apart.

Inhale:

Allow your abdomen to rise and fill with air.

Exhale:

Tighten and flatten your abdominal muscles and lift your hips off the floor. Do not tighten your buttocks or arch your lower back. Think of the tops of your thighs as the highest point, and your spine as a straight, diagonal line. Inhale.

Exhale:

Again, tighten your abdominal muscles and roll your spine, one vertebra at a time, back to the floor.

Total:

Six times.

KNEE ROLLS

This exercise feels wonderful for the lower back, and helps to tone your waist.

To Start:
Lie on your back, with your knees close to your chest. Place your hands, palms down, out to the sides, just below shoulder height.

Inhale:
Roll your legs to the right side. Try to keep your knees high and your left shoulder down toward the floor.

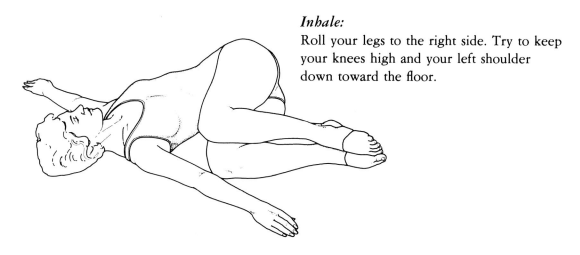

Exhale:
Tighten and flatten your abdominals as you roll your upper back, waist, and lower back to the floor, returning to the starting position.

Total:
Six times to each side, alternating sides.

ARM CIRCLES

If done slowly and with deep, full breaths, this exercise can feel wonderfully relaxing for the upper back and shoulders.

To Start:

Lie on your back, with your arms out to your sides below shoulder height.

Bend your right leg toward your chest and cross it to your left side. Let your right foot rest on the floor.

Keep your fingers on the floor as you circle your right arm above your head and down past your right hip. Stretch your shoulder open and lengthen your arm as it moves.

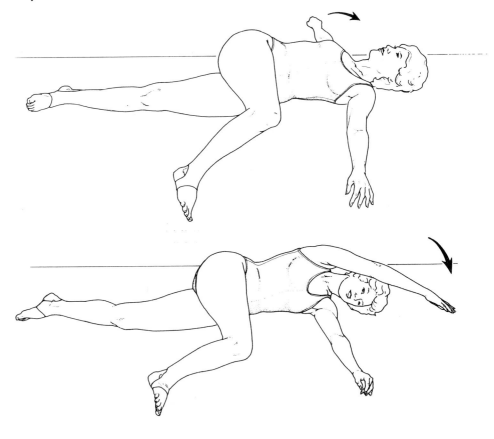

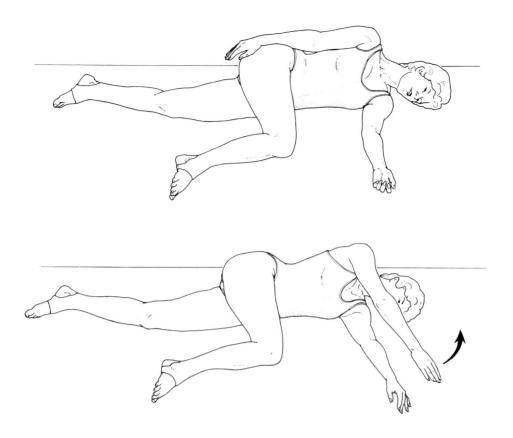

Now reverse direction and circle your arm
across your body and over your head.

Roll your hips back to the floor and
straighten your right leg next to your left.

Total:
Three times each side.

LEG CROSSOVERS

This is a total body movement, working the legs, abdominals, and waist all at the same time.

To Start:
Lie on the floor, with your legs straight and your arms out to the sides, just below shoulder height.

Exhale:
Lift your right leg toward the ceiling, but keep the left leg stretching along the floor.

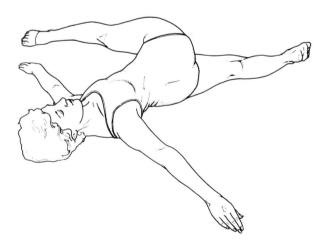

Inhale:
Stretch your right leg across your body. Allow your right hip to leave the floor, but try to keep your right hand in place.

Exhale:
Tighten and flatten your abdominals as you lift your right leg back toward the ceiling, your hips and back completely on the floor. Stretch both legs even longer.

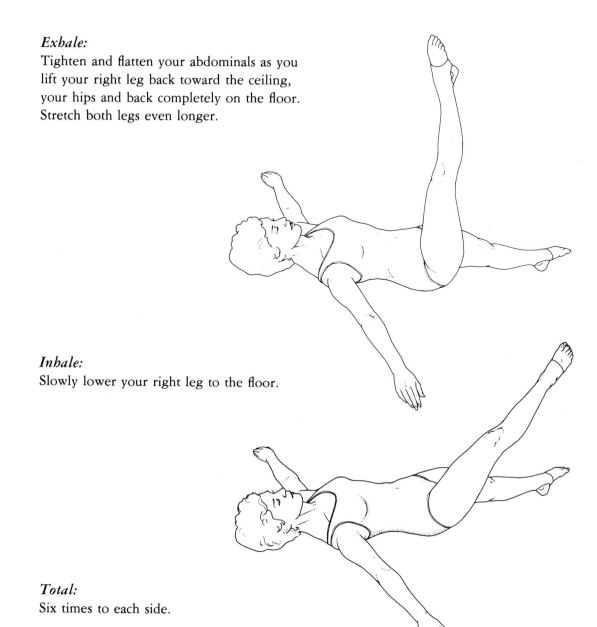

Inhale:
Slowly lower your right leg to the floor.

Total:
Six times to each side.

THE CAT

Again we end with the cat. It relaxes the lower back and increases the flexibility of the muscles all along the spine.

To Start:
Support your weight on your hands and knees—hands directly under your shoulders, knees slightly apart and directly under your hips.

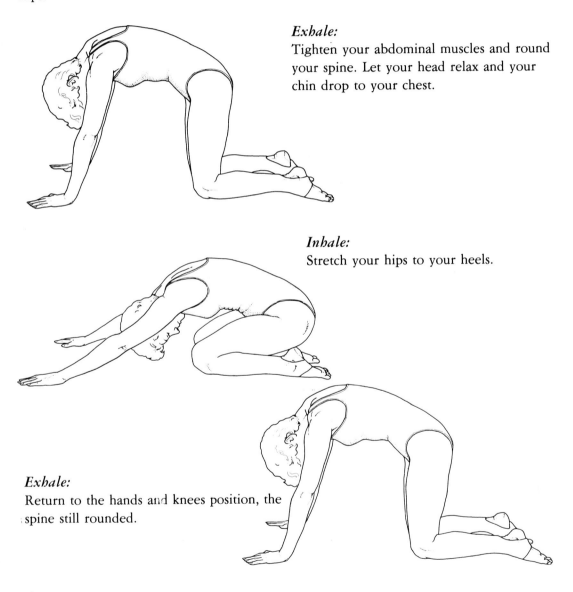

Exhale:
Tighten your abdominal muscles and round your spine. Let your head relax and your chin drop to your chest.

Inhale:
Stretch your hips to your heels.

Exhale:
Return to the hands and knees position, the spine still rounded.

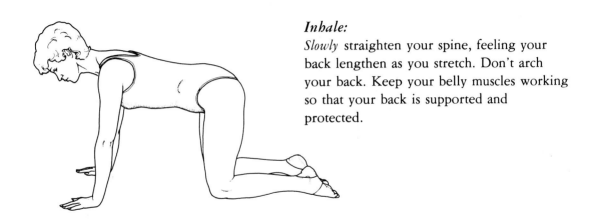

Inhale:

Slowly straighten your spine, feeling your back lengthen as you stretch. Don't arch your back. Keep your belly muscles working so that your back is supported and protected.

Total:
Six times.

SOME FINAL SUGGESTIONS

If there's one last thing we can tell you about the postpartum period, it's that you should think of yourself. Taking care of an infant and recovering from childbirth are your most important tasks right now, and they both take tremendous amounts of energy. You must think of yourself and how to make this time of your life enjoyable and easier. Think of frozen dinners and take-out food and any store that delivers. Think of dog walkers, housekeepers, and cleaning help. Think of insisting that your husband take his vacation time now to help you, think of inviting your mother for a visit, and think of asking for assistance from anyone who can help you.

This is not the time to worry about extravagances or driving to three different supermarkets to cash in coupons. Conserving your time and energy is much more important than saving money. No matter how much you wanted your child or how prepared you were for the change in life-style, you must acknowledge that caring for a newborn is a burden. If you don't pamper yourself during these first three months, your emotional and physical health will suffer. Your enjoyment of the baby is directly related to how much energy you have and how well you feel.

There are two common psychological pitfalls in child rearing that can undermine your energy, commitment, and pleasure: the issues of control and guilt. Control means that you believe you should be able to keep your baby happy all the time, and guilt is what you feel when you can't. Certainly, you have control over the environment to the degree that you change, bathe, and feed your baby. But if he wants to fuss, or fall asleep during visual-stimulation time, there's very little you can do. Some babies are active, whereas others are placid; if you can accept your child's personality early on, you'll be way ahead of the game. Avoid trying to control your child's behavior and blaming yourself for everything that goes wrong. These are nonproductive behaviors that work against your vitality and the enjoyment of your baby.

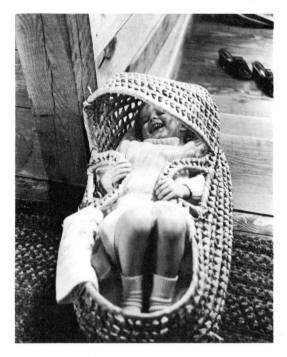

CHAPTER 15

The Second Baby

*I*t's common knowledge that having a baby is the most momentous step in your marriage. While it's true that the first child more radically alters your life-style, the decision to have a second is perhaps more profound because it is an informed choice, one that is made with your eyes open.

If you have one child, any subsequent pregnancies are going to be quite different from the first. The first time is like no other because of the excitement and the wonder of creating a human life. The second time can be thrilling, too, but it's tempered by experience and the knowledge that pregnancy is just a means to an end. Physically, the second time is usually more tiring, and minor complaints can seem more bothersome. From an emotional standpoint, it's easier because you're much less anxious about the normal aches and pains of pregnancy and you're more confident about taking care of an infant.

During your first pregnancy you were probably absorbed in yourself and your symptoms. This time you're probably focusing less on bodily changes and more on how you will integrate the new baby into the family. One of the big preoccupations of second- or third-time mothers is organization and scheduling. This time you won't be daydreaming about the layette, you'll be concentrating on trickier matters, such as how can I get child number one to nursery school by 8:30 if the baby is just waking up? Can I manage both of them at the pediatrician or should I make separate appointments? How will I get anything done around the house if their nap times are different?

Despite the tangled logistics of two children's schedules, we believe the addition of child number two is a smoother process than the incorporation of the first one. This is primarily because you've done it before and, having lived through night feedings, colds, and teething, you know these are developmental hurdles, not life-threatening crises. Your threshold for anxiety has been raised considerably, and this new tolerance is accompanied by a greatly increased ability to enjoy your baby. In addition, you're spared the trauma of completely changing your lifestyle because that wrenching process already occurred after the birth of your first baby. Second-time parents are much less bothered about not going to the movies every week or not sleeping late, for they know the rewards of parenthood outweigh the sacrifices.

There will probably be less friction this time around between you and your husband because he is not going to feel as insecure as he might have the first time. He realizes that having a new baby is an exciting experience, not an alienating one, and most likely he'll be very involved in helping your older child to adjust to the new sibling. Both of you are going to be infinitely more relaxed with the second baby, and this should enhance your relationship. First-time parents are inclined to argue about each other's burping techniques or whether the baby is hungry or tired, but this sort of thing rarely happens again because you're both more secure—and busier.

Although your husband may be more helpful with the second child, he's likely to act a bit casual about the pregnancy, as will the rest of the world. During the first pregnancy, you caught everyone's fancy—the butcher, your co-workers, and your mother-in-law all marveled at your expanding girth and glowing demeanor. Unfortunately, the mystique is now gone. This time you're old hat, and people are apt to take a ho-hum attitude, or even a negative one if your pregnancies have been closely spaced.

The thing to do in this case is to pamper and indulge yourself as much as possible, because you need it, no matter how many times you've been pregnant. Don't be too hard on your husband if he's not eager to run out for pizza or wake up in the middle of the night to massage a cramped muscle. The excitement of the first pregnancy is unique and can't be repeated. The second time can be great, but it's not the same. To compensate, go to exercise class, buy some new maternity clothes, get a facial, read some new pregnancy books, or do anything that makes you feel special, even though you've been pregnant before.

PHYSICAL CHANGES

During the first pregnancy, you experienced considerable stretching of the abdomen, ligaments, and muscles of the pelvic floor and uterus. For this reason, you may carry lower and show earlier with the second and each subsequent pregnancy. At the end of a first pregnancy, the baby's presenting part—usually the head—engages or drops down in the pelvis, allowing a little more room around the diaphragm. This doesn't occur during later pregnancies because the abdominal muscles are not as taut and the uterus bulges out instead of being pushed down by those muscles. Engagement may not occur until you go into labor.

In addition to weaker stomach muscles, you will also experience less stability in your pelvis due to a greater softening of the cartilaginous joints, particularly around your pubic bone. This phenomenon creates the sensation that the baby is literally falling out of you, and it can make walking or extended standing quite uncomfortable.

You will probably feel much more tired during a second pregnancy because you have to take care of your first child. Some women claim that even though they worked until the end of their first pregnancies, they were considerably more fatigued during later ones spent at home. This is not surprising; everyone knows a two-year-old is more demanding than the most tyrannical boss.

First pregnancies are infamous for food cravings and eating binges. There seems to be a fat woman lurking inside most of us, but many women are reluctant to let her out again because the memory of post pregnancy dieting is still painfully fresh. Many second-time mothers also don't eat as well as they did the first time because of lack of time and energy. For breakfast, they're likely to share some eggs with their child, then grab lunch at McDonald's, and later whip up something easy for dinner. We know you are probably feeling worn-out and overwhelmed, but you've got to remember the importance of feeding the baby that is growing inside you. This baby's dependence is as real as your older child's because he is also relying on you for nourishment.

LABOR AGAIN

Your attitude about your second labor is going to have a lot to do with your feelings about the first experience. In general, women handle labor more easily because they know what a contraction feels like and are secure in the knowledge that they've gotten through it once already. Although second or third labors are not known to be less painful, they often seem so because they are half as long and because the intensity of the pain is not as shocking as it was initially.

Some couples are so unconcerned about labor—or so intent on blocking out their first experience—that they don't feel the need to take a refresher course in Lamaze. The problem with this approach is that without the course, they'll be unlikely to practice, and preparation is as important as it was the first time around. We recommend a refresher seminar if you had your last baby more than two years ago. It can be offered as part of a regular Lamaze series or as a distinct entity by itself. Refresher courses generally concentrate on reviewing the breathing patterns and describing recent changes in hospital procedures. Very little time is spent on anatomy or describing the process of labor and delivery. Review chapter 5 of this book, which instructs you in all the breathing and relaxing techniques.

We strongly recommend a refresher for several reasons:

+ It keeps you up-to-date on the latest developments in obstetric practice
+ It affords some camaraderie with other couples, which should help your morale

LABOR AGAIN

♦

"The Lamaze refresher course took on a whole new perspective because we had actually been through a Lamaze birth with our first baby. I took the breathing exercises more seriously the second time."

♦

"So many things were better about the second time—shorter labor, shorter hospital stay. Even the things that were worse *seemed* better. The first time my episiotomy bothered me for months. The second time I had both an episiotomy and tearing, but I felt great in about a week. I think my attitude was so much better for the second delivery that it colored my perceptions of everything."

♦

"It took a third as long as the first time. It was sheer heaven, and left me with enough energy to enjoy the whole experience."

♦

"The first time was nice, but this time was the greatest. It was a short, manageable labor and exciting delivery. We really got to know my daughter right away because she roomed in with me."

♦

"I was very depressed because I realized this would probably be my last baby."

♦

"From experience, I knew what to expect and I felt better prepared. I knew my strengths and weaknesses and what I needed to stress."

♦

"I was very pleased with the entire birth experience the second time because I spoke up for what I wanted—and got it. I was much more confident of my abilities and secure in the knowledge that what I wanted was not unreasonable."

continued

"The first time I was not prepared for the degree of concentration and the effort required; the second time, I was."

- ◆ It can help work out any lingering doubts or questions you have about your first birth
- ◆ It will start you thinking about the birth and reviewing the breathing and relaxation exercises you should be practicing

Many couples take a refresher course because they had a bad or mediocre birth experience the first time and now they're seeking a new approach. They may have changed doctors or hospitals and they are restudying the method in order to use it to better advantage. Often, refresher courses are undertaken with the bittersweet attitude that the upcoming birth may be the last, making it a final chance to fulfill a fantasy. Whatever your reasons, a refresher course will spark your enthusiasm and get you in the proper frame of mind to have your baby.

Even though you have already given birth, you can't predict what kind of labor you will have. If you had back labor, or had to be induced, or if your water broke hours before contractions began, there's no rule that says it will happen that way again. It's also possible that you may require a cesarean delivery this time. About 10 percent of all second-time mothers who previously delivered vaginally have C-sections, usually for placental or umbilical problems, and you should prepare yourself for this. Labors are as individual as the children they produce, and you shouldn't set yourself up for one particular type of experience.

Although every birth experience is different, there are some common characteristics between first and second vaginal births:

- ◆ The time spent in labor is generally half as long as the first time. This also holds true for the expulsion phase. If your pregnancies are spaced more than ten years apart, however, this does not apply.

- False labor is more common during second pregnancies, and Braxton-Hicks contractions can seem stronger.
- Babies are much more likely to arrive on time or early, and they usually weigh a few ounces more than their siblings did at birth.
- If you had telescopic labor the first time, you're likely to have a very fast labor the second.
- Second-time mothers are less likely to develop toxemia (unless there is a different father).
- Dilation and effacement often occur earlier in the pregnancy because the Braxton-Hicks contractions are stronger and the cervix is more pliable.

VAGINAL BIRTH AFTER A CESAREAN (VBAC)

In 1916, Dr. Edward Craigin made a speech to the New York Medical Society in which he stated, "Once a cesarean, always a cesarean." At the time, the national cesarean rate was less than 1 percent, and the classical or vertical incision was the only one performed.

Craigin's axiom ruled the practice of obstetrics for nearly seventy years, and to a great extent it still does. In 1982 the American College of Obstetricians and Gynecologists reversed its long-standing policy and stated encouragement for attempted vaginal delivery after a cesarean. The National Center for Health Statistics estimates, however, that only 5.7 percent of the women who are eligible for a VBAC are actually having them. (This figure, based on statistics gathered in 1984, is considered only an estimate, because it is determined by hospital-discharge data, which can be incomplete or imprecise.)

The justification for performing repeat cesareans is fear that the uterine scar may rupture. While this possibility is greater with the now rarely performed classical incision, it is much less with the low-transverse or bikini cut—0.25 to 0.5 percent. Even if rupture of a low-transverse scar occurs, it rarely happens before labor begins and it is unlikely to be catastrophic. It may even go unnoticed, since the rupture is usually incomplete.

Today many women are aware of the possibility of vaginal birth following a cesarean, thanks to the work of Nancy Wainer Cohen, who coined the term *VBAC* (vaginal birth after cesarean). The mother of three, Cohen has experienced two VBACs, one a homebirth, and has counseled thousands of women on how to have a normal delivery after a cesarean. She has written, with Lois Estner, *The Silent Knife—Cesarean Prevention and Vaginal Birth After Cesarean,* a book stating a convincing case for the safety and correctness of VBAC.

Working with women who desire VBAC, Cohen anticipates that more than 90 percent of them can be successful in their goal. Although there are many factors outside one's control, she tries to instill a sense of spirituality and confidence in women, who frequently believe their bodies have failed them. In her book she says, ''We believe that most of the cesareans that are performed could and should be prevented. We believe that there is an attitude in our country on the part of most health professionals that birth is impossible without tools, tubes, chemicals, drugs and machines. In our country, we have come to believe that Doctors Deliver Babies, not that Women Give Birth. . . . Women come to their births believing that someone else will get their baby out for them, rather than trusting in themselves and their body's ability to open and actively birth their babies.''

In response to the great interest in VBAC, some doctors are now permitting a cesarean mother to undergo a trial of labor to determine if vaginal delivery is possible.

Cohen doesn't believe in this approach, because it can ''undermine a woman's confidence'' and because a VBAC candidate shouldn't be treated any differently from a normal woman in labor. Many doctors, however, would consider her attitude to be overly casual and would insist on the following criteria for a woman attempting a VBAC:

+ Electronic fetal monitoring
+ Frequent readings of maternal pulse and blood pressure
+ An anesthesiologist, operating room, and blood bank on hand
+ A single baby to be delivered (multiple births are thought to overly distend the uterus)
+ An intravenous in place

It is also important that the obstetrician be with his or her patient; this is not a labor that can be managed by phone from the office.

VBAC is one of the most exciting developments in childbirth in the past decade. Its implementation gives real hope to lowering the escalating cesarean rate while allowing many women who might never have had the chance the joyous experience of a natural birth. If a woman has had a cesarean done by a bikini incision, VBAC is a safe practice. Many doctors, however, are slow to change their ways, and for this reason you may have to search a bit before finding a doctor who believes in VBAC.

LABOR BEGINS

As you know from your first experience, labor can start anytime, anyplace. Although you are familiar with the sensation of a contraction, this knowledge doesn't necessarily give you the ability to know when you are in labor. Many second-time mothers often think they are merely having gas pains or normal backache and, just like the first time, have difficulty recognizing that labor has begun.

Your sense of the intensity of labor and how long to stay home will be guided by what happened during your first experience. Women who felt they should have waited at home longer the first time tend to delay, and that's fine. You should be prepared, however, to leave at the drop of a hat, because things can change abruptly during second labors. To determine when to leave for the hospital, you should use the standard of regular minute-long contractions, four to five minutes apart, guided by your instinctive feeling about the right time to get going.

For second-time mothers, anxiety about the onset of labor is generally not about the labor itself, but rather about the baby-sitting arrangements for the first child. We urge you to call the baby-sitter as soon as you have the slightest inkling you are in labor. (This obviously does not apply if your older child is accompanying you to a birthing center.) Even if you don't go to the hospital for hours, it will be a relief to have your backup on call, and it will permit you to concentrate on the contractions and rest in preparation for the birth. You shouldn't be a martyr and delay calling the sitter or your husband, because things can take off very quickly the second or third time.

AT THE HOSPITAL OR BIRTH CENTER

Once you get to the hospital, the admission process should be about the same as last time. The only difference is that your first examination may be done by your doctor, since he'll be at the hospital much sooner, in anticipation of a quicker birth. In general, everything should run more smoothly. Husbands tend to be better labor partners the second time around, since they're less intimidated by hospital procedures and by labor itself. The two of you have already worked successfully as a team, and your husband shouldn't have any nagging fears about passing out at a critical moment.

As we said before, labor is usually not less painful, it just goes faster, because the cervix is more responsive and less resistant. Women often do not need medication for a second labor because dilation progresses much more rapidly and because the pain does not seem as shocking as it did the first time. Also, there may be more motivation to avoid taking anything if there was a previous negative experience. For example, many women who filled out our questionnaire reported great disappointment with Demerol; it did little to reduce pain and lessened control and they said they would never take it again. Typically, pain relief is requested during transition, and even a well-motivated woman may feel she needs something at this time. In general, however, it's easier to avoid an anesthetic during transition the second time, because this phase consists of just a few contractions and lasts no more than ten to fifteen minutes.

You will spend much less time pushing. In fact, your doctor or midwife may even allow you to push lightly during transition. This is because if the head is still high and the cervix is pliable, this expulsive motion may ease the pain and bring the baby into proper place. If you plan on using a delivery room, you will probably not be permitted to push in the labor bed. As soon as you start to push, you will be transferred to the delivery room.

Doctors and midwives are also usually more relaxed in dealing with a woman who has given birth before because her body has proved it can do the job. Often a conservative doctor who does not generally favor birthing rooms will allow a second-time mother to deliver there since she is no longer considered an untried pelvis. There's also more latitude in that women who've previously given birth require less medication, thereby decreasing the risk of complications. The birthing room is always a good choice, but it is even better for a second delivery: You're generally more aware and more in control than you were the first time. The delivery is less of a procedure and more of an experience. Women commonly watch the births of their second children (remembering their glasses), and they are more conscious of their surroundings. A typical first-time attitude is, "Let's get this thing over with," while the second or third time, there's a greater tendency to savor and enjoy the delivery.

In a certain way, the second birth can be more exciting, because the sex of the baby has become more significant. Many couples with a boy long for a girl, and vice versa. If you get the sex you want, the birth is especially joyful. Scores of the people who filled out our questionnaires described the highlight of their second child's birth as seeing that it was the boy or girl they desired. If you don't get your choice, you may suffer a sense of disappointment and will have to adjust your expectations, but usually this isn't difficult. A healthy baby offers great consolation, and soon becomes exactly the baby you wanted.

POSTPARTUM

Although labor and delivery are normally easier the second time around, the immediate postpartum period isn't always. There are likely to be more difficulties with the delivery of the placenta, along with an increased risk of developing high blood pressure. This is because the uterus may be a bit stretched out and less able to contract efficiently, expelling the placenta. Women who have had several children are at more serious risk for placental problems. You are much less likely to require an episiotomy, however, and if one is performed, it will be done along the line of the old one. (Your doctor may use this opportunity to repair the scar of the original one if it was sewn improperly.)

After the birth of a second baby, your uterus is quite stretched out and has to work hard to return to its normal state. Afterbirth pains are apt to be much stronger than the first time. In fact, they may be severe enough to require medication for a day or so following delivery. Some good news is that your milk will come in much sooner, approximately twenty-four to thirty-six hours after birth as compared with forty-eight hours the first time, and breast-feeding is easier to initiate and enjoy when you've had prior experience.

In general, the postpartum period in the hospital should be more relaxed and pleasurable the second time around. Some women actually look forward to their hospital stay; it affords them a break from chores and an opportunity to focus exclusively on the baby. Once you're home, it's a different story: You'll be meeting the demands of two or more children, and you will probably be more tired than you were following the birth of your first child.

This postpartum experience will be radically different, however, in your ability to enjoy your newborn. It's a rare second-time mother who checks her baby's breathing every ten minutes or calls the pediatrician to report a case of hiccoughs. This child will be a pleasure because you

♦

"I was able to enjoy this baby more because we were so relaxed the second time around and maintained a good sense of humor."

♦

"My four-year-old was full of questions and observations. Many times the three of us would get into the bathtub and share feelings of happiness and frustration that a new member brings to the family. It created a basis for many discussions we've had since then."

♦

"It took us ten days or so to coordinate a four-and-a-half-year-old, a twenty-one-month-old in diapers, and the new one. Diapers, diapers, diapers!"

♦

"My two-year-old was constantly hitting the new baby and pinching and pushing him when I had my back turned."

♦

"I found that people help you more with your first baby. They figure that by the third time around, you don't need any help. Actually, you need it more, because there's more to do."

♦

"My sister-in-law came for one week with her son, who is my son's age. She was great, and it was nice for my son to have a playmate his age when I brought a new baby home, even if the house lost some quiet."

♦

"My two older children, ages four and six, constantly wanted to be holding, touching, playing with, and doing things for the baby. It was difficult making them

continued

see that he was a person in his own right, who needed at times the same kind of privacy and quiet they needed."

♦

"It was nice to have an infant again."

♦

"I was surprised at how intense my love for the new baby was, since I didn't feel that way about my first for months."

♦

"I had a hard time finding the chance to sleep. My two-year-old daughter took naps, but not when the baby was asleep. He woke up a lot at night, which made it worse. Everyone said my daughter would be jealous, but she wasn't. She had her own baby, and we nursed our babies together."

♦

"My three-year-old had trouble adjusting to her for about two months. He needed extra personal attention. We focused on the things he could do because he was a big boy. He loved her but was afraid at the same time."

know how to diaper him, you know that newborns twitch and grimace, and you know that despite your inexperience your baby will survive.

HOW TO PREPARE AN OLDER CHILD FOR THE BIRTH OF A SIBLING

One of the greatest differences between a first and second pregnancy is the shift of your emotional focus. The first time you are completely self-absorbed, noticing all the small and wondrous changes of your body. The second time you become less preoccupied with your own emotional state and more concerned about the feelings of your older child.

We know the inclusion of a new baby into the family is of great concern to any mother, whether it be her second or her seventh child. To gather some suggestions for this tempestuous time, we consulted Joan Solomon Weiss, the author of *Your Second Child.* Weiss has encountered this very situation—she has two sons—and she's written a practical book dealing with the decision and implications of adding to a family.

A new baby has great impact on any sibling, whether the spacing is thirteen months or ten years. Many parents expect older children to be better equipped to handle the adjustment, but often their hopes are dashed by rebellious or aggressive behavior. Any child, according to Weiss, needs to be prepared and given time to adapt to the new situation. It's not a matter of simply buying a few children's books about sibling rivalry; parents must actively involve themselves in the adjustment. To guide you in this effort, Weiss has outlined four positive approaches that lead to acceptance of a new baby, as well as four negative ones that can impair family integration.

Tactics That Encourage Acceptance of a Sibling

- ◆ Try to talk factually about the baby. It's unwise to paint a misleading picture of a rosy future with brother or sister, because the child will feel duped once the new baby comes home. You should talk about the crying and the feeding demands of a newborn. By speaking realistically to your child, you will afford him a chance to discuss his own fears about the new baby. Some people may accuse you of implanting negative thoughts, but that's not so, you're merely being realistic.

- ◆ It's very important to reassure your child that once the baby comes, you'll love your first child and respond to his needs as usual. To make this clear, give concrete examples, such as, "I will still read to you every night before bed," or "We will always eat breakfast together in the morning." Talk about how things will be different with a new baby, but always emphasize that your affection and care will remain constant.

- ◆ Make the baby's birth real by providing tangible symbols of the event to your child. You can point out newborns whenever you see them, or arrange to visit friends or neighbors with a new baby. You might drive past the hospital or birth center to show your child where the baby will be born. Setting up the baby's room or special area in the house will help your child prepare emotionally for the event.

+ A dress rehearsal with a borrowed infant can provide some insight into your child's future behavior with a sibling. This can best be accomplished by baby-sitting for a friend's baby, creating a situation in which you must be responsible for meeting the baby's needs. This staging may give your child a chance to express some feelings and concerns he might have.

Tactics That Discourage Adjustment to a Sibling

+ Don't push your first child ahead developmentally to make it easier for you to deal with the new baby. Every mother would like to have her first child weaned, toilet trained, and sleeping in a bed by the time the next baby is born, but that's not always possible. If you pressure the older child, he will feel it and then blame the baby. This resentment will be nourished when your older child sees the baby enjoying bottles he still desires or sleeping in the crib that he still considers his. It's best to follow the child's developmental clues and allow his maturation to continue at its own pace.

+ Don't shower your first child with treats and toys in the weeks before the baby arrives. Many parents believe that new playthings and special outings will cushion the jolt of adjustment, but that's a fallacy. He is likely to become suspicious about all the fuss and may believe that something terrible is about to happen.

+ Don't delay in telling your first child about your pregnancy. The more time he has to work out his feelings about the new baby, the easier the adjustment will be. There's a good chance your child may overhear a conversation about the pregnancy and not fully under-stand what is being said. He may then feel anxious because there's something mysterious in the air, or may just be confused.

The moment you tell the world about your pregnancy is a good time to explain things to your child. This can be done matter-of-factly, by saying something like, "You are going to have a baby brother or sister. Right now the baby is growing inside of me in my uterus. In October, Susan Jones, the midwife, will help deliver the baby."

+ Don't tell your first child that he'll be loved just as much or more than the new baby. This approach sets up a competition before the baby has even arrived and raises the possibility that the tables may turn someday. Comparisons are a divisive technique, and you shouldn't get into the habit of articulating them. Explain how you can love both children in the same way your child loves both parents. If the child asks how you'll feel after the new baby comes, you might say something like, "You'll both be very special to me, each in your own way."

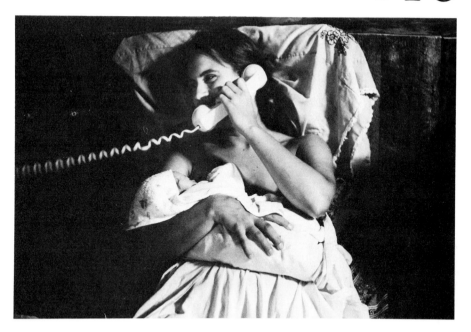

CHAPTER 16

Birth Reports

*A*lthough we think we've done a good job preparing you for labor and delivery, there's no substitute for hearing the accounts of real childbirth experiences. We can tell you second births are generally easier because they're shorter, but unless you've talked to several women who've had three-hour labors, you may remain unconvinced. For this reason, we've devoted an entire chapter to birth reports, the stories of thirty-seven labors and deliveries told by the men and women who became parents in the process.

Throughout this book we've tried to impress upon you that there is no average birth; each one is unique. The variety of the birth reports proves this. The reports were culled from the responses to our question-naire and from the experiences of friends and clients. We didn't have to seek diversity, it simply exists in the nature of birth.

This chapter is organized into seven sections: uncomplicated first births, births aided by Pitocin, forceps deliveries, a breech baby deliv-ered by cesarean, cesarean births, stillbirth, and second births. We in-cluded the account of a stillbirth because it's something many expectant couples dread, wondering how they would handle such tragedy. Discus-sion of stillbirth also helps acknowledge that there are some things beyond our control.

We feel these reports are eloquent, engaging, and very true to life. The stories are vividly told and express the profound joy of giving birth and becoming parents. This is a fitting last chapter, moving birth from the theoretical realm into the real world. We've wanted this book to be authoritative as well as very practical, and all the people who shared their experiences have made that possible. Their stories express the joy and excitement that is the miracle of giving birth.

UNCOMPLICATED FIRST BIRTHS

I felt my first contraction at 5:00 A.M. I thought it was false labor, took a shower, and put on my favorite maternity dress to wear to my baby shower at 3:00 P.M. By 11:00 A.M. the contractions were eight to ten minutes apart, and I figured I'd better let them know I wasn't going to make it to my party (though I said to myself, "This isn't bad, I could probably manage").

John was with me for most of the morning. He had an important business meeting at 1:00 P.M., and he left for a while. As soon as the door closed, the contractions got closer and more intense. I felt more fright-ened alone and felt it was so silly to have encouraged him to go. John called around 2:00 P.M. and he then made a mad dash home. It was so much easier with him there.

Sometime in the afternoon I started the early breathing. We hadn't gotten film for the camera, so John said, "Let's take a walk." So around 4:00 P.M. we took a fast stroll through Central Park, me panting at every bench. I'll always wonder how we managed that walk—I think contrac-tions were four to five minutes apart and pretty intense. But we kept remembering that our Lamaze instructor told us to be active.

By 6:00 P.M. I was good and scared and wasn't sure I could handle it; I was afraid it would go on for hours or days. The doctor reluctantly agreed to see us. He said all was going fine and predicted our baby would come around midnight. He said we could go home for a while or go to the hospital. Our class had given us this bias against hospitals so with the validation that labor was progressing, we opted for home.

We watched T.V.; I slept between contractions; lots of very painful and scary back labor. John was there—his voice really did keep me going. A couple of times I lost it, but John's voice and touch brought me back where I should be. John's telling me that I was doing well and that the contraction was almost over gave me strength. So we sat on the couch, would move to the bed . . . I remember more of the pain now as I write. When the baby comes, all memory of the pain fades. And that's what's magic about pain: when it's gone, there's no pain left.

By 9:00 P.M. there was water and blood everywhere, and I was terrified. I called the doctor, but he was out at a restaurant and said to call him in half an hour. At this point I realized I was being too good a patient. I was scared and I wanted the hospital. We called back and said we were on our way. We had the sweetest cab driver in the world, and at the hospital it was pleasant and I was upstairs fast.

The doctor was there and asked if we wanted the birthing room or the labor room. I felt I'd never get through this without medication, but I was too embarrassed to say that. The doctor asked again; I said, "Just choose—I need a place to lie down." So he directed us toward the birthing room.

I went to the bathroom, but the nurse wanted me back. I told her I needed to have a bowel movement; she said, "Don't push too hard or you'll have the baby in the toilet." (I still didn't realize how close to transition I was!) We settled in the most comfortable bed I've ever been in. John was there. I was breathing without thinking about it. I kept hearing the steadiness of John's voice, and it just kept me doing what I was supposed to do. When I started to lose it, my nurse just found my eyes and breathed with me. I followed her, and we were okay. No IV, no shave, no enema. Just a brief monitor.

Time to push. I kept remembering my Lamaze teacher saying to push the baby up and out, but I kept breathing out instead of holding my breath. I looked in the mirror and saw the difference when I breathed right. I watched our baby's head—I didn't push hard enough and it went back—harder push—more head, more hair—we're here!

We were all crying—our baby was wrapped up and placed on my belly. Tears—we were so happy. I forgot to ask if it was a boy or girl, and the doctor said "Look!" So I unwrapped our baby, with blood and cord and other stuff—a boy! We all relaxed, glowed. Later John cut the cord.

We all spent another one and a half hours in the birthing room (we'd gotten there at 9:20 P.M., and Daniel arrived at 10:40 P.M.!) Peaceful, quiet, it felt like just the three of us. The hospital people weren't intrusive. There was a phone there, so John didn't have to go anywhere to let people know, and I could talk, too. Our baby was here.

Now that Daniel is two and a half months old, I can't believe there was a time when he wasn't in our life. The most important thing about labor is it gives you your baby, no matter what kind of birth experience you have. But we were lucky—the process leading up to Daniel's arrival went smoothly, and we got to welcome him with all the joy that his being has come to give us.

On a Friday a week before I was due, I was at the doctor's office for a prenatal visit. The baby was supposed to be engaged already, but he thought he felt a head further up, so he sent me for a sonogram. I had the sonogram, and on Monday he told me the results—that I was going to have twins! There hadn't been any indication. I hadn't gained that much weight (twenty-three pounds), the pregnancy had progressed very normally, and I was taking exercise classes up to the very end. I honestly thought he was joking when he told me the results. He didn't think a cesarean would be necessary because both the heads were down, and one was already engaged. I was worried—I really didn't want to have a cesarean, and I hoped the babies would stay put.

In the morning of April 5 I started feeling pains, but I wasn't sure if it was real labor or false labor, so I went to see the doctor. I was one centimeter dilated, and he sent me home rather than spend the whole day in the hospital. By the end of the day I called again, but he said that even though it was probably labor, I'd be a lot more comfortable at home than in the hospital. He said to wait until the contractions were four or five minutes apart for an hour. A little after one in the morning I started bleeding a little, and I called the doctor once more. This time he said to go to the hospital, and by the time I arrived, I was five centimeters dilated. Then I was seven in an hour, and then the easy part stopped. After that, it was about an hour a centimeter. Even so, I didn't take any medication.

At 8:30 in the morning, Dr. K. left, and Dr. L. had to come on. Dr. K. was sorry to leave, since he really wanted to deliver the twins, but it was a good thing he left, because even after I was fully dilated, I pushed for four hours, finally delivering at 1:00 P.M.

I never did feel the urge to push. The doctor kept coming in, and the nurse would say, "It will be another hour or so." I fell fast asleep for the three or four minutes between contractions. I couldn't keep my eyes open. But I was glad they let me keep pushing. Apparently, the contractions weren't strong enough to make the pushing work, so toward the end they gave me a shot of Pitocin. That seemed to help a lot.

Once the first twin was out, I couldn't believe I still had to push some more. But it was only about three pushes, and he came right out. At that time, I had the urge to push. People say it's easier the second time around, and it was!

*F*rom 10:00 A.M. to 4:30 P.M., I was very comfortable. My doctor had me enter the hospital at noon, since I was dilating quickly. There weren't any labor rooms available, so I was put in the recovery room. I really think all of the activity and confusion helped divert my attention. I also had a brand-new labor nurse. She, too, was nervous and confused, but great!

From 4:30 to 5:30 P.M., one of my doctors was waiting for another to get to the hospital, so he spent this time with me and my husband. We played cards in between my breathing. The relaxation techniques helped a lot!

From 5:30 to 6:05 P.M., when I asked my doctor for some pain relief, he said I was ready to deliver. The pushing was *hard,* because the baby was ten pounds two ounces, and his shoulders were wider than his head. The doctor who had waited with us delivered my son, which I appreciated. It was a vaginal delivery with *no* medication!

*W*hen I found out I was pregnant, I had mixed emotions. I loved the idea of having a baby, but I had heard from my relatives how painful labor was going to be. My grandmother said, "That is the worst thing you'll ever have to go through. It's a pain that's the next thing to death." Boy, did that scare me. I had these thoughts for about six or seven months until my doctor explained the Lamaze method to me.

I thought that if my husband went to these classes with me and saw that other men were actually excited about witnessing the birth of their child, that he would become enthusiastic about it, too. He agreed to go, and we enrolled in the classes. During the first one, we got to know the other couples and found out that they had the same fears we did. It was really comforting to know that we were not the only ones experiencing these feelings. The classes really helped, and my husband did become excited—almost as excited as I was.

At 1:45 in the morning, two weeks after my due date, something woke me from what I thought was a deep sleep. I lay there waiting for it to come again, and it did, exactly five minutes later. The pain that had awakened me was somewhat like menstrual cramps, only harder. I got up and sat in the living room, timing myself. The pains were exactly five minutes apart. I woke my husband, and we sat anxiously waiting for the pains to become closer together or for my water to break. We finally decided to go to the hospital. We arrived there about 3:30 A.M. If I had it to do over, I probably would have waited about three or four more hours at home and relaxed.

I was taken to a prep room where I was weighed. My blood pressure was taken, I was given a pubic clip, given an enema, and asked what seemed like a thousand questions. Then I was taken to a labor room, where I was joined by my husband.

The pains became steadily harder, and I became more tired. I was glad I had brought socks, because my feet got cold. I was hooked up to an external fetal monitor, which made changing positions a bit awkward, but it was reassuring to know that my baby's heartbeat was being monitored as my pains became harder. A thought that kept going through my mind was that if I was experiencing these intense pains, what was my baby feeling?

My membranes hadn't ruptured by the time I had dilated six centimeters, so the doctor broke them. The pains became a lot harder after that. It was about this time that I felt an *incredible* urge to push. It was so intense that I had to cling to my husband's shirt. He suffered fingernail marks on his arms as a result of my clutching at him. But I will never forget that urge. To me, not pushing was the most difficult part of the entire process.

By the time I had dilated eight centimeters, I was begging the doctor to let me push. I knew that I had to wait until ten centimeters, but I was desperate. After what seemed like ages and hundreds of pains and a continuous urge to push, he told me to push, but very easy, and it was to be a short one. Even though it was a short one, it felt glorious. It was only a short time after this that I heard him telling a nurse, "She's ten, let's move her into the delivery room."

Finally! It was almost over! During the transition phase, I had become nauseated and vomited. I was still a bit queasy, but when I heard this, nothing else mattered except to be able to push and give birth.

In the delivery room, my spirits zoomed higher. In a short time, I would have my baby and be able to hold her (or him). After what seemed like a thousand pushes and a thousand breathing corrections, my baby was born. Did it ever feel fantastic! She's a girl. She was born at 11:04 A.M. and weighed eight pounds eleven ounces and was twenty-two inches long. She was so beautiful to my husband and me. Never had I seen so much emotion on my husband's face. Tears of joy were streaming down his face, and he said, "I wouldn't have missed this for the world."

She woke up about 1:30 in the morning and said, "I think something's coming. I'm going into the living room, but why don't you stay asleep?" Then I woke up at 5 A.M. and she was still out there, making a chart. Her contractions were about seven minutes apart. She ate a little toast and some orange juice, but that was about all.

Her water broke in the cab, and we were stuck on the Brooklyn Bridge. When we got to the hospital, they did a check and said to my wife, "You know, you are fully dilated and you're ready to go." And I had just finished unpacking all my little goodies!

The nurse was terrific, just supporting her in a very nice way when the doctor couldn't and I didn't know what position or breathing might be needed. Lamaze made it much easier. It was much less frightening to know what we were doing.

Lindsay found pushing difficult. The contractions weren't very strong, and they were four or five minutes apart, so the baby wasn't coming down fast enough. We went into the delivery room and did some more pushing and finally the doctor said, "Maybe I'd better give you a little Pitocin to get you more contractions or we'll be here all day." So that was it—it was amazing. We never got to pant-breathing. It was nine hours altogether.

*M*idnight: I woke with diarrhea and accompanying cramps. It was four days before my due date, but I assumed I was coming down with the flu. At 1:00 A.M. the diarrhea had long subsided, but the cramping had continued. A pattern had established itself for the last hour, and it dawned on me that this might be labor. We went to the hospital. At 2:00 A.M. I was examined and was six centimeters dilated. My contractions were two minutes apart, but I had to breathe through them. I still assumed I was in early labor and anticipated it would be *many* hours before birth.

Three A.M.: In labor room now. I was too involved with my labor to talk to anyone, and at times couldn't perceive what was being said around me. My contractions were coming rapidly and were severe. I assumed I was in active labor. After forty-five minutes I was surprised that I felt the urge to push and that the strong pain had subsided. The doctor was not available to examine me, and the nurse said if I felt like pushing, go ahead. I still thought I was in active labor and was totally confused at this instruction from the nurse. Minutes later, they wheeled me into the birthing room.

Four A.M.: Just got settled in birthing room. Was mentally prepared to be there *awhile*. Felt exhausted. Did not feel contractions, but nurse at monitor said I was having them and instructed me when to push. Soon the doctor said to start blowing. I thought she was crazy. I started blowing, but soon the urge to push became too powerful. I pushed, and the baby was born at 4:15 A.M.

*D*espite the fact that Kathleen and I had taken two sets of pregnancy classes, my first comment when she told me something was "leaking out" of her on Friday night, April 19, was *"Oh my God!"* Not panic, but more shock. This was around 6:30 P.M. I asked her if it was clear and odorless, she said yes—and we sort of knew that her water bag had broken and that *this was it.* Kathleen put off calling the doctor until around 7:30, giving us time to eat dinner (salad) and for her to pack her Lamaze bag, which she hadn't done yet despite the fact that our official due date was two days away. Actually, I think she put off calling the doctor until around 8:30, and meanwhile she said she felt some mild cramps, like she was getting her period. Over the course of an hour the cramps intensified into definite but mild contractions and they were coming fairly close together—maybe four minutes apart.

The doctor said we should come in and Kathleen should go on the monitor to see what was going on—so off we went. Arrived at around 9:15 P.M., went smoothly through admitting, she still feeling pretty good, though a little worried that contractions might cease. They didn't. Doc examined her, said she was only one centimeter dilated, that the water bag had in fact broken, that she had "a long night and a lot of work ahead of her," and that we should go home and, unless anything changed dramatically, stay home until nine next morning.

Back at home, the contractions soon began to come on a lot stronger and they seemed *very* close together—maybe three minutes. Kathleen was vomiting and trembling, and this got us a little scared. It seemed to be dramatic enough change for us, so, after calling doc, we were back at hospital by midnight or so. He was right, however, we did have a long night ahead. They made us walk up and down the halls and told us to check back with the nurses every half hour so Kathleen could go on monitor. So we hit the halls, Kathleen beginning to look pretty grim, vomiting intermittently (that damned salad), but doing her breathing and keeping it together. By 2:30 A.M. or 3:00 A.M. she really wanted to be in bed in labor room, and the nurses had no objection. At some point—I think when she first got in bed—she had some Demerol. Nothing much happened until around 7:00 A.M.—she lying propped up in bed, doing early labor breathing, not talking much, found good focal point on picture on wall; me coaching, watching the contractions and listening to heartbeat on monitor, drifted off to sleep for a minute or so. At 6:00 A.M. I went home to walk the dogs—back before 7:00. All this time Kathleen was not dilating much, and we thought we were in for long haul, but around 7:00 A.M. the doctor, much to our (and his, I think) surprise, said she was fully effaced and the dilation would begin to go more rapidly now. This was a real turning point, and from here on things started to go *very* fast. They put her on Pitocin around this time to hasten the process, and the contractions were pretty strong. But at each internal exam she was more dilated—two centimeters, then four, then at some point I remember them saying seven centimeters, and that was really thrilling. Kathleen had shifted into more shallow breathing, really grim now, concentrating fully. Around 10:15 or so she started saying with edge of desperation, "Get me some *help* now! I need help. I can't take this anymore," and I ran out and told nurses we needed help pronto. They sent in a resident, and Kathleen said, "I really feel like pushing." Resident did an internal—nine centimeters! The end was in sight. A really bright, bouncy nurse came in and said, "I'm going to teach you how to push." I went out to change to scrub suit. By the time I got back, Kathleen had been through two pushes and was really pushing with all her might. The next thing I knew, we were all in the delivery room under those bright lights and there was a little piece of the baby's head showing, about as wide as a paperback book. Nurse then announced, "On the next push, you're going to have your baby"—but I didn't believe it. How could this be possible when there was so little of the head showing? But she was right! Kathleen gave a mighty push, and little Emily Ann slid out in what seemed to me like one smooth motion. I was looking at her face, saying, "It's a boy! Look at him! Looks just like me!" when I heard the nurse saying, "You have a baby girl." Kathleen smiled for the first time in about twelve hours and said, "Hello there, baby" to her little (six pounds even) daughter on her stomach.

*M*y membranes ruptured at 5:20 A.M. As per instructions from my doctor and my Lamaze teacher, I drank four ounces of castor oil followed by a quart and a half of water at approximately 6:00 A.M. Contractions started about an hour later, about thirty seconds long and twelve to fifteen minutes apart. Contractions lengthened to about forty-five seconds long and three to four minutes apart at noon. It was apparent I had back labor. Dr. P. said to go to the hospital in about an hour and a half. Contractions were still three to four minutes apart as I started my Lamaze breathing in the cab to the hospital. Upon arrival at 1:30 P.M. the examination showed that I was 90 percent effaced, one centimeter dilated, and the baby was at 0 station. I started active-labor breathing at about this time.

By 3:30 P.M. I was five to six centimeters dilated, and the doctor was called. I continued using second-phase breathing throughout my labor. At about 4:30 Dr. P. said he had to turn the baby around. I was to start pushing. The baby was turned in about half an hour. I was instructed to go to the birthing room, and the baby was born at 5:41 P.M. No episiotomy was performed.

Problems arose when the doctor tried to remove all the afterbirth. The placenta had separated, and he had to manually remove the sections that remained. For this reason I was taken to the recovery room, and an IV of Pitocin was needed. But I felt fine and was sipping champagne later that evening. John Edward had arrived!

*B*egan at 7:00 A.M. Extreme excitement! I felt a tremendous need to get the nursery in order before we left. I was not at all anxious to go to the hospital.

At 7:45 P.M. we left for the hospital, and I was found to be six centimeters dilated, so this phase was not too long for me. Most of it was spent enduring shave and enema and getting somewhat adjusted to the imposing armamentarium. I tried to keep walking during this time. My son was lying posterior and either did not want or was not able to be born in that position, so transition was long, difficult, and trying. The doctors threatened forceps several times, but I violently refused. So, I suffered the nurse's exercises and prodding as she manually turned him (externally). He was finally born at 3:08 A.M. I felt extremely tired. I had back labor the whole time. I wondered if it would ever end—not because the pain was anywhere near unbearable, but being in a strange place and situation and surrounded by impersonal strangers, I longed for reality again.

I thought I was having false labor. My water bags broke at 4:30 A.M. and 5:00 A.M. My contractions didn't start until 8:30 A.M. and were five to twelve minutes apart. All I felt was cramps—light and then hard and felt better and more comfortable walking around the house. I was at the doctor's office around 9:30 and the hospital about 10:00 or 10:30. I felt fine, only light cramps. I wanted to walk, but the nurses asked me to stay in bed. Coming close to transition my "cramplike" feeling was harder. Not painful, just uncomfortable. I couldn't lie still and had trouble getting comfortable in bed.

The boys were six weeks early, and I was a little worried about complications. Having my husband there and knowing he was by my side, I knew I could get through any problems that might occur. Also, I seemed to block out the nurses and doctor! I mainly remember hearing my husband telling me or talking me through the different breathing techniques.

I was surprised how fast the birthing went, and relieved to finally get rid of the crampy feeling of my contractions. I went into the delivery room at noon, and my first son was born at 12:15, my second son nine minutes later.

I wasn't sure I was even in labor. I felt nauseated and crampy, like a period. It never even registered that I had had two days of diarrhea before the birth and that my "cramps" were actually the first phase of labor.

My water broke at 9:15 A.M. when I was at work. The contractions were strong, and I felt as if things were going a bit fast. I got to the doctor's office about 10:00 A.M., where, upon examination, he discovered that I had already dilated to seven centimeters.

I walked to the hospital, which was across the street from the doctor's office. I got up to the labor room and I pushed for about forty minutes. Then, when they were about to hook up the monitor and IV, the doctor came, examined me, and said there was no time for that, just get me to delivery. I used a table that was set at a forty-five-degree angle, which I was told was brand-new (didn't make me feel better, knowing I was the first to use it!), and after a few more pushes, a tear, and an episiotomy my son was born at 11:52 A.M. (just in time for lunch). I never went through transition in the sense that I got angry or mean, as I was warned could happen.

I was very excited when my wife went into labor. The first thing I did was take a shower, because I didn't know when I'd get the chance again. Then I began timing the contractions until they were five minutes apart. We gathered our things for the twenty-minute ride to the hospital in the rain.

I was excused from the labor room while she was prepped and given a gown for the delivery room, then returned to push on her back for back labor and to calm her down when she tensed against the contractions. We continued timing and watching for the baby to crown, which he soon did. Her waters were broken in this phase.

An overpowering urge to push hit her immediately after the waters were broken, and the next half hour was hard and fast. She was tired by now and begged me to get the doctor to give her something so she could sleep. I only pretended to look for him. We were soon given a healthy baby boy.

I had begun to think that my labor would never begin! Although I had been two centimeters dilated and partly effaced for two weeks, I was twelve days "late" when the baby actually appeared. When I woke up that Thursday morning with contractions about thirty seconds long every three minutes, I didn't want to jump to conclusions since I had been having contractions for two weeks. It was the bloody show that made me realize that this was finally it. I went back to sleep and told my husband when he awoke that I thought I was in labor. The contractions stopped after Peter called the office and told them he was staying home. So I vacuumed the entire apartment, trying to get them started again! It worked, but they were still irregular. Peter and I decided to take a walk around 1:30 or 2:00 P.M. The walking made the contractions stronger, and by the time we got to the restaurant, I had to start doing some of the breathing. I called the doctor, who said to wait until the contractions got to one minute long (they were about three to five minutes apart and thirty seconds long), and to call by 7:00 P.M. We never made it that long! When we got home from the restaurant, I lay down for a while and began to concentrate on the red spot Peter had put on the wall earlier so that I could practice. By 4:00 P.M. the contractions started getting stronger, and I was now doing the breathing pretty regularly. I tried to watch a movie with my husband but ended up turned the other way on the sofa.

We called my mother at 5:00 P.M. to tell her that she could finally make her plane reservations, but at that point I was finding it difficult to talk during my contractions. It was impossible when my father called about forty-five minutes later to say good luck, so we decided to call the doctor, who said to come to the office. We got there about 7:00. Peter shuffled me through the waiting room into a back office, where I lay on the sofa. I was having some problems by then, because I was hyperventilating, and my husband kept reminding me to slow down. The contractions were *very* intense by now. When the doctor examined me, I was already six centimeters dilated! He sent us directly to the hospital, but warned us it was very crowded.

That was an understatement! I ended up in the recovery room during most of my labor. (So much for the birthing room, but I could have cared less at that point.) Dr. Y examined me, broke my membranes, and hooked me up to a fetal monitor. I don't remember the contractions getting that much stronger, as I'd been told would happen. In fact, nothing really went as I thought it would. My contractions were still only about thirty to forty-five seconds long, but they were doing the trick, because an hour later I was told I could start pushing. Before I was allowed to push, I'd managed to throw up a couple of times, but I never got to the point where I was yelling at Peter or anything. I was scared at one point because both doctors were at the foot of the bed conferring about something, and I was convinced I was going to have a cesarean. I asked them, and they reassured me that everything was going great. I just had one small part of my cervix that wasn't fully dilated, and I would have to push the baby past that.

Everyone was so encouraging, and the doctor was so reassuring when I saw her sitting at the side of my bed. Peter and the labor nurse were fantastic. They were like a cheerleading team and kept telling me how well I was doing. I needed that, because I ended up pushing for one and a half hours, and that was hard work! Once I got the hang of pushing, I felt better, but it seemed that before I could get my breath after one contraction, another one would start. I would get about three and a half pushes out of each contraction. The nurse kept telling me how well I was pushing and that the baby would be there soon. At one point I began to wonder, although my time sense was distorted by then. I remember telling Peter that I wasn't sure how long I would be able to do this, but deep down inside I knew it would be over soon, and that I was going to get through without any medication.

Eventually I got taken to a labor room, but we only lasted there for about ten minutes when the nurse said I was ready for the delivery room. If I'd had any doubt about what it feels like to push, I certainly knew by then. It was an overwhelming sensation, and I knew it was doing some good because they could see the head, and the baby was not going to be bald! It really hurt, though, and I was getting tired. It helped to grunt when I pushed, and Peter grunted with me.

I was pleasantly surprised by the delivery room. The nurse said she liked to keep the lights low to make it romantic, and the only light was the one over the table and over the warmer for the baby. They asked me if I wanted to see everything in the mirror, but I didn't feel comfortable looking, so they moved it. After four or five pushes, the baby's head appeared (I could see it through my legs). My husband later told me that the cord was wrapped around the baby's neck. I guess that's why Dr. Y. told me to blow at that point. One more push and the baby squirted out, literally, at 10:00 P.M. It was a strange sensation. Peter said, "It's a girl. No, a boy. No, a girl!" We both started crying because we were so happy that she was okay.

They put her on my stomach briefly. She was very slippery, covered with blood and such. I felt delirious, but so happy to be holding my daughter. Then they took her to the warmer to do all the things they do and started beating on her to warm her up. That worried me. I asked Peter why they were beating up my baby! Everyone kept saying how beautiful she was. Meanwhile, I became overcome with the shakes, which were unbelievably strong. At least I'd read about them, but Peter later told me how scared he was. They covered me with surgical leg coverings, and then the doctor started to sew me up. I think that hurt most of all.

She'd had to do an episiotomy because I wasn't quite wide enough to get the baby out, and my daughter's head was not small. Peter held our daughter, and she was very quiet and alert. She didn't have any of the birthmarks I'd worried about, or a cone head. She was beautiful, and I remember I couldn't stop believing she was out! After a group picture, I was wheeled down the hall back to the recovery room. Everyone congratulated us as we went down the hall.

In the recovery room, we opened the champagne, and then Peter went to make some phone calls. My mother later told me that Peter told them we had a "pretty, pink little girl." He was gone quite a while and missed my first attempt at breast-feeding her. The doctor and nurse helped me —I was so nervous holding her and moving her around. It felt so funny, those little tugs at my breasts. She had no problem, though! It was a very exhilarating feeling to nurse her. When my husband came back, we both kept going over all the details. It's hard to believe you have just been through what you have been through, and you want to keep talking about it.

After a while they took the baby away, and Peter and I went to my room. We ran into Dr. Y on the way, and she said how happy she was. We all kissed and embraced, and I have never felt better about a doctor in my life. I am so happy that she was able to deliver the baby. In my room, Peter and I kept hugging and kissing. I think that night was the happiest night in my life, and I will never forget it. Nor have I ever felt closer to Peter. He was so wonderful throughout the entire experience, and I couldn't have done it without him. Despite all his initial fears about labor and fainting, he was so excited by the whole thing and was most supportive of me. But that had been true through my pregnancy, from all the backrubs to just washing my face with a cool washcloth during labor. I wish the intensity of those emotions you feel after all this could stay forever.

We did it, and it was glorious! I wouldn't have changed a thing. One funny anecdote: My husband, who'd become my nurse in the last few days before labor, had baked me a peach pie to cheer me up. This was Sunday night around 9:30 P.M. We'd had a real good dinner, and I was looking forward to pie à la mode. Well, I took one bite of the mouthwatering pie and went into labor! And knew I couldn't eat another mouthful! What a surprise!

Everything progressed at a fairly rapid pace, though I had expected those first contractions to last through the night and into the morning. But by 11:00 a loud pop (internal) was heard and waters broke. So we were off to the birthing center—a foggy, misty, quiet Sunday—on our way into the mystery of it all. Little did we understand that we would not walk back into that house as two individuals.

Everything was set up for us at the cottage—it was just like home, only not our home, and I was proceeding to get frequent and stronger contractions. Our midwife let Bob and me work on our own for the first two hours there, and I don't think we were doing the best kind of breathing. I was working too fast and getting tired. She came down from a nap around this time, and with my husband behind me massaging my back and just being supportive, I hooked on to her eyes, and we breathed together for the next few hours. She really was strong and steady and earthy and she got me through the rough time of transition. I don't think

I've ever breathed so low. And then I was fully dilated. It had taken about four hours. So she called the rest of the team, another nurse, the doctor, and my friend to come on over. And she said I could begin to push.

Well, I didn't feel like pushing. I had considered during our prenatal classes the idea of breathing the baby out, but I think it would have taken hours. So I began to push and just couldn't get down low and *out* enough in the beginning. But eventually she must have shifted down even more, and then I began to feel how to get there. I really needed to use my voice —low, guttural grunts and later scream-pushes. As it turned out, she emerged with her hand next to her ear, and so it *was* really harder than ordinary. And I did tear a little on the outside, despite the massaging the midwife was doing. And that final push—well, I do remember feeling so much burning that ambivalence swam over me. I didn't want to push anymore. But then she was there, and I was okay. My-goodnessing all over the place, and any exhaustion I had was quickly exchanged for an incredible adrenalin burst that lasted for three days—(very little sleep, just watching and marveling). And so everything went, as far as I can really feel, beautifully, and I wouldn't have changed or exchanged any of those feelings, pain or otherwise. It was the best.

We remained at the cottage until the following afternoon, me awake and high and Bob trying to get some rest. He couldn't sleep in the bed next to both of us, the energy was too charged. So he made a space on the floor and tried to rest that way.

And then we were going home. Everything was different—the air, the colors, and the smells! And we both said to each other, as we drove home on a hazy afternoon, that it sort of was like going to the store and getting a baby!

*A*t my wife's request, I read some material and talked to some people who had experienced home deliveries. We "helped" in one of the couples' deliveries, and after seeing this, I was motivated and convinced this was the best way to have children. I would have panicked at the childbirth if I had not prepared. I would have been worse than useless to my wife in a high-stress situation.

During early labor, I was shocked at my wife's joy and composure. She woke me at 7:00 and told me she was going to the grocery store and the baby would be born today. I went to school, came home, and she was fine. I was excited.

Later on, I watched her very closely, because the contractions were more intense. She started to slow down. I was getting more serious. She was glad I was there and she held my hand. I was there for her to "focus" on and I coached her.

The birth was beautiful—joyous—Laura did great. The midwife was cool. I was ecstatic. After the birth, Laura and the baby were in the bed after a warm bath, and we were so happy—that was a high point in my life.

During my pregnancy Dave and I would arrive at the center for my regular prenatal checkup. We'd get my chart and write down how things had been since the last visit. Then I'd weigh myself, get a urine sample, test it for sugar and protein, and fill in my chart. My husband would then take my blood pressure and record that. The midwife would come in and listen to the baby's heart and then spend at least thirty to forty-five minutes just talking. So that by delivery we really knew the midwives, and they really knew us. They could offer moral support. We trusted them, and trusting the care providers is very important.

Contractions started at twelve midnight. Contractions were five minutes apart, so we went to the birthing center. As it turned out, our daughter was born twelve hours after we got there. We got rather bored. I would use the word *monotonous* to describe it.

Because they monitored the baby by hand, I was able to be up and walking around, eating and drinking, taking a whirlpool, making Dave's lunch, etc. Once the contractions got stronger, I spent quite a bit of time in a rocking chair, which, I found, provided me movement without me going anywhere. Right before transition started, I moved over to the bed and sat on the edge until the contractions got too strong, which is when I lay down.

My water was finally broken by the midwife as the head presented, and after just eighteen minutes of pushing, Laura was born. Once she was out (5:12 P.M.), they placed her on my stomach and put warmed blankets on top. Dave then got to cut the cord while she nursed. She had had the cord once around the neck, so she was rather blue, but a little oxygen and she pinked right up. Dave then took Laura and weighed her on a dresser right in the room. Then she came back to me for another suck while they stitched me up. When the baby was three hours old, she got her more complete physical with erythromycin ointment in her eyes, etc. All done on the bed next to me. Then the three of us slept in the same bed that I'd delivered in. Actually, the baby slept while we marveled over how amazing she was—how God could get all the pieces together so perfectly. Seven-thirty the next morning we left the center and came home.

I think labor is potentially a very violent experience in terms of pain. No matter how much you welcome the contraction or think of the pain as warmth, you can't make the pain stop, you can only try to get on top of it in some way. It just keeps coming, and it gets bigger and worse and more intense.

What helps is to keep thinking it's temporary. I kept thinking to myself, this will be over today, and something wonderful is going to come from it. I felt spiritually that I was joining a sorority of women throughout the world who have been through this, and that was really a nice feeling. I used that to help me a lot.

I'm the kind of person who likes to be in control, so when I talk about being out of control, it's a big thing for me. So it was nice to know that I had some techniques to have a handle and have a direction. Knowing the options, and yet I didn't choose a lot of them—I could have them if I wanted them.

A week before I gave birth my closest girlfriend and I had lunch. She's never had a child, but we were talking about it, and she said that everyone she knows had an epidural. Well, that registered in my mind as a challenge! And I used that. And my doctor—he has a real way of challenging me—he'd say, "Oh, Lynn, I can see you're not very athletic." Well, he knows very well that I work out all the time. So, of course, it helped me push harder. I felt I was in touch with who I was and what worked for me.

I went in with a very open mind about medication. That there are things that can help me if I'm in too much pain for me. And I left it feeling that I would say to any woman, "Whatever you need to do, do it." Don't be a heroine and don't try to prove anything. Do what you need to do for yourself and be proud of going through it any way you do. I would never say to anyone, "Try to do it without anything," because everybody's an individual. It wouldn't have been the same experience without Dr. D. But I knew that when I went in. I was very careful about picking him years ago with the idea in mind that I might have a child someday. The doctor can be very helpful—and should be!

I've said to people who have visited me that Lamaze, taught in the right way, can make a big difference. The way it was taught to me, insisting that the conditioning be done, was great. I knew what was going to happen, and it happened. I knew exactly what was going on.

*T*he baby was two weeks overdue, so I was impatient for my labor to begin. Even so, I was surprised at how strong the actual contractions felt—I had been definitely overconfident beforehand!

I had about five hours of contractions, which stopped early on Sunday morning; this was very disappointing. Mark and I took a long—slow!—walk on Sunday afternoon to take our minds off it, and the pains began again at around 4:00 P.M. By 6:00 P.M. they were coming fairly regularly, every twenty minutes or so. Still, it wasn't until halfway through the night that I was convinced that this was true labor.

At around 1:00 A.M. the contractions were five minutes apart, so Mark phoned our midwife as instructed—and she said, "Wait two more hours, or until they are three minutes apart." This was frustrating to me (I had expected to be called right in to the hospital), and so the contractions slowed to about eight minutes apart.

The midwife also suggested that I have a bowl of cereal to give me more strength. She said this would slow down the contractions so that I could sleep in between, besides giving me more blood sugar. This was again frustrating advice, because I really wanted to get it all over with —but I ate cereal anyway.

I found that the Lamaze breathing helped tremendously, although I think I may have departed from the use of varied breathing techniques. I was so surprised by the intensity of the pains that I found using the slightly accelerated breaths, all through just nose or mouth, worked best. We also discovered that if I squeezed Mark's hand hard during contractions, it helped us both—me with the pain, and he was glad to be able to share it a bit. He also counted out every fifteen-second mark for me

—I missed this during the few contractions through which I allowed him to doze off! I dozed continually in between.

By 3:30 A.M. the contractions were back on track, so Mark phoned again, and we were reminded that I should be drinking juice (not water, which has no nutrition), so he ran out for some. Thank goodness for New York City hours!

Only in retrospect do I realize which stage of labor I was in at what point. I was in active labor when Mark phoned in again at 7:00 A.M. As he spoke to Suzanne, the midwife, I suddenly felt a new sensation: "Tell her I feel like *pushing*!" I said, and when he did, she said "Okay, I'll see you at the hospital."

I thought I might have the baby in the cab: I spent the whole ride breathing the fast, shallow breath with one hand squeezing Mark's and the other over my face, as instructed. I never felt I was hyperventilating, so I think I was doing it right. The cab driver was terrific (his wife was seven months pregnant), so we gave him a huge tip.

The elevator in the hospital took forever. Our midwife arrived a half hour or so after us and was with us until the end in the birthing room. I was eight to nine centimeters dilated when I arrived, and she suggested breaking my membranes to speed dilation a bit. By 9:45 I was fully dilated—finally! I found transition the most difficult stage to control, partly because one nurse told me to stop panting and breathe long, controlled breaths, which confused me—but also because my body really wanted to take over by then.

It was a relief to push, but I pushed for a good hour on my left side, and then in a sitting position without a lot of progress—even though Sue said I was pushing like a pro. She suggested I sit on the toilet—which worked very well, and quickly! Then, when I went back to the bed, she suggested pushing in a kneeling position. After two hours of pushing, Anastatia came out, and we realized why it had taken so long. She was nine pounds three and one-half ounces, two pounds bigger than expected.

We are convinced that Suzanne did a superb job delivering Anastatia —who didn't do so badly herself: her Apgar was 9/10!

I had been effaced to 70 percent and dilated to three centimeters for three weeks. My water broke, and this started the labor. I was overjoyed at the fact that I was finally going to have this baby. I was two weeks overdue. When I reached the hospital, contractions were five minutes apart and not very intense. I was coaxed to walk the halls (five hours) and try nipple stimulation. I was given a shot of Demerol for my back labor, but it didn't help.

My labor picked up after about ten hours. I was given an enema and an IV. I was allowed to take a shower to help with my extreme back labor. My spirits were decreasing. My doctor said he'd see me in a couple hours and had to yell at me to make sure I comprehended. When transition happened, it was as if my cervix popped. My nurse had left for supper and said that she would check me when she came back. The fill-in nurse refused to check me when I told her I needed to push, because, she said, it was too early yet. My coach insisted that she check me, and when she did, all she could say was, "There's no cervix." My nurse was called, and my doctor was called forty-five minutes after he said he'd see me in a couple of hours.

My world had opened up, and my social distance had expanded. I told my coach to quit yelling in my face because I could talk now. Two pushes, and my baby crowned. They took me to delivery, and I was told to quit pushing because the doctor wasn't there. After two contractions he arrived. He gave me an episiotomy, and two pushes later my baby was born. I was ecstatic. It was a miracle. The biggest highlight was when I gave that last push and felt her tiny little body leave mine. It was an indescribable experience and feeling.

BIRTHS AIDED BY PITOCIN

*M*y water broke at 7:00 A.M. on December 9, with no contractions. At 5:00 A.M. on December 10, I had a few contractions on my own. They were bearable and regular. I was bored and anxious awaiting the inevitable and relieved when they began. I was allowed a hot shower before they put the Pitocin in, and I could have stayed in there forever and delivered. I almost did! I kept thinking, "This isn't too bad."

Because I had a Pitocin-stimulated delivery, the active, middle, and end phases blurred into one stage. Things go very quickly. . . . I went to second-stage breathing *(a-he)* within ten minutes after the Pitocin was injected. I coped, but I thought at the time, I was going to die. I kept thinking, "He did this to me" and "Who would do this a second time?" I really wanted drugs, even asking my husband to go into the streets if he had to!

Transition was the "good girl" stage. If you're a good girl, during the worst part, you get to push. I kept thinking about the end, which you're not supposed to do, during the most painful part. All the descriptions and expectations cannot fully prepare you for the monster of transition. During the worst part, my friend said to me, "This is nothing, wait till the kid hits adolescence." Somehow the pain wasn't too bad.

Well, right on my due date the water broke. There was meconium in the fluid, so I went right to the hospital, arriving around noon. The doctor said she could see my belly contracting, but I wasn't feeling any contractions. I got an enema and I walked some, but four hours later I still wasn't in labor, so around 3:30 or 4:00 they plugged me in to the Pitocin. I went into labor immediately and had a real hard, fast, three-and-a-half-hour labor.

Once they hooked me up, contractions started about two and a half minutes apart and about a minute and a half long. It was almost like going right into transition. I kept saying, "This is intolerable," and the doctor kept saying, "This baby is going to be born any minute." By the time I was really in agony, I was six centimeters dilated.

One of the things that really pushed me over the edge was when the baby's heartbeat dropped and they took me off the Pitocin for a while. I had the experience of what regular labor feels like. The contractions were identical, but the thirty-second rests in between were really relaxing. When I was on the Pitocin, there were no rests, and I realized that the labor never stopped. There never was a thirty-second gap—it was always a lesser or a greater contraction. Off the Pitocin, for thirty seconds I wasn't in labor, and that's all I needed. So I started screaming, "Turn the machine off. Can't you give me a minute between contractions? You're in control, stop it!" When you are induced, there is a feeling that you are not in control—that it's not your body doing it. I felt like I was having surgery more than having a baby.

My husband was there the whole time, coaching and breathing and hyperventilating. I made him breathe with me for every contraction. There's absolutely no way I could have made it without the breathing.

I don't think if I hadn't taken the course I would have breathed—I don't think it's a natural thing to do. I felt like it took a tremendous amount of concentration and willpower not to scream in pain and to do other things. The last thing you want to do is ignore the pain. It almost made me angry that I had to work so hard. I kept saying, "I don't want to do this," but if you do give in to the pain, it just gets worse.

My husband breathed with me, stroked my forehead, and kept me calm. He kept saying things like, "You're doing fine, everything's all right," and I kept saying, "I can't go through ten hours of this!" He'd tell me to forget about that and to just work on the next contraction. He held my hand, kept me breathing, and kept me focused on what I was supposed to do. I focused on his eyes and watched his face.

There wasn't a sense of labor progressing. It was almost the same all the way through. When the doctor said to push, I didn't feel like this was the end. Pushing hurt until I got into it. There was something about initiating pushing at the beginning of the contractions that was like self-inflicted pain. But then the second or third push in the contraction wouldn't hurt, and I could push. Pushing took about twenty minutes. Because of the meconium, I couldn't hold the baby immediately. They took him over to the side and aspirated him really carefully to make sure he hadn't swallowed any of it. They took him away for a while, but they brought him back to the recovery room, and we had him for about half an hour.

I hardly slept at all that night. I was really stunned! I had been so scared about the meconium and scared of the induction. It's so amazing that it all worked out okay. I never thought I'd have a three-and-a-half-hour labor. Everything I wanted to avoid I got—an internal fetal monitor, an induced labor, stirrups—but I think I made exactly the right choices. I'm really glad I didn't go to a maternity center, because I would have been assigned to a doctor I didn't really know. I had as much control as I possibly could.

FORCEPS DELIVERIES

I was unprepared. My wife went into labor a week early, and I didn't have any champagne or film for the camera. We had thought that we'd have a week to clean up all the loose ends, so when contractions started, I was surprised. Also, I was afraid of overreacting to early labor. I didn't want to rush off to the hospital and find out we had eighteen hours to go, so I was skeptical at first. About 2:30 in the morning I called the doctor and told him the contractions were about three minutes apart and pretty substantial, and he said, "Well, that means you waited too long"—but that's how they started out!

I was very nervous driving to the hospital. I had had these thoughts that there'd be three million tankers going into the Lincoln Tunnel and then crosstown traffic, but none of that materialized. I made incredible time and even found a legal parking space.

Early on, she was walking all over the hospital. She was missing a button of the hospital gown, so she was flapping in the breeze, walking all around—it was hysterical. Later, she wanted some Demerol. I was holding out, trying to encourage her to hold out, but then she said, "I just can't keep doing this, I can't keep going on like this," and she was hyperventilating. It made me feel really helpless, that as the coach, I couldn't control the situation—like I was losing my grip, too. But the Demerol really worked wonders. It enabled her to relax in between the contractions. She slowed her breathing, and a couple of times she dozed between contractions.

It was difficult to judge Anna's mood, difficult to know how firm to be and how much to let her have her own head. Even after she had had the Demerol she was restless and couldn't find a comfortable position. She wanted to walk around, and yet she was out of it. I didn't think she should be walking around in this condition, but she really wanted to, so I'd traipse along behind her, just in case she collapsed.

Time moves incredibly slowly and yet incredibly fast. Those fifteen-second intervals seemed to take forever sometimes, and then when she was having particularly bad contractions, the clock just crawled. But then, when you think back on it, it seemed like time had gone so quickly in the end. It's almost like being in a car accident, where everything happens in slow motion.

There were times she said, "Okay, that's it, it's time to leave, and I don't want to do this anymore." You just have to ride it out, you have to be cool, you've got to walk that fine line. It was difficult to know when to be firm, especially at the end. She was about two centimeters away from crowning, and you could see, when she would push, her vagina would bulge and kind of open like a flower, and you could see the head there. On the initial push there was progress, but then everything would sort of slip back, and she'd be right back where she started. After about an hour and twenty minutes she was really running out of gas and wanted to quit. So I said, "Listen, just give it another twenty minutes, just take it to 11:30, and then let's see where you are." Dr. D. had already told her she didn't have to keep doing this if it was too frustrating, so we went for another ten minutes, and she said, "I just can't do this anymore."

The idea of forceps and an episiotomy as an alternative to a cesarean seemed like a perfect middle ground. So at that point I said, "Let's go." The doctor was wonderful. I was surprised by the forceps. They are huge, and the pressure that is used is scary. His hands were shaking from the amount of pressure, but I had total confidence in him. I just knew that he knew what he was doing, that the forceps were going in the right place, and that it was the right thing to do. It was very comforting.

Looking back, there wasn't anything we would have changed. For what it was, I thought we did fine. It was like a bronco at a rodeo or something—there were a couple of falls, but she took them well. It's great being a father. You don't think about the larger things anymore, because you just gradually make your adjustments, and it becomes part of your routine. I took a week off and then went back to work. Now I just feel like I'm cheating at both ends. I'm not giving 100 percent either way, and it's a little bit of juggling. But it's working out. You just take it day by day.

My water broke Saturday night about midnight. We were totally unprepared—we had heard stories of so many women who were late, we thought we'd be late, too. We went back to bed, but then all of a sudden I started getting contractions every three minutes, lasting for about sixty seconds, and pretty intense. Jerry immediately called the doctor, who said, "I think you waited too long." And my husband told him, "But we didn't wait!"

I pulled on a pair of maternity pants with no underwear, and we jumped into the car. By the time we got to the hospital, they were soaked through, because every time I had a contraction, water would run down my leg. We parked the car, and on the way to the hospital, every two minutes I'd have to stop and fixate on a street sign. People would walk by and say, "Oh, my goodness, did you see that woman?"

We didn't have to go to admissions. When we walked in, a man started coming toward us, and I said, "I can't talk to you now," and we just went right up in the elevator to the labor floor. Dr. D. was already sitting at the nurse's station. In the labor room he said, "I know how this seems to you, but you're not as advanced as you think you are, and I don't think this will be as fast as you hope it will be." He was right. I really did think that with contractions every three minutes we'd be in and out in an hour. He examined me, and I was two centimeters dilated.

I couldn't find a comfortable position, so I took what I thought was the position of least resistance—sitting with the bed rolled almost completely up. About every fifteen minutes I would decide I needed to get out of bed, and I'd walk around the floor, the hospital gown flapping in the breeze. Everybody would look at me and say, "There she goes again." My personality had totally changed, and Jerry was calling me Mr. Hyde. I was so nasty to so many people, I can't believe it. The head resident still remembers when I threw him out of the room. It was like one long transition. I kept thinking, "These people all have their nerve —they have no idea what this is like!"

I felt like I was in classic transition. A few times I just wanted to get up and leave. I'd say to my husband, "I'm getting out of here, I'm just not going to put up with this anymore." And he'd say, "Honey, you can't just leave!" He'd tell me I was doing really well, and I'd say, "That's easy for you to say—you're not lying here!"

But I did the breathing religiously, and I would never have gotten through it if it hadn't been for the breathing. I used the slow chest breathing for a long time until I couldn't use anything but the short breaths. I don't know how anyone could do it without the breathing. Actually, I do know, because there was a woman down the hall screaming throughout her whole labor, which is exactly what I would have done. But the breathing really helps—it makes the time go by, it takes your mind off the pain, and it forces you, on some level, to calm down.

By this time I'd long lost track of the baby. Every two hours or so we'd hear a baby cry, because someone would have theirs, but I just didn't believe we'd ever get to the end of it. At around 4:00 A.M. the doctor said he didn't think I'd have the baby before noon, and I thought, "Noon! I'll never be able to make it to then—out of the question." I couldn't believe he could be right, and thought he was making a gross miscalculation; that by 6:00 he would say, "Oh, sorry, I was off by six hours." I just kept watching that clock in the labor room and thinking, "There will never be a baby."

God bless Demerol. It didn't help the pain at all, but in-between contractions I was really able to relax. The Demerol allowed me to sleep between contractions, which I never would have believed possible. I think it's the greatest stuff.

At ten in the morning, Dr. D. finally said I was ten centimeters. But it had no meaning, really. I thought, "Hooray! Now I can do what everyone says will make me feel better." But it was totally different than I had expected. It didn't feel good, and it was the worst part of the whole thing. Pushing is the one thing you can't practice. You can't do it in advance and think, "This is how it feels, this is how I'll handle it." I tried to squat, but I kept falling over because I was so exhausted. I fought them every step of the way. It was painful, and I kept saying, "I can't," and I lost control a couple of times. I'd be in the middle of pushing, and they'd want me to push again, and I'd stop. I pushed on and off for about an hour and a half.

Dr. D. came in and said, "I can't let you push indefinitely. You're frustrated, and I just want to tell you there are things I can do." I said, "What?" And he told me he could do an episiotomy and use forceps. Part of me said, I can't do that, and the other part of me said that's the most wonderful thing I've ever heard. I pushed for another five minutes, but then said, "I just can't push this baby out." And the doctor said, "Well, then, let's help him out."

We went into the delivery room, and I got a local for the episiotomy. I pushed, and Dr. D. tugged a couple of times, which was pretty intense, but then he got the head to a certain place and took the forceps out, and said, "Now look in the mirror." I looked, and for the first time I reacted to what was really happening, and I pushed him out that last step of the way. The baby was born at 11:38. All of a sudden, I noticed there was light in the delivery room and I couldn't believe it was daytime.

I was admitted around 3:30 on Tuesday afternoon and delivered at 1:00 on Wednesday afternoon. It was a long haul.

My water broke, and because I was three weeks late, and because I thought I'd had that leakage since Sunday (it all looked the same to me), the doctor said, "I think you should go in to the hospital right away. We're going to put you on Pitocin." I was started at two drops per minute and then went up to fourteen, and back down to twelve. I went up to five centimeters after a couple of hours, and barely to six by 8:00

the next morning. The contractions weren't bad—I used the slow breathing for a *very* long time.

The doctor was really concerned that it was taking so long, so I got an epidural. I must have relaxed, because I went to seven centimeters pretty quickly, and by 12:00 I was ten centimeters dilated.

The doctor tried everything. At one point he said C-section, and although I was upset, I thought, "If this doctor is saying that, then it's absolutely necessary, because that's the way he is." But he really hung in there. He was at the hospital the whole time I was, checking me and then waiting until I was fully dilated. He's a really good guy.

I had no feeling that I wanted to push, but I tried a few times in the labor room just to be able to figure out how to do it. In the delivery room the doctor said he'd have to use forceps, and I was able to push the baby out with the forceps. When they put him on my stomach, he almost crushed me, he was so big (ten pounds three ounces)!

During labor, I thought, Oh my god, they couldn't put one more thing in me, what with the Pitocin, the epidural, and the monitor, but the baby came out, and it was fine.

At 8:28 A.M. on Tuesday, November 6 (my due date), I had my first contraction. This being my first pregnancy, I was not positive that I was, in fact, in labor. The duration of each contraction was between forty and forty-five seconds, and they were coming approximately every six minutes. They persisted for about thirty minutes. Later that morning, I noticed the "bloody show." I called my doctor, and he told me to call him when the contractions resumed. The contractions resumed at 8:26 P.M. that evening; however, they were neither extreme nor consistent. They continued all evening. My doctor called me around 10:00 P.M. and told me to have a large glass of wine, and if the contractions continued, I was to call him back. I went to bed at around 10:30 P.M., but could not fall asleep. (My husband did; he was so sure I wasn't in labor—no one has a baby on their due date!) I woke up my husband around 1:30 A.M., and we continued to time the contractions and started the breathing technique. They were painful, coming at an average of five minutes apart and lasting about sixty seconds; however, some were as close as three minutes apart. We called the doctor at 3:00 A.M., and he instructed us to leave for the hospital.

We arrived at the hospital around 3:45 A.M. To my surprise, I was only three centimeters dilated (I assumed that I was almost ten centimeters already—I was in such pain). The doctor broke my water and discovered that meconium was present and immediately inserted an internal fetal monitor. The baby was in posterior position, giving me back labor and making the pain hard to tolerate; however, I could not have my medication until I reached five centimeters. My husband, who was standing by my side throughout the whole experience, was very comforting. He made sure that I stayed relaxed and remembered to breathe through contractions. We tried pressure and ice packs on my back, but the pain was too intense. At around 6:00 A.M. my contractions started coming further apart, directing the doctor to administer Pitocin to speed up the labor. We continued the breathing technique until I was able to receive Demerol at around 7:00 A.M. At about 8:00 A.M. he increased the dosage of Pitocin, and within the next hour I had fully dilated and the baby was in the birth canal. At this point, the fetal monitor indicated that the baby's heartbeat had dropped drastically.

I was then transferred to the delivery room, strapped to the table, and prepared for the birth. An episiotomy was done, because forceps were needed to turn the baby from its occiput posterior position. Once the baby was turned, I pushed a few times, and the head was out, and at 9:17 A.M. on Wednesday, November 7, our daughter was born.

A BREECH BABY DELIVERED BY CESAREAN

I had a terrific pregnancy right up to the eighth month, when my OB was doing a routine exam, gave an exasperated sigh, and said, "Damn! It's a breech. I'll have to do a cesarean. What a mess!" I knew what a breech was, but I didn't consider it a drastic problem and I didn't understand what was upsetting him—but I was fast getting the idea that I should be upset, too.

I walked out of the office totally depressed and confused. I felt totally uneducated about the problem. Even Dr. S. had said that it was a complicated issue, but that he had just received the most recent advice on breeches in the mail and it advocated X-ray pelvimetry or cesarean. But he, from the old school, would be willing to try a vaginal birth. Anything to avoid the section. I bought three books on avoiding C-sections and went home to read them. Each one had something on cesareans for breech, and the literature in general was saying one thing. *Don't have a cesarean unless you absolutely have to! it's risky for the mother! the baby might have respiratory problems!* The books also said that there were exercises to do that might turn the baby and that external version was an excellent technique for preventing a cesarean when indicated by a breech position. I set out to turn the baby.

I was able to get the name of Dr. C. at Saint Luke's Hospital in New York. I called Dr. C., who said that he would want to have a consultation with me before doing a version "to explain the risks" and see if I was a candidate for the procedure. My husband and I went in the next day to hear his incredibly sane explanation of breech position—cause and effect—and his thoughts on version. It came down to this: He wouldn't do it if he thought the baby would turn back, be harmed, or if the cause of the breech was the shape of my uterus. In order to make that judgment, he needed to do a sonogram. If the sonogram was okay, and if the baby was "feeling well" (good heart rate in response to stress), he would go ahead. He had never had a complication after something like three hundred versions. But he cautioned that a large percentage don't turn or turn back within days of version. We said we would be back for the sonogram the next day.

I went back to Dr. S. for a regular visit and told him that I was going to have a version. He did not appreciate my amateur research. He was on the defensive from this point on and went over his position, this time adding that breech babies are sometimes defective and that in some cases water on the brain causes the breech. He pointed out a book he had read (a novel) wherein the princess, upon learning that her baby was born breech, dashed its head against the rocks, knowing it would never be normal. This was the last straw. I decided to change doctors (with exactly four weeks to my due date!). I should add that Dr. S. and I were quite close as patient and doctor, and as a GYN he is excellent. But under the stress of finding out I might have a C-section, he was less than helpful and quite nervous. I'm not sure this was foreseeable, but I'd be more careful choosing an OB next time.

I went back to Dr. C. the next day, somehow believing Dr. S. and thinking that something was wrong with the baby. Dr. C. did the sonogram, said the baby was extremely healthy and, from all appearances, very normal. His emphasis on the *well* aspects of the baby was a great relief. But Dr. C. said that he would not perform a version. The uterus was normal, but he had the feeling that the baby was in a position it preferred, and his guess was that it would turn back. My RH-negative blood was also a factor, should a hemorrhage occur (the fetal blood would be more likely to mix with mine, possibly causing antibody formation). He showed me the placenta, which, because it was located in the upper-right-hand side of the uterus, formed a pillow for the baby's head and, apparently, was too comfortable for the fetus to give up. He said that the exercises would be good to continue and wished me luck, but recommended that I just go for a cesarean.

At this point I was spending two hours a day doing three different exercises to turn the baby. In the morning I did the ironing board (twenty minutes on the board, put at a forty-five-degree angle with head down) and twenty minutes with my feet and rear propped up on pillows and twenty minutes on my knees with my head down and rear in the air. I played music, thought good thoughts about babies getting born, and meditated on turning actions—somersaults, cartwheels, etc. Same thing each night. Nothing happened, although the baby moved a lot during these periods. Usually, if the exercises are going to work, they work right away, as long as there is plenty of amniotic fluid in the uterus. I knew from Dr. C. that I still had fluid there, but he had also said that this would rapidly diminish. Still, I had four weeks to go!

I now had to find a new doctor. Fortunately, I had called the woman whose breech baby had turned and found her very optimistic and talkative. She said that she had gone to Drs. B., P., and S., a group practice. She was delivered without an episiotomy and felt the practice was excellent. My husband, meanwhile, had asked his doctor and gotten a recommendation to the same group. We decided they must be good. I made an appointment.

This was the turning point in my breech problem. Up until now, I had not been able to get a straight answer about whether to try a vaginal delivery or not, whether X-ray pelvimetry was smart (some studies have shown it may cause childhood leukemia), whether a C-section was an acceptable alternative. Dr. P. began to explain the situation and then called in a partner to assist. First, she explained, there were excellent chances of the baby turning on its own right up until birth and even during labor. Second, she was interested in trying breech deliveries (vaginally) if four conditions were present: (a) the labor was booming; (b) X-ray pelvimetry was done and showed a good cephalo-pelvic proportion; (c) the breech was a frank breech; and (d) that the baby did not weigh over eight pounds. She discussed the risks of pelvimetry—it was dubious whether this was, in fact, a cause of leukemia; nonetheless, she would not want to have one done until the last minute, because things in the pelvic region change a lot during labor and any prelabor X ray would be inaccurate. It was worth having if I wanted a vaginal delivery. Dr. S. was more conservative. He said that if the patient were his wife, he would just go with a section, unless the labor were really booming. He added that it would be different if this were my second baby and I had a proven pelvis, but chances were that my labor would not boom. In the end, as he put it, what is our goal? Our goal is to have a healthy baby. Any risk, no matter how small, is too large a risk. And having a breech baby vaginally presents some risk. Much more risk than a section presents. They encouraged me to keep the exercises up, feeling that a turn was likely prior to birth.

The following week I went back. The baby had not turned and it was growing at a more rapid pace. Dr. B. said, "This is going to be a good-sized baby, about seven and a half pounds." I asked if I could go into labor even if I declined to have an X ray. They said that I could but that no doctor in New York would allow a vaginal delivery without one, so that if labor boomed, I would still have to have it. Then I asked what the chances really were of my having a vaginal birth. She pulled out a statistic that made up my mind for me: *Even with good position, booming labor, and good cephalo-pelvic proportion, my chances were still under 30 percent.* In other words, after all that trouble, I still stood a 70 percent chance of having a cesarean. I left that day thinking that now I knew enough and that my choice was to have a section, but to go into labor first, so that I could wait the longest possible time before giving up, just in case that baby decided to turn. I also felt it would be healthier for the baby to call its own shots and to have some of the preparation for life on the outside that is one of the benefits of labor.

I went into labor on August 7, at about 2:00 A.M.—very mild cramps. I wasn't even sure it was labor, so I just puttered around, watched some TV, and then tried to sleep. At 9:00 A.M. the contractions were coming every fifteen to twenty-five minutes. My husband went to work, and I decided to take care of some last-minute errands. I walked around the neighborhood for about two hours. By the time I got home, I was counting contractions every twelve minutes on the button and couldn't talk during the middle of one. My husband rushed home. I was starved and wanted to eat, but thought that since I had to have a section, I wasn't supposed to eat. I called my doctor. He asked a few questions and said, "Go straight to the hospital!" I suddenly panicked and said I didn't want to go yet and that actually it wasn't that bad. Dr. S. wasn't fooled by this! My husband spoke to him and learned that the best anesthetist was on duty until 5:00 P.M., so we really should come ahead. I asked for another hour to do last-minute things, and we left for the hospital.

When we got there, I was taken right in for a sonogram, to see if the baby had turned and to look at its general position. The doctor announced to the residents that I was an expert on breeches and should be informed of everything going on. The fetal monitor was put on—and it looked like my contractions were coming every five minutes now. I was only three centimeters dilated, though, and no waters had broken; the baby had not dropped. Not a booming labor. It was time for the epidural and time for the cesarean.

All of this was very easy to take. The epidural was interesting; the surgery was exciting, scary, not unlike a vaginal birth. My husband was there the whole time and gave me great support. I felt the tugs of the doctor trying to get the baby out, heard the doctor exclaim, "My god, the cord's wrapped around its neck four times!" and then suddenly the whoosh and the words, "It's a girl!" and the cry of my daughter. I saw her right away, a feisty little redhead, extremely alert, pink, and healthy. I burst into tears of happiness. I watched her on the warming table, getting cleaned off and worked on by the pediatrician.

I sent my husband over to hold the baby and comfort her, and this enabled me to relax. Afterwards I held the baby and breast-fed her. I had rooming-in. I felt good about the birth. My only complaint about the surgery was the freezing temperature in the operating room and, of course, the recovery days, which were quite painful. In fact, it was very painful and depressing, and I began to realize why women campaign so hard against the section. But I also thought, after all the scary literature that I had read, that the section is a valid procedure. In my case, the doctor said that I was very lucky. With the cord around her neck, my daughter would not have survived a version, not to mention a vaginal birth. One thing not covered by any book or doctor: How possible is it that doing the exercises to turn the baby caused the cord to get wrapped around the neck?

Lessons learned from this experience: The most important was that not having natural childbirth is not a disaster. With all the (good) emphasis on having natural childbirth, there has been too much emphasis on the horrors of cesarean, so that the pregnant woman feels trapped and inadequate when a section is indicated. This should not be so. At the same time, you have to be optimistic about breech presentation. Accept the likelihood of a section, but don't give up until the last minute. The vast majority of breeches turn, exercises do help, version is possible and safe when performed by a conservative, experienced doctor. As for vaginal delivery, I expect that even if I had met the conditions, I would have chosen a cesarean. Because the bottom line will always be minimizing risks to the baby. No birth is risk-free, but vaginal breech births are riskier and, in my case, might have been fatal. And one thing I read somewhere that really helped: If you choose the section, you are choosing the alternative that is most risky to you and the least risky to the baby —that's just a basic part of motherhood in human and nonhuman life. It comes down to instinct: You try to protect the young. It helps to rationalize like that. I don't know if I'd feel the same way about a section that was performed for other reasons, but for breeches, I can see why the current trend is toward cesarean birth.

CESAREAN BIRTHS

*A*t 4:00 A.M. I woke up with a start, urgently treaded toward the bathroom, where I passed the mucous plug, and said to myself, "This is it. There's no mistake about it, I'm in labor." When I got back to bed and could recognize a pattern to the contractions, and admitted to myself just how uncomfortable they were already becoming, any doubts I had, however remote, vanished. I can't describe just how excited I was. Ten long months of waiting and I was soon going to be able to meet that little person I had been nurturing, that person who already had a room, but no name; that person who already had a space in our lives and our hearts, but no face. I *couldn't wait* to meet *him/her.*

After laboring at home for about seventeen hours, the hospital nurse told us it seemed like time to come in. At the check, I was about two centimeters dilated. I could go home or stay—my choice. I chose to go home but stayed there (home) for about two hours and went back because I continued to have some unusual bleeding, which remains unexplained. I was admitted and remained in the birthing room for the next twenty-one hours of labor, during which time every possible method of stimulating the progress of my labor was tried. Even after ten hours of Pitocin, several hours of transitionlike contractions, I was "five, maybe six centimeters dilated." It is almost impossible to make this long story short. Nonetheless, after thirty-nine hours, we decided on a cesarean. During that hour of preparation for the surgery, my contractions resumed their pre-Pitocin, feeble level. I asked for, and got, the type of incision I wanted, but not without a little hassle from my doctor. We decided on a general, and my son was born about forty hours after I knew he was on his way.

How did I feel about all this? Briefly, like a failure. I had prepared for this event for so long and so well because I was determined to give my baby every possible advantage. I had asserted my control over every aspect of my pregnancy over which it was possible to assert my control. For ten months, I ate "by the book," exercised, avoided harmful substances, which wasn't always easy, and did whatever I could to give my developing baby the best possible environment in which to grow. Then, when it seemed to count the most, my body failed me and held me hostage by refusing to do what I wanted to do. I had prepared for a birth that was as free of medical intervention as possible and ended up getting nearly every kind that was available.

*T*hat morning I had really good contractions five minutes apart, and for a few hours they continued. Some were even three minutes apart, and then they went away. I had a high leak, so around noon I went to the hospital. A few hours later the contractions started on their own again, but then my water really broke, and there was meconium. But they weren't really concerned. I wasn't thrilled about it, but they were all pretty calm, so I stayed calm. When the doctor examined me, I wasn't dilated at all. My doctor wasn't there, his partner was. I had met her before and had liked her and had even hoped she'd be on, but she turned out to be really obnoxious. She'd come in and say, "Ah, doesn't look good! It doesn't look like she's going anywhere." She was very clinical about the whole thing.

They didn't start the Pitocin until about three in the morning. The thing about the Pitocin was that I'd be doing really well, and then I'd have a hypertonic contraction, lasting three or five minutes. Every time they'd increase the Pitocin, I'd have these contractions and they'd be so concerned with the baby's health they'd decrease it again. And when they decreased the Pitocin, the contractions would slow down. I wasn't having any contractions on my own at all.

Finally around eight, my doctor arrived. He has such a wonderful bedside manner. He came in and said, "Oh, the baby is doing so well! You have such a strong baby." He gave orders to up the Pitocin, and as long as the baby's heartbeat was good, they let me go on. My doctor said he had a meeting and that he would come back around twelve. They finally got the Pitocin regulated, and my contractions were finally forming a pattern. I kept wanting someone to go out to the board by the nurse's station to change the word *irregular* to *regular contractions.* I was really pleased. All night I had been walking around seeing *irregular contractions* on the chalk board. Contractions were around two or three minutes apart, and I had some back pressure, so I was feeling pretty good. My legs started to shake a little, so I thought, "This looks pretty good." My doctor came back around twelve and thought so, too, but I pleaded with him not to examine me yet, but to let me go longer, because I didn't want to be only three centimeters dilated. I wanted him to come back at two and say, "Okay, time to push!" He said okay and came back an hour later. Then he examined me, and there had been no progress.

At that point I fell apart. I was hysterical. Just thinking about it makes me want to cry. They turned off the Pitocin. But the doctor was very good and told me it was okay that I should feel that way. But at that point my water had been broken a long time, I was two weeks late, and there had been meconium staining. They decided to do a cesarean. They didn't want to give me an epidural, so they gave me a spinal. I hated the feeling. I knew I'd be numb, but I didn't expect to be paralyzed. I couldn't even move my toes. Not having any feeling was bizarre.

The worst part was that Lonnie couldn't be in the room with me. That was the worst part of the whole thing, since we had been through so much all along. Even though my doctor says next time I could deliver vaginally, I won't go to a hospital where they don't allow the husbands.

I couldn't believe how fast it was before the baby was out. But they showed me the baby for only a second, and then whisk, the child was gone. But it was so exciting for that second, "Oh, it's a boy!" They did give the baby to Lonnie, and they brought me the baby right away once I got to my room.

At first I felt really depressed about taking Lamaze classes, that I went through all that, but I think now that they're wonderful and that it really helped. Also, once I had rooming in, I felt much better about everything.

*A*lthough my wife experienced very little labor, once a C-section was decided upon, things started to move very rapidly. I could sense her tension and fears building and made an extra effort to appear calm and supportive. We both waited anxiously for news on whether or not I would be allowed to be present during the delivery. When she learned that I would be with her, she became much more relaxed (while I secretly was having a nervous breakdown). The highlight was the very moment I first saw my daughter. I had never before witnessed anything so beautiful, and the love I felt then for both her and my wife will be forever unsurpassed.

A STILLBIRTH

I was thirty-four years old and thrilled to be pregnant. It was a perfectly normal pregnancy, but I had had the amniocentesis done to ease my mind. The report came back that I had a healthy boy. I continued to work throughout my pregnancy. I felt fine, went to all my doctor appointments, watched my diet, and did everything you are supposed to do.

On February 2, my due date, I saw the doctor, and he said that everything was fine, that I hadn't started to dilate and not to worry, since many first babies are late. About three days later I returned for another visit, and then on February 8 I went into labor. My mucous plug came out, and I started having regular contractions. After about an hour and a half I called the doctor, and he suggested that I come to his office so he could check for any dilation. I remember the baby was moving and kicking and how excited we were.

I was with a group of doctors, and the senior member was the one who saw me at the office. He put a fetoscope on my belly to listen to the baby, handed it back to the nurse and asked for another pair, listened again, and asked for a third pair. After the third try he said to me, "I can't get a heartbeat. It doesn't mean the baby has died, but I want you to go right to the hospital. Two of the other doctors are already there and they will meet you. We'll see what's happened." At the hospital, a nurse was waiting for us and took my husband and me right up to the labor floor.

They put me in a labor room, and one of the other members of the group came in with a portable sonogram machine. He kept pressing very hard on my belly to see if the heart was moving. After a couple of minutes he turned to us and said, "I'm really sorry."

I was in a state of shock. Intelligently I knew that people lost babies, but I thought that once I was past the third month, I was home free, that I would never have a problem. The baby's room was all set up. I guess ignorance is bliss, but now I know why there's an old wives' tale not to get everything ready.

At that point my labor had stopped, since I was in such a state of panic. I was only one centimeter dilated, and the doctor said he would administer Pitocin and other drugs to make me "comfortable," and that they would deliver me as quickly and painlessly as possible. The doctor left us alone, and I don't know where I got the strength from, but I turned to my husband and said, "We have to make some phone calls." So they gave us a private room, and we called our families and a girlfriend of mine who happened to be a therapist and who had lost two children (genetic problems) herself. We also called a close friend of my husband's and gave him the whole list of all those wonderful people I was supposed to call from the hospital about the birth. In my mind I was hysterical, but outwardly I was very rational.

They started the Pitocin IV and gave me some Demerol. The contractions got really painful, so they gave me more Demerol, and I remember looking at my husband and saying, "I'm so dizzy." The next thing I remember is waking up in bed and having my husband and my friend there, along with two of the doctors from the group. My husband told me, "I was there for the delivery, I never left your side. He was eight and a half pounds and he was beautiful. There was nothing wrong with him."

The nurses told me I had to see the baby then or not at all. I don't know how long it had been since he had been born and I suppose they didn't have the facilities to keep him. But I was scared. I didn't know what I had given birth to. Even though they told me there was nothing wrong with the baby, I couldn't believe it. I thought that he had to have been a monster, that there was something drastically wrong with him, because he had died. They tried to hand the baby to me to hold, but because I felt so drugged (I was seeing double and triple), I was afraid I would drop him. The nurse came over and held the baby in front of me, I touched the baby's face, and then they took him away.

Once the baby was gone I started asking my husband about memories I had, and he kept saying, "I don't know how you know that." He told me that I had been in so much pain and was so agitated (I still don't know what I was doing—probably screaming), they gave me scopolamine. The result is that I had incredibly bad nightmares and pieces of my memory are missing that I still to this day can't put together. Personally, I would have preferred to have all the memory rather than just some.

I had an awful hospital experience. They wanted me done and out of the way and they didn't care whether I was rational or not. They forced us to decide whether we wanted to bury the baby or give him to them to dispose of, and whether we wanted an autopsy done. The only good thing was that my doctors arranged to have a cot brought in for my husband, since neither of us wanted to be alone, and sleeping pills for us both. At least it got us through the first night.

The nursing staff didn't know how to deal with me. The only one who talked to me was a nurse who had lost a child herself. That was helpful —to see someone who had lived through it, because I didn't know how I would. My doctor told me that stillbirths were very rare, that he hardly ever saw them, and that I shouldn't worry about having another child. He tried to be reassuring, but all he did was make me feel like a freak. I felt like I had failed myself and, even more, that I had failed my husband. I apologized to him a hundred times. And it broke his heart to hear me. To him it was a tragedy that happened to both of us, but I felt it was something that was wrong with me. I later found out that this doctor's first child had also been stillborn and he never told me. If only he had said to me, "This happened to me and my wife on our first child," I would have felt a lot better.

The hospital never took a picture of the baby, nor a footprint. I've since found out that this is a very important thing. I have the feeling the hospital dealt with the baby by pretending it never existed. But I learned that a picture is taken just before the autopsy, and my doctor found it for me. The slide isn't pretty, because the autopsy wasn't done for a few days and the baby hadn't been cleaned off. It's something no one else should see, but it's the only thing I have to prove to myself that the baby existed. Because I have no memory of seeing the baby, it's easy to start thinking that it never happened. My husband was at the birth and has a memory of what the baby looked like, so he doesn't like looking at that slide, but I do.

My husband and I decided that we would bury the child because to us, he lived. We also decided to name the child and to have an autopsy done because we wanted to know what had happened. But there were no answers. The doctors even said to me, "We hate to admit it because we are scientific people, but we can't come up with any reason. He was a perfectly healthy male child, and there was a normal cord and normal placenta." It was hard for us to accept that reply, and we had a number of doctors look at the report. We couldn't believe that there wasn't something someone could find and say, "Ah! There was this reason."

After many months and long-distance phone calls I located a support group, the National Council of Jewish Women (but it's nonsectarian). I received phone counseling first and then attended their six-week session. After the six weeks I felt so much better and had gotten so much moral support from the other women that I decided to become a counselor myself. I feel it is important to do some kind of volunteer work, and this is a way I can honor that child. If he hadn't come, I wouldn't be able to do this work. I went through their training program, and I am now doing phone counseling and co-leading groups.

My husband left the decision about having another child up to me, but I decided I wanted to try again. I knew if I didn't try to get pregnant right away, I'd never have the guts, so as soon as I got the doctor's okay, we tried. I conceived immediately. As it turned out, the due dates for both babies was the same—February 2, one year apart.

During the second pregnancy I treated myself like a princess. If I was careful the first time, I was ridiculous the second. I had a sonogram practically every month past the fifth month. I even had a cardiogram done of the baby just in case the first one had had a small heart defect that wasn't picked up. I wanted to make sure there wasn't something I was overlooking. The amniocentesis results were fine, and I was told it was a little girl. Now it doesn't matter, but at the time I was glad it was the opposite sex. If I had been repeating the pregnancy with the same sex child, it would have been too much the same. At least this way I felt my fate could be different.

I didn't want to go past my due date. I felt that if I went to February 3, this baby might die, too. As we got closer to the day and I wasn't softening or dilating, we started consulting with a number of doctors about whether we should try to induce labor. Then I called my Lamaze teacher, and she suggested I come to her for a visualization. I had been to the doctor on a Friday and was told the cervix was closed, and I went for the visualization on Saturday. When I went back to the doctors on Monday, they said the cervix had begun to change and then on Tuesday I lost the mucous plug and went into labor.

We all wanted the baby born as quickly as possible, so I went directly to the hospital. They broke my water and put both internal and external monitors on. This was fine with me—I was too scared to move, anyway.

They gave me Pitocin. I dilated very quickly, and they didn't make me push too long. The doctor used low forceps, but they made no marks; just a small lump I felt later.

After she was born, I was incredibly relieved that I had had a successful birth, that she was alive. I remember standing at the nursery window for the first time after I had delivered her and looking at Allison and all the other babies and thinking that every one of those babies is an absolute miracle. I used to take it so much for granted that everyone could have a baby who wanted one, but now I see birth as an absolute miracle. I think I'm a different mother than I would have been without the experience because I really cherish my daughter more. I probably tend to be a little overprotective, but I think that's just a by-product of feeling she's so special to us.

SECOND BIRTHS

*L*abor began about 10:00 P.M. with a stomachache and diarrhea. I went to bed and slept until 1:30 A.M. My mucous plug came out then. There were no regular contractions until I woke up. The contractions were finally about three minutes apart and getting strong, so we went to the hospital at 4:30 A.M. I was two to three centimeters when we got to the hospital. The contractions stopped for a while when we got there, so I walked the halls until they came back. They were strong, but I could still handle it. I did jogger's breathing, sat up in bed, and talked to my husband and the nurses. The pain was not bad. I was able to keep up with my breathing. It was like very, very bad menstrual cramps. It almost felt hot and burning.

Just before transition started, I went to the bathroom and had diarrhea again. I thought I was going to have the baby. When I got to the bed, the doctor broke my water since the bag was bulging. The contractions were very strong then, but I had an internal monitor so I knew when a contraction was coming.

I had had Demerol with my first labor, and it made me too tired—I could not do my breathing and wasn't alert. This time I didn't want it if I could help it. During transition at the end I wanted something, but my doctor told me to push instead. I felt better immediately!

I had wanted to use the birth chair, but someone else was using it. The delivery table was comfortable, because one end tilted so that I could somewhat sit up. I could feel my hips widening, and my bones all felt loose as the baby came out. I just stared at the mirror watching the baby's head come out. The doctor was very helpful, as were the nurses and my husband with encouraging words.

My doctor was excellent. My husband and I felt so relaxed and at home even in the delivery room. He and my husband didn't wear green gowns and masks. That made me more comfortable to see faces and smiles!

I felt like I was floating around. Everyone was so excited, and then we started talking about a movie we'd all seen on TV, which made me laugh. What a thing to talk about while you're waiting for the placenta to come out.

[The highlight] was when my son came sliding out of me—the pain was gone, and we started to cry and laugh at the same time.

*I*ntense "gas" pains, pains in back woke me at 3:00 A.M., approximately four to five minutes apart, lasting about a minute. Pains quickly became two to three minutes apart, lasting about one and a half minutes. Very intense back labor, very painful. This went on for hours. I kept busy walking, visiting neighbors, and more walking. Ten P.M. (that evening), nineteen hours of labor, I have become very tired and discouraged. Who says the second baby comes faster? We decide to go to the hospital to see how far dilated—the answer is seven centimeters —how discouraging—decide to check in. More walking, more pushing on my back, my brother takes a lot of pictures—12:00 A.M., 1:00 A.M., 2:00 A.M. Pains are becoming constant—no more curve—just a constant, horrendous pain.

Finally decide to get into bed—lying on my side—everyone takes turns pushing on my back—my husband holds my face, eye contact to help me concentrate. I begin to feel huge amount of pressure—we put the bean bag behind me—nurse comes in and announces the head has crowned—what a surprise! Doctor comes in just as the water breaks, sits down just as she starts to come out all the way—all of us start cheering, yelling, laughing, crying—who said we were tired? The end went so quickly.

The highlight was holding our daughter to nurse for the first time while my husband cut the umbilical cord and handing her to my mother and brother and seeing their faces after being included so actively in the whole birth.

*I*t was a Wednesday night that I was starting to feel kind of crampy, but I went to sleep. I thought I might be in labor, but I had had a couple of bouts of false labor and I had already dilated to four centimeters, so I wasn't sure if it was the real thing. I also started to get diarrhea that night, but I didn't know whether that was connected or not. In any event, I went to sleep from about eleven to one and then I woke up with continued crampiness, but nothing really more. I went back to sleep and woke up about 2:30 A.M. I decided to time what was going on and found that the contractions were coming every three minutes for forty-five seconds. I didn't have to use my breathing yet at that point.

I called the midwife, and she said it was hard for her to tell whether I really should come on in to the hospital. The concern was that since I had started out four centimeters and since I was a ways from the hospital, whether I should come in right away. But I told her I would give it a couple of hours to see whether the contractions got stronger, which is what I did.

By 5:30 I could feel there was a difference, so I called the midwife back and told her I was going to go in to the hospital and have them check me out. I called my mother, and she got here about 6:00. Then we woke Jakey, my first child, and told him. His reaction was, "Today?" Like he thought maybe it would be a year from now! We told him we were going to have the baby today and that my mother was there. He wanted to go in to our bed and that's what he did. I told him that visiting hours were at 3:00 and that he could come see me later in the day and that I would call him after the baby was born. He tried to be stoic, keeping himself from crying.

We got to the hospital around 6:30, and the midwife was there, which was a surprise—I didn't know she was going to be there. She introduced us to the nurse that she was working with and took us into a birthing room. I wasn't using my breathing yet, and even though the contractions were more painful, I could manage without. I was five to six centimeters dilated, which disappointed me because I felt like I had gotten so far with just the false labor, and these contractions seemed like so much more.

The midwife felt it would be a while. They hooked me up to to fetal monitor to get an idea of how the heartbeat was and to measure and time the contractions. Then she said I could walk around. I walked for a while, but I went back to the room and went to lie on the bed. At 7:30 I was about seven centimeters. At around 8:15 I sent my husband out for a minute because I needed him to make a phone call for me. When he got back, I really felt the urge to push. The nurse came in at that point, and I said to her, "You know, I'm bleeding, and I feel the urge to push." She said, Yes, I was bleeding but ignored the fact that I needed to push. So Andrew went to get the midwife, and when she examined me, I was ten centimeters dilated. She lowered the bottom part of the bed and told me I could start pushing. I was semisitting with my legs up toward me. She didn't even have time to put her gloves on, which she enjoyed a lot, being able to really feel the baby. And out came this little guy!

Teddy was having a little trouble breathing. He was very blue, so they gave him oxygen and aspirated him. But it was weird, because at that point you could have told me that the bomb was being dropped—I just couldn't connect or worry about anything being wrong. They took the baby out, but came back about ten minutes later to say that his temperature had dropped and that once they warmed him up, he was fine. It was nice that they came back right away to let me know. I was washed and taken to the recovery room for a while, and got our baby back once I got upstairs to my room around 9:30 or 10:00 in the morning.

*M*y first hospital birth had been extremely unsatisfactory, and I had not prepared for that birth. I felt that anything other than the drug-loaded first birth experience (Demerol, ?, lidocaine) was bound to be substantially better for both myself and my subsequent child/children.

Light contractions began at 5:00 and lasted until 3:00 P.M. When pains were still light and easy to control—unpredictable lapses between contractions, and sometimes small twinges, sometimes no pain at all associated with contractions.

Arrived at hospital, examined, and was told that I was five centimeters dilated, 50 percent effaced, bag of waters intact, however child's head was not engaged. Was told to walk around and come back for exam at 5:00 P.M., at which time I was admitted at still five centimeters dilated

75 percent effaced, baby's head at −3 station. Pains were there but very controllable with my breathing techniques—pain relief I declined. (There was) excitement, fear, expectations about the upcoming labor and delivery, having experienced it before. I felt very much in control of my contractions and breathing techniques during this whole time. I hated having to lie down in bed on my back and having first external monitors and then internal monitors hooked up to us.

At seven centimeters my bag of waters was ripped (under protest), and baby went from −3 to +3 immediately! Contractions came in waves with no more than thirty seconds between and the baby's heartbeat decelerated dangerously, so I was rolled on to my left side and put on oxygen for the remainder of transition in the labor room. This was the absolute worst of the whole birth experience, and I believe it was due to the manual breaking of my bag of waters by my obstetrician with his hook. I immediately lost control, as contractions came boom, boom, boom! Not only did I lose all control over breathing, but I refused to allow my husband away from my side (even to the other side of my bed!) I slapped my husband, pulled the doctor down to my face, and shouted that I had to push at eight centimeters (he was very gallant and gentle with me at this point, unlike the other OB resident on duty at the time). My head felt like it was swarming with a million bees, as did my arms, which were rigid and in the air, although I believed them to be relaxed and by my side. I had received no pain relief. As far as I know no pain relief will be given once transition has been reached in military hospitals —I think that this is a great policy.

Ten minutes before the birth the heart rate was good again, and I was taken off oxygen. Being able to push finally was terrific. I was given an episiotomy (lidocaine), and after five good pushes we heard her first cries. I was awake, aware, and overwhelmed with the total experience.

*E*ven though I was having true contractions, they were not regular. When we got to the hospital, the nurse didn't think I would be admitted, because my contractions were not regular (even though I knew they were true contractions). After she gave me an internal, I was dilated to four centimeters and effaced to 90 percent. I was admitted and taken to the birthing bed. Every time I had contractions, my husband helped me breathe, and in between them we joked and laughed. It was pretty easy. [Then the] contractions were harder and stronger. If I didn't have the Lamaze, I surely would not have been able to handle the pain.

I wouldn't dilate past nine, because my bag of waters was stopping it. I asked the nurse if she could call the doctor and ask him if he could break the bag because I was hungry and wanted to make it to my room for breakfast. He came, broke it, and with the next contraction I was ready to push. He was born six minutes later! I think the hardest part of labor and most painful is when one must blow out when you want to push.

Even though I was disappointed with him being a boy, I love it when they gave the baby to me to hold! I didn't want to give him back. I think holding him and actually seeing him come out are tied for being the highlight. I'd love to have a hundred more.

The Lamaze method really helped out a lot. No one could emphasize how important it is to take it seriously and really practice. I love my children and I love giving birth. Just the thought of it gets me excited. We are going to try for one more. The expenses can kill you, but the love they have inside them (no matter how much they fuss), and to watch them grow is so exciting. I wish I could have more! They are great, and so is the birth.

*A*fter making two false runs (and being admitted the second time) I wanted to make sure this was the real thing. It was—the contractions began to hurt a little. I was excited, happy, joking—couldn't wait to hold the baby. I wondered why I wanted a second baby!

The baby was in a breech position, that was known six weeks or more before delivery. I was "allowed" to deliver naturally as long as everything was going perfectly. Labor was going a little slower than the doctor liked, so there was concern that I might have to have a C-section. I was *bored*. They made me stay on the delivery table from the time my water was broken. I really didn't mind, I just wished I had a magazine or something. I was still cracking jokes and talking with the nurse. The pain really wasn't really bad until transition, when it became a steady ache with moments of extra pain. Until then it was just ninety-second stitches to be gotten through.

The doctor gave me a pudendal—all it numbed was the birth canal. I couldn't believe how my hips hurt! I just wanted the kid to be born. I felt worse for him than I did for myself! I also *seriously* considered telling everyone good-bye. The only thing that kept me on that delivery table was the fact that the nurse would've probably bonked me over the head. I just wanted to go home and go to bed. The only thing that helped me push was when the doctor said to push as if I were having a bowel movement. After she had said it three or four times, I thought, "Fine! She wants it, she's got it!" Boy, did I surprise myself!

*F*or the second birth, we took a VBAC class because we planned a vaginal birth after the first one, which was a C-section. I had read about VBAC classes and finally found one in a city thirty miles away. Our instructor was a young OB labor and delivery nurse who is at home now caring for a three-year-old and an eighteen-month-old, both of whom were born cesarean because they were breech. She was charismatic, informed, and planning herself to one day be a VBAC mom.

Early labor began Friday afternoon around 5:00 P.M., fifteen to twenty minutes apart. Like cramps. I walked and breathed deeply through the contractions. Didn't sleep well. On Sunday, early-evening contractions were five minutes apart. I was tired, and it was hot, and it was harder to walk through the contractions. I kneeled on stairs. Went to the hospital around 11:00 P.M.

I had back labor with both girls. With my first, I was on my back, hooked to a fetal monitor, and that slowed my labor. The second time, I kept moving, went to the hospital later, postponed insertion of internal fetal monitor (even though I was considered "high risk") and stayed on my hands and knees.

[My partner was a] confidence builder. My husband is the eternal optimist without being "rah-rah"! He was calm, supported my wishes, rubbed my back, argued with the doctor in charge of our "case" while I was in the labor room, took pictures of the birth while helping me push. I couldn't have done it alone.

Between 2:00 and 3:00 A.M. before the birth at 4:36 I "lost it." I was exhausted, had back labor, and screamed "no" through the contractions. I was on my hands and knees with my husband rubbing my back.

I got a beautiful, healthy, red-headed girl, and I "gave" birth to her; I got to hold her on my chest before she was cleaned off and see her take her first look at the world. A joy and a privilege. We delivered normally . . . against many odds. It was a great feeling.

Appendix:
The Birth
Questionnaire

Name:

Age:

Number of Children:

Note: If you have more than one child, please indicate which birth you are describing _____

_____

_____

Prepared Childbirth

1. What prepared childbirth method did you study?
   - _____ Lamaze   _____ Dick-Read
   - _____ Bradley   _____ other:

2. What was your purpose in studying prepared childbirth?

3. How did you select your prepared-childbirth course?
   - _____ Doctor/midwife referral
   - _____ Friend or relative recommended
   - _____ Other:

4. How did you feel about your chosen method of prepared childbirth (a) while taking the classes; and (b) after giving birth?

5. What were the strengths and weaknesses of your instructor?

Labor and Delivery

6. How long was your labor?
   - _____ One to five hours   _____ Twelve to eighteen hours
   - _____ Six to twelve hours   _____ hours

7. Can you briefly describe the course of your labor and your reaction to each phase?
    a. Early or beginning phase:
    b. Active or middle phase:
    c. Transition or end phase:

8. How painful, if at all, was your labor and can you describe it?

9. What helped you to cope with pain?
    _____ Breathing techniques
    _____ Maintaining a focal point
    _____ Walking
    _____ Vocalizing
    _____ Stroking abdomen
    _____ Music
    _____ Partner's support
    _____ Massage (where?)
    _____ Body position (which one?)
    _____ Specific images (visualization) (which ones?)
    _____ Other:

10. If you had back labor, can you describe it and how did you deal with it?

11. What was your attitude toward medication (a) prior to labor; and (b) now that you have given birth?

12. In what ways, if any, was your partner helpful during labor?

13. Can you describe pushing in one sentence?

14. Did techniques or specific images help you push?

15. Where did you give birth?
    _____ Delivery table   _____ Birth chair or stool
    _____ Labor bed   _____ Other:
    _____ Birthing bed

16. How did you feel about giving birth in this manner?

17. How did you feel about having any of the following procedures?
    _____ Enema:
    _____ Pubic shave:
    _____ External fetal monitor:

_____ Internal fetal monitor:

_____ Intravenous:

_____ Rupture of the membranes:

_____ Pitocin stimulation of labor:

_____ Pitocin induction of labor:

_____ Oxygen:

_____ Fetal-scalp sampling:

_____ Analgesia (Demerol, Valium, other):

_____ Anesthetic (epidural, pudendal, paracervical, spinal, caudal, nitrous oxide, general, other):

_____ Episiotomy:

_____ Forceps:

_____ C-section:

18. What in your Lamaze bag proved useful?

_____ Socks   _____ Heating pad or hot-water bottle

_____ Lollipop   _____ Cold pack

_____ Lip gloss   _____ Picture or object for focus

_____ Breath spray   _____ Other:

_____ Tennis balls

Doctor/Midwife

19. Who attended your birth?

_____ Obstetrician   _____ Lay midwife

_____ General practitioner   _____ Other:

_____ Nurse-midwife

20. How did you select this person?

_____ Your gynecologist

_____ Referred by gynecologist or family doctor

_____ Referred by friend or relative

_____ Other:

21. Did you discuss what you wanted from your birth experience with this person prior to labor and delivery? Yes_____ No_____

22. In what ways did you get what you wanted and in what ways were you disappointed?

Birthplace

23. Where did you give birth?
    _____ Hospital   _____ Home
    _____ Birth center (out of hospital)   _____ Other:
    a. Why did you choose this setting?
    b. Would you select this setting again? Yes_____ No_____Why?

Postpartum

24. Can you describe your feelings immediately following your baby's birth?

25. How long were you with your baby following birth?

26. Can you describe in one sentence your feelings during the first three months of your baby's life?
    a. What did you find most difficult during this period?
    b. What was most pleasurable?

27. What kind of household assistance did you have, if any, for the postpartum period? Was it helpful?

Summation

28. Can you describe one moment that was the highlight of your birth experience?

    Please feel free to add any further observations you may have about Lamaze or any aspect of your baby's birth.

Questionnaire for Partner or Support Person

1. Why did you study prepared childbirth?

2. Did you find the training helpful? Yes_____ No_____ Why?

3. What did you like or dislike about prepared-childbirth classes?

4. What fears did you have, if any, about childbirth before witnessing it?

5. Can you briefly describe the course of labor and your reaction to each phase?
    a. Early or beginning phase:
    b. Active or middle phase:
    c. Transition or end phase:

6. How do you think you helped your partner in labor?

7. Can you describe in one sentence the first three months of your baby's life?

8. Can you describe one moment that was the highlight of the birth experience?

Please feel free to include any additional comments about any aspect of the birth on the back of this sheet.

Sources

American Academy of Husband-Coached Childbirth (Bradley Method)
P.O. Box 5224
Sherman Oaks, California 91413
800-423-2397

American College of Nurse Midwives
1012 14th Street N. W. Suite 801
Washington, D.C. 20005
202-347-5447

ASPO/Lamaze
1840 Wilson Boulevard Suite 204
Arlington, Virginia 22201
703-524-7802

C/SEC, Inc.
22 Forrest Road
Framingham, Massachusetts 01701
617-877-8266

ICEA
International Childbirth Education Association
5636 W. Burleigh Street
Milwaukee, Wisconsin 53210
414-445-7470

La Leche League
9616 Minneapolis Avenue
Franklin Park, Illinois 60131
312-455-7730

NAPSAC
National Association for Parents and Professionals for Safe
Alternatives in Childbirth
P.O. Box 267
Marble Hill, Missouri 63764
314-238-2010

National Council of Jewish Women
9 East 69th Street
New York, New York 10021
212-535-2900

National Foundation/March of Dimes
1275 Mamaroneck Avenue
White Plains, New York 10605
914-428-7100

National Organization of Mothers of Twins Club
5402 Amberwood Lane
Rockville, Maryland 20853
301-460-9108

National Sudden Infant Death Syndrome Foundation
2 Metro Plaza, Suite 205
8240 Professional Place
Landover, Maryland 20785
301-459-3388

References

Chapter 1

Lamaze, Dr. Fernand, *Painless Childbirth: The Lamaze Method* (New York: Pocket Books, 1974), pp. 13, 14.

Feldman, Sylvia, *Choices in Childbirth* (New York: Grosset and Dunlap, 1978), p. 106.

Bradley, Dr. Robert, *Husband-Coached Childbirth* (New York: Harper & Row, 1980), p. 133.

Bradley, p. 148.

Chapter 3

Sagov, et al., *Home Birth: A Practitioner's Guide to Birth Outside the Hospital* (Rockville, Md.: Aspen Systems Corporation, 1984), p. xiii.

Mehl, Lewis, M.D., Ph. D., "Home Delivery Research Today: A Review," presented at the annual meeting of the American Foundation for Maternal and Infant Health, New York City, November 15, 1976.

Sagov, et al., p. xii.

Centers for Disease Control, *Journal of the American Medical Association.*

Rothman, Barbara Katz, *In Labor: Women and Power in the Birthplace* (New York: W. W. Norton & Company, 1982), pp. 17, 18.

Bennetts, Anita B., CNM, Ph. D., and Ruth Watson Lubic, CNM, Ed. D., "The Free Standing Birth Center," *Lancet* 1:8,268: 378–380, February 13, 1982.

Chapter 5

Brewer, Gail Sforza, *Nine Months, Nine Lessons* (New York: Simon & Schuster, Inc., 1983), p. 43.

Chapter 7

Davis, Elizabeth, *A Guide to Midwifery: Heart and Hands* (New York: Bantam Books, 1983), pp. 146–147.

Shapiro, Dr. Howard, *The Pregnancy Book for Today's Woman* (New York: Harper & Row, 1983), p. 377.

Morley, G. W., "Breech Presentation: A 15-Year Review," *Obstetrics and Gynecology* 30:745, 1967.

Nathan, Dr. Neil, "Muscle Tension May Affect Breech Presentation," *Ob. Gyn. News,* 16, no. 22 (November 15, 1981), p. 15.

Henricksen, Adrienne, CNM, "Prolonged Pregnancy: A Literature Review," *Journal of Nurse-Midwifery,* 30, no. 1 (January/February 1985), p. 38.

Rayburn, William F., M.D.; Motley, May E., L.P.N.; and Zuspan, Frederick P., M.D., "Conditions Affecting Nonstress Test Results," *Obstetrics and Gynecology,* April 1982 (Vol 59, no. 8).

Davis, p. 140.

Chayen, Benjamin, M.D., Tejani, Nergesh, M.D., and Verman, Uma, M.D., "Induction of Labor Using An Electric Breast Pump," from The Department of Obstetrics and Gynecology, Nassau County Medical Center, East Meadow, NY, and the Health Sciences Center, S.U.N.Y., at Stony Brook, NY.

Chapter 9

Zuspan, Frederick P., M.D., and Quilligan, Edward J., M.D., editors, *Practical Manual of Obstetric Care* (St. Louis: C. V. Mosby Company, 1982), p. 234.

Ibid., p. 234.

Banta, David, M.D., and Thacker, Stephen B., M.D. "Electronic Fetal Monitoring: Is It of Benefit?" *Birth & Family Journal* 6 (Winter 1979).

The 1980 Task Force on Cesarean Section, convened by the National Institute of Child Health and Human Development, Washington, D.C., September 1980.

Chapter 10

Odent, Dr. Michel, *Birth Reborn* (New York: Pantheon Books, 1984), p. 47.

Ibid., p. 53.

Kitzinger, Sheila, *The Experience of Childbirth* (Great Britain: Penguin Books, 1981), p. 234.

Banta, David, M.D., and Thacker, Stephen B., M.D., "The Risks and Benefits of Episiotomy: A Review," *Birth,* 9:1 (Spring, 1982), p. 29.

British Medical Journal, 288 (June, 1984) pp. 1971–1975.

Chapter 11

Carrington, Reid, M.D., and Ledger, William, M.D., *Obstetrics and Gynecology* (St. Louis: C. V. Mosby Company, 1983), p. 415.

Shapiro, Dr. Howard, p. 194.

Floyd, Cathy C., RN, MS, ACCE, "Epidural Anesthesia: Use or Abuse?" *Genesis* (August/September 1984), p. 12.

Hoult, I. J.; MacLennan, A. H., and Carrie, Les, "Lumbar Epidural Analgesia in Labor: Relation to Fetal Malposition and Instrumental Delivery," *British Medical Journal,* January 1, 1977, p. 14.

Avard, Denise M., Ph. D., and Nimrod, Carl M., M.B., F.R.S.C., "Risks and Benefits of Obstetric Epidural Analgesia: A Review," *Birth* 12:4 (Winter 1985), p. 223.

Dripps, Robert D., M.D., Eckenhoff, James E., M.D., and Vandam, Leroy D., M.D., *Introduction to Anesthesia: The Principles of Safe Practice* (Philadelphia: W. B. Saunders Company, 1982), p. 227.

Chapter 12

Shapiro, Dr. Howard, p. 374.

Marieskind, Helen A., D.P.H., "An Evaluation of Cesarean Section in the United States," Washington, D. C., Department of Health, Education and Welfare, June 1979.

Massachusetts Department of Public Health Study, 1984, as reported in the *Boston Globe* (October 26, 1984), p. 57.

The 1980 Task Force on Cesarean Section, convened by the National Institute of Child Health and Human Development, Washington, D. C., September 1980.

Chapter 14

Kitzinger, Sheila, p. 272.

Chapter 15

Cohen, Nancy Wainer, and Estner, Lois J., *Silent Knife: Cesarean Prevention and Vaginal Birth After Cesarean* (Massachusetts: Bergin & Garvey Publishers, Inc., 1983), p. 2.

Weiss, Joan Solomon, *Your Second Child* (New York: Summit Books, 1981).

Glossary

Active Labor During this second phase of labor, the cervix will dilate from four to seven centimeters. It lasts an average of three to four hours, during which time contractions are one minute long and occur every three to four minutes.

Amnestic A drug that causes amnesia, or loss of memory. Scopolamine is the most common one for childbirth, but these drugs are now rarely used.

Amniotic Fluid The clear, odorless, sterile liquid that surrounds the baby in utero. It is continually absorbed and replenished during pregnancy. The average amount at term is one quart.

Amniotic Sac A bag that lines the uterus, enclosing the baby and the amniotic fluid, also known as the membranes or bag of waters.

Amniotomy The artificial rupture of the amniotic sac. This can be done manually or with a plastic hook.

Analgesia Medication that offers relief from pain without loss of consciousness. Demerol is the most common analgesic used during labor.

Anesthesia A local or regional anesthetic obliterates feeling to a limited area; a general anesthestic induces a loss of consciousness.

Anterior Position The position of an unborn baby when he is facing the mother's spine.

Apgar Score Named after Dr. Virginia Apgar, it is a general assessment of the condition of the newborn at one and five minutes after birth.

Bradycardia When the baby's heart rate is below 120 beats per minute.

Braxton-Hicks Contractions Contractions that occur throughout pregnancy, increasing in frequency and strength as labor nears.

Breech Presentation A position in which the baby's feet or buttocks are presenting first. It occurs in only 3 to 4 percent of term pregnancies.

Cephalo-pelvic Disproportion (CPD) A condition in which the mother's pelvis is too small to accommodate the baby. Though statistically it should be a rare occurrence (roughly 2 percent), this is one of the most common reasons given for cesarean sections today.

Cervix The muscular neck of the uterus located at the top of the vagina. During labor, the cervix will efface and dilate, allowing the uterus and vagina to form one continuous birth canal.

Cesarean Birth Delivery of the baby through an incision in the mother's abdomen and uterus. Either a general or a regional anesthetic is used.

Colostrum A clear, yellowish fluid that is rich in proteins and the mother's antibodies and precedes true breast milk.

Cord Prolapse A condition that occurs when the umbilical cord slips down into the vagina ahead of the baby's presenting part. This is especially common if the baby is presenting as a footling breech.

Crowning When the top of the baby's head is visible at the vaginal opening, both during and between contractions, just before delivery.

Diaphragm The muscular sheath located just below the lungs that controls respiration.

Dilation The widening of the cervical opening caused by uterine contractions. During labor, dilation is complete at ten centimeters, or five fingers.

Early Labor This is the first phase of labor. Contractions are usually mild, thirty to forty-five seconds long, and occur every five to fifteen minutes. It lasts an average of eight to nine hours, during which time the cervix will completely efface and dilate to three centimeters.

Edema Fluid retention that causes body tissues to swell. Though this is a common occurrence during pregnancy, it can also be a sign of preeclampsia.

Effacement The process by which the cervix thins and flattens. This is measured in percentages, with 100 percent describing total effacement.

Effleurage A light stroking on the abdomen, legs, feet, or back, or counterpressure to the back or lower abdomen.

Engagement Also known as zero station, lightening, or dropping, engagement occurs when the baby's head descends into the pelvis. This can occur two or three weeks prior to labor, or during labor itself.

Epidural The most common form of regional anesthesia, in which medication is injected into the epidural space outside the spinal canal.

Episiotomy   A surgical incision into the perineum to enlarge the vagina opening and speed the birth of the baby.

External Rotation   Movement during which the baby rotates to the side position after the head is delivered, in preparation for the delivery of the shoulders.

External Version   The manipulation of the fetus from outside the abdomen from a breech to a head-first presentation.

False Labor   Braxton-Hicks contractions, which precede true labor. They are usually mild, short in duration, and irregular, and are often mistaken for early labor.

Fetal Distress   A condition that occurs when the baby's oxygen supply is compromised. There can be many causes, but it is reflected by a fetal heart rate above 160 or below 120 beats per minute or one that lacks beat-to-beat variability.

Fetal Monitor   Equipment used to monitor the relationship between the fetal heart rate and uterine contractions. There are both internal and external fetal monitors.

Fundus   The top of the uterus.

Hemorrhoids   Swollen blood vessels around the rectum.

Hypertension   High blood pressure.

Hyperventilation   A change in the pH balance of the blood, usually caused by abnormally forceful breathing. Symptoms include a feeling of being light-headed and a sensation of tingling in the fingers and lips.

Hypotension   Low blood pressure.

Induction   The attempt to begin labor by artificial means, usually by amniotomy or Pitocin.

Internal Rotation   Movement during which the unborn baby rotates within the mother's pelvis, usually to a position facing either the mother's spine or her belly.

Intravenous   Also known as the IV, this is the introduction of fluids directly into a vein.

Involution   The process in which the uterus returns to its nonpregnant size.

Jaundice   A common newborn condition caused by the inability of the liver to break down and excrete excess red blood cells in the blood.

Kegal Exercise   The tightening and relaxing of the pelvic floor to maintain tone and elasticity.

Leboyer Method of Birth   A method of birth originated by French obstetrician Frederick Leboyer that includes low lights, delayed clamping of the umbilical cord, soft voices, no routine suctioning, skin-to-skin contact, and a warm bath for the newborn.

Lithotomy Position   The position in which a woman lies on her back with her legs apart and supported by stirrups. This is the standard position for gynecological examinations and hospital deliveries.

Lochia   The postpartum discharge of blood and tissue.

Meconium   The baby's first bowel movement.

Membranes   The amniotic sac.

Mucous Plug   A mass of capillaries and mucus that fills the cervical opening during pregnancy, helping to protect the unborn baby from infection. The amniotic sac, however, is the more important form of protection.

Narcotic   A type of analgesic used to decrease the perception of pain. Demerol is the most common narcotic used during labor.

Nitrous Oxide   A gas that can be used either for analgesia or anesthesia in the delivery room.

Nonstress Test   A prenatal check for fetal well-being that compares the reaction of the fetal heart rate to movement. A rise in the heart rate concomitant with fetal movement is a good, reactive test.

Oxytocin   A natural hormone that causes the uterus to contract.

Paracervical   A form of regional anesthesia, rarely used today which deadens the sensation of a contraction. The injections are given on either side of the cervix.

Pelvic Floor   The muscle that supports the pelvic organs—the uterus, vagina, and bladder. The Kegel exercise tones the pelvic floor.

Pelvis   The bony structure that encloses the pelvic organs, composed of the pubic bone, the sacrum, and the ilium.

Perineum   The area between the vagina and the rectum.

Pitocin   A synthetic hormone that produces uterine contractions and is used to induce or augment labor.

Placenta   An organ, also known as the afterbirth, that transfers oxygen and nutrients from the mother to the baby and waste products from the baby back to the mother. The placenta is created during pregnancy and is expelled once the baby is born.

Placenta Abruptio   A rare, but serious condition in which the placenta partially or completely separates from the uterine wall, decreasing the oxygen supply to the baby. This is sometimes recognized by the sudden onset of uninterrupted and localized pain.

Placenta Previa   A rare, but potentially dangerous condition in which the placenta partially or completely covers the cervix, impeding the baby's passage into the vagina.

Posterior Position   The position in which the back of the baby's head is against the mother's spine. Women with babies in this position usually experience back labor, in which contractions are felt in the back rather than the lower abdomen.

Postdate Pregnancy   A pregnancy that continues past forty-two weeks.

Postmaturity   A situation in which the placenta ceases to function efficiently, causing the baby to lose weight. This occurs in approximately 4 percent of all pregnancies.

Pre-eclampsia   Also known as toxemia, this is a dangerous condition heralded by a trio of symptoms: edema, high blood pressure, and protein in the urine.

Premature Birth   The delivery of a baby, weighing less than 5½ pounds, between the twenty-eighth week and the end of the thirty-sixth week of pregnancy.

Premature Rupture of the Membranes (PROM)   Rupture of the membranes prior to the onset of labor contractions.

Presenting Part   That part of the baby's body that is closest to the cervix.

Pudendal Block   A form of local anesthesia administered by injection into the pudendal nerves on either side of the vagina. It numbs the vagina, vulva, and perineum.

Saddle Block   A type of spinal anesthesia, rarely used today, which numbs the vagina, perineum, and upper thighs.

Spinal Anesthesia   A type of anesthesia usually only used for cesarean sections. It is administered by injecting a local anesthetic medication into the spinal canal in the lower back. Spinals numb and paralyze the lower half of the body, from the chest to the toes.

Station   A term that describes the baby's position in relation to the mother's pelvis. Minus five is the very top of the pelvis; plus five is at the bottom of the vagina (crowning).

Tachycardia   When the baby's heartbeat is above 160 beats per minute.

Toxemia   See *Pre-eclampsia.*

Transition   The period of labor when the cervix dilates from eight to ten centimeters. This is the third phase of labor and usually lasts about an hour. Contractions are strong, long, and close together.

Umbilical Cord   The lifeline that connects the baby to the placenta.

Uterus   The muscular organ that encloses the baby, the amniotic sac, and the amniotic fluid.

Vacuum Extractor   An alternative to forceps, this is a machine that uses suction to help deliver a baby.

Vernix   A creamlike substance that covers and protects the baby's skin in utero.

Index

Fever, *see* Temperature
Fibroids, 155
First stage of labor, *see* Labor, the first stage of
Fluids, 182, 194, 312
    after cesarean section, 298
    in early labor, 175
    withholding of, 60, 196–97
    see also Alcohol; Food
Flying during last month, 148
Focal point, 91, 193
Food, 194
    after cesarean section, 298
    in early labor, 176, 312
    during second pregnancy, 368
    before sleeping, 148
    withholding, during labor, 60, 196
    see also Fluids
Food and Drug Administration (FDA), 186–87
Football hold, 296, 298
Foot circles, 300
Footprints, 152, 234
Foot pumping, 300
Footwork, 114
Forceps delivery, 8, 59, 199, 202, 222, 241, 271–76
    anesthetics and, 254, 256, 259, 262, 264, 276, 323
    avoiding a, 276
    birth reports, 404–10
    comments on, 273
    episiotomy and, 231, 273–74, 323
    indications for, 274–75, 322–23
    midwives prohibited from performing, 46
    the procedure, 273–74
    risks of, 275
    types of, 272
    vs. vacuum extraction, 277, 278–79

Formula, 342
Frank breech presentation, 153, 154, 159
Friedman, Dr. Emanuel, 275
Full relaxation, 126, 130–33, 137
    visualization exercise, 132–33
Future of Lamaze, 20–22

Gaskin, Ina May, 165
Gas pains, 298
Gate theory, 4
General anesthetics, *see* Anesthetics, general
Genitals, baby's, 240
Glossary, 441–46
    of body parts, 74–76
Goal in using Lamaze method, 13
Gonorrhea, 241
Gown, hospital, 194, 332
Group practice, 30, 33–36, 144
    comments on, 37–38
Guided relaxation, *see* Visualization
Guide to Midwifery, A (Davis), 142
Guilt, 364

Harper's Bazaar, 9
Head, baby's, 274
    shape of, 240
Headache from anesthetic, 263–64
Head circles, 118
Hearing disorders, 275
Heartbeat:
    of fetus, 163, 186, 222, 265
        fetal monitoring of, 194, 198–202, 262
        patterns of, 198–99
    maternal, 372
    of newborn, 252

Heart disease, 231, 275
Heating pad, 180
Help during postpartum period, 145–46, 340, 347–48, 364
Hematomas, 276, 278
Hemorrhage, 196, 244, 285, 288
Hemorrhoids, 230, 332–33
Heparin lock, 197
Hepatitis, 299
Herpes, 285
High blood pressure, *see* Hypertension
High-forceps delivery, 272, 275
Holding your baby:
    after cesarean section, 289, 290, 295, 296, 324
    premature baby, 336
    after vaginal birth, 33, 234, 235, 242, 323
        feelings immediately after birth, 235–38
    see also Seeing your baby
Holistic Psychotherapy and Medical Group, 158
Home Birth: A Practitioner's Guide to Birth Outside the Hospital, 48, 50
Homebirths, 45, 47–48, 50–57
    comments on, 52–53
    guidelines for safe, 56–57
    importance of your choice, 48–50
    percentage of planned, 50–51
    reasons for choosing, 52, 53–56
    unattended, 50, 51
    see also Birth Centers; Hospital delivery
Hospital affiliation of doctor, 29–30, 143–45
Hospital classes in Lamaze method, 18–19, 20–22
Hospital delivery, 47, 48, 51, 60–72

New York Medical Society, 371

Nine Months, Nine Lessons (Brewer), 102

Ninth month of pregnancy, *see* Last month of pregnancy

Nipples:
    care of, when breast-feeding, 333
    stimulation of, 163, 165, 204, 244, 284

Nisentil, 249

Nitrous oxide (laughing gas), 273

Nonstress test (NST), 162, 163, 286

North Central Bronx Hospital, 46

Nurse anesthetist, 255

Nutritional counseling, 43, 57

Ob. Gyn. News, 158

Obstetrician, *see* Doctor(s)

Obstetrics and Gynecology (Wilson, Carrington, and Ledger), 246

Odent, Dr. Michael, 176, 220, 221–22

Office hours, pediatrician's, 144

Office of pediatrician, 144

Office of Technology Assessment, 200

Operating room for cesarean delivery, 289–94, 372
    partner in the, 32, 289

Oregon, 51

Os, 75

Ottolini, Dr. James, 278–79

Overview of Lamaze method:
    beginnings of Lamaze, 8–10
    childbirth before Lamaze, 4–8
    classes in Lamaze, 20–22
    the future of Lamaze, 20–22
    for natural childbirth, 10–14
    teachers of Lamaze, 14–19

Oxygen, baby's, 202, 286

Oxytocin, 85, 184, 187

Packing:
    your Lamaze bag, 150, 193
    your suitcase, 151, 193

Pain, 134, 246
    of active labor, 190–92
    of back labor, 177–82
    of cesarean section, 298–99
    gas, 298
    neuromuscular relaxation during labor, 134
    partner's help in working through the, 319
    recognition of, in childbirth, 13–14
    relief of, *see* Medication
    of second labor, 374
    of transition, 208–11, 317

Painless Childbirth Through Psychoprophylaxis (Bonstein), 9

Paracervical, 255, 265

Parents magazine, xv

Partners:
    during active labor, 189–93, 194, 204, 313–17
    attending Lamaze classes, 20, 307–10, 368–70
    at cesarean section, 32, 289, 294–95, 323–24
    after cesarean section, 295, 296
    comments by and about, 304–5, 306, 315–16, 318, 319, 326
    cutting the umbilical cord, 235, 322
    in the delivery room, 66, 221, 223, 234, 260, 320–22, 323
    doctor's view of role of, 30
    at doctors visits, 152, 307
    during early labor, 311–12, 313

fears about childbirth, 305–7
forceps deliveries and, 322–23
getting to the hospital, 189–93, 311
guide to labor, 328–29
hospital procedures and, 194
in the last months, 310–11
medication decision and, 317–20
midwives' relationship with, 43–45
the postpartum period, 326–28, 344–51
practicing Lamaze breathing, 308–10
premature babies and, 336
reasons to attend the birth, 303–5
relaxation techniques practiced with, 126, 128–29, 131, 134–36
role in back labor, 182
second baby and, 366–67, 373–74
seeing your baby, 235, 294–95, 304–5, 323, 324–26
during transition, 210, 317, 318
as wife's advocate at the hospital, 312–13, 320

Pattern-paced breathing, 95–96, 107

Payment schedule, 30

Pearse, Dr. Warren, 51

Pediatrician, 240–41, 294, 295
    selecting a, 143–45

Pelvic inlet and outlet, 75

Pelvic tilt, 115, 300

Pelvis, 367
    description of the, 75
    engagement and station, 79
    Kegel exercises for pelvic floor and organs of the, 124, 232, 332, 352

Temperature (*cont.*)
    fever after cesarean section,
        299, 332
    newborn's, 252
Tenth month of pregnancy,
    163–66
    natural ways to help trigger
        labor, 165–66
    see also Postmaturity
Tetracycline, 241–42
Thacker, Dr. Stephen, 200, 231
Thank You, Dr. Lamaze (Kar-
    mel), 9–10
Third stage of labor, *see* Labor,
    the third stage of
Thrombosis, 296
Timing within the contractions,
    90–91
Tour of the hospital, 63–64
Toxemia, 186, 231, 288, 335,
    371
    cesarean section and, 287
Traction, 274, 277
Tranquilizers, 253, 266–67
Transition, 82–83, 106–7,
    208–11, 246, 262, 317,
    318, 328–29, 374
    breathing for, *see* Patterned-
        paced breathing; Pyra-
        mid breathing
    comments on, 209
    symptoms of, 208–11
Transverse presentation, 184,
    287
Travel in the last month, 148–
    49
Tuberculosis, 299
"Twilight sleep," *see*
    Scopolamine
Twins, *see* Multiple births
Twist, 119

Ultrasound, 155–57, 161
Umbilical cord, 163, 198, 201
    color of the, 234

cutting the, 83, 234–35, 322
    late-clamping, 235, 243
    Leboyer method and, 33
    description of the, 75–76
    forceps deliveries and prob-
        lems with, 274–75
    prolapsed, 154, 159, 183–
        84, 286
    short, 222, 274
U.S. Department of Health,
    Education, and Welfare,
    282
University of Michigan Hospi-
    tal, 154
University of Minnesota School
    of Medicine, 158
Upper-body circles, 118, 354
Ureter, injury to the, 288
Urination, 230, 260–61, 332
    frequent, 146–47, 332
    incontinence, 124
Urine:
    protein in the, 287
    sample, 194
Uterus:
    abnormalities of the, 153,
        155
    contractions of the, 76, 87,
        274
        in active labor, 82, 89,
            188–89, 202, 203,
            204
        in early labor, 81, 82,
            89, 170–71, 172–
            74, 175, 176, 311,
            312, 373
        epidural's effect on, 256
        to expel the placenta,
            83–85, 235, 243–44
        induced labor and, 185,
            186, 187
        monitoring, *see* Fetal
            monitor
        in pushing stage, 83,
            217–18, 222
        stress test, 163

    timing within the, 90–
        91
    in transition, 82–83,
        208
    description of the, 75
    involution of the, 331
    prolapse of the, 124, 233
    after second birth, 375

Vacation, delivering during doc-
    tor's, 30, 35
Vacuum extraction, 59, 276–79
    cesarean section and, 278
    vs. forceps delivery, 277,
        278–79
    improvements in, 276, 277–
        78
    indications for using, 276
Vaginal delivery:
    of breech baby, 159–60
    pushing, *see* Pushing
    the second baby, 370–73
        after a cesarean, 371–73
    see also Labor
Vaginal examination, 152
    in active labor, 194–95, 207
Valium, 253
Valsalva maneuver, 102
Vernix, 240
Version, *see* External version
Visits to the doctor:
    in last month, 152
    length of, 30, 144
    schedule of, 30, 152
Vistaril, 253
Visualization, 130–33, 158,
    276, 284
    exercises:
        for full relaxation, 132–
            33
        for good posture, 125
Vocalization while pushing, 221
Vomiting, 197, 208, 251, 296

About the Authors

BEVERLY SAVAGE is a free-lance writer and the mother of Elizabeth, born in 1982, and Matthew, born in 1986. She graduated from Barnard College and worked for four years as a reporter for the *Star-Ledger,* New Jersey's largest newspaper.

DIANA SIMKIN, M.A., is an ASPO/Lamaze-certified childbirth educator and the director of Family Focus, Inc., in Manhattan, a center for pregnancy, childbirth, and parenthood. Prior to co-founding Family Focus, she was the director of exercise and Lamaze instructor at the Elisabeth Bing Center for Parents. She is the author of *The Complete Pregnancy Exercise Program* and *The Complete Baby Exercise Program.*

About the Photographer

MARY MOTLEY KALERGIS has been a professional photographer for the past fourteen years. She is currently on the faculty of the International Center for Photography in New York City and is a regular contributor to the *Manchester Guardian* in London. She has photographed more than sixty births and has received critical acclaim for her book, *Giving Birth* (Harper and Row, 1983). Most recently, thirty-five of her birth photos appeared in *New Parenthood* by Cecilia Worth (McGraw-Hill, 1985). Her latest book, *Mother: A Collective Portrait,* will be published by E.P. Dutton in May, 1987. Mary is the mother of three boys.